慢性病长期用药处方

国际发展研究与借鉴

中国药师协会　组织编著

中国医药科技出版社

内 容 提 要

慢性病已成为严重威胁我国居民健康的重大公共卫生问题。国际上部分国家实行慢性病长期用药处方服务模式，在平衡药品可获得性、用药安全性以及加强医药合作等方面取得了很好的社会效果。本书比较系统地研究 7 个国家和中国台湾地区慢性病长期用药处方项目，分析其相关法规与操作流程、信息技术支撑、制度运行风险防范等问题，并附以具体实践指导或图表的中文版及英文原件，便于读者查阅和参考。期望本研究能助力我国深化医药体制改革，助力实施慢性病综合防控战略。

本书可以协助医药卫生政策制定者、卫生管理者、医疗专业人士更好思考慢性病防控宏观战略，切实管理和开展长期用药处方项目，也为研究人员提供很好的理论素材、案件材料、操作规程及深入研究的线索等。相信读者将从本书所介绍的研究内容中受益。

图书在版编目（CIP）数据

慢性病长期用药处方国际发展研究与借鉴 / 朱珠，（美）张海莲主编；中国药师协会组织编著. — 北京：中国医药科技出版社，2017.6

ISBN 978-7-5067-9354-4

Ⅰ. ①慢… Ⅱ. ①朱… ②张… ③中… Ⅲ. ①慢性病 – 用药法 – 研究 – 世界 Ⅳ. ① R452

中国版本图书馆 CIP 数据核字（2017）第 127401 号

美术编辑 陈君杞
版式设计 也 在

出版 **中国医药科技出版社**
地址 北京市海淀区文慧园北路甲 22 号
邮编 100082
电话 发行：010 – 62227427　邮购：010 – 62236938
网址 www.cmstp.com
规格 710×1000mm $\frac{1}{16}$
印张 27
字数 360 千字
版次 2017 年 6 月第 1 版
印次 2017 年 6 月第 1 次印刷
印刷 三河市万龙印装有限公司
经销 全国各地新华书店
书号 ISBN 978-7-5067-9354-4
定价 **68.00 元**

编委会

医疗没有国界；不同国家和地区的医疗服务方式虽有差异，但所遇到的难题和公众需求存在共性。慢性非传染性疾病的患者占全球人口的比例越来越高，这些患者的诊疗、复查与随访、多次地就诊和取药，极大地占用了医疗资源和交通资源，隐性成本较高，尤其给老年患者及其家庭带来诸多不便。

2016 年 8 月 19~20 日在京召开的"全国卫生与健康大会"上，中共中央总书记、国家主席、中央军委主席习近平强调：要把人民健康放在优先发展的战略地位，以普及健康生活、优化健康服务、完善健康保障、建设健康环境、发展健康产业为重点，加快推进健康中国建设，努力全方位、全周期保障人民健康，为实现"两个一百年"奋斗目标、实现中华民族伟大复兴的中国梦打下坚实健康基础。2017 年 1 月国务院办公厅发布的《中国防治慢性病中长期规划（2017–2025 年）》（国办发〔2017〕12 号），为加强慢性病防治工作，降低疾病负担，提高居民健康期望寿命，努力全方位、全周期保障人民健康，依据《"健康中国 2030"规划纲要》，制定了周密的规划；其中特别提及高血压、糖尿病患者规范管理率要从目前的 50% 逐步提高到 2020 年 60%、2025 年 70%；在"完善保障政策，切实减轻群众就医负担"的举措中，要求"老年慢性病患者可以由家庭签约医生开具慢性病长期药品处方，探索以多种方式满足患者用药需求"。

本书所研究的正是慢性病长期用药处方，在美国、英国、澳大利亚、日本等国以及中国台湾地区是针对病情稳定的慢性病患者已实行的处方开具、调配与管理方式。在中国台湾地区，习惯称之为"慢性病连续处方笺"。研究表明，这是方便患者维持长期药物治疗、减少患者为取药而往返医院就诊次数的便民举措，也是节约医生诊疗时间、控制诊疗成本、减少到医疗机构开药的患者数、降低医疗机构拥挤程度的有效措施之一，是优化医疗资源、急慢分治、分级诊疗、灵活开展便民服务、提高公立医院医疗资源利用效率的可行措施之一。育龄妇女的长期避孕需求，在部分国家也借用了长期用药处方的发药服务模式。

本书重点研究和概述了七个国家和我国台湾地区实施慢性病长期用药处方的情况，侧重其法规依据、操作与管理方式、适用患者范围、适用的药品范围、存在风险、风险防范措施等；各个国家或地区的相关法规和实践规范，以附件形式放在每章之后，其英文原文放在全书之后的附录，便于读者查阅和参考。荷兰、芬兰、爱尔兰、新西兰等国也有少量文献，本书未能囊括。总之，期望本研究助力我国深化医药卫生体制改革，助力落实防治慢性病中长期规划、贯彻医改的三医联动和分级诊疗。限于水平，书中难免存在疏漏，敬请批评指正。

编　者

2017 年 5 月

目 录

第一章　慢性病长期用药处方及其国际发展概论

第二章　美国慢性病长期用药处方项目的研究与借鉴

第五章　日本慢性病长期用药处方项目的研究与借鉴

第六章　瑞典慢性病长期用药处方项目的研究与借鉴

第七章　澳大利亚慢性病长期用药处方项目的研究与借鉴

第八章　新加坡慢性病长期用药处方项目的研究与借鉴

第九章　中国台湾地区慢性病长期用药处方项目的
　　　　研究与借鉴

附录

第一章 慢性病长期用药处方及其国际发展概论

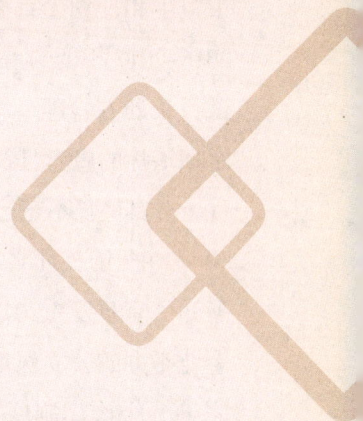

国务院办公厅在 2017 年初发布的《中国防治慢性病中长期规划（2017–2025 年）》中提到：老年慢病患者可以由家庭签约医生开具慢性病长期药品处方，探索以多种方式满足患者用药需求[1]。这是我国政府首次提到"慢性病长期药品处方"的概念。

此前据媒体报道，2015 年 4 月浙江省医改的便民措施之一是试行慢性病长期用药处方，处方有效期 84 天，每次取 4 周的药量，试点时间三年[2]。北京市卫生和计划生育委员会等四部门于 2016 年发布《北京市分级诊疗制度建设 2016–2017 年度的重点任务》（京卫医（2016）113 号），提及"在社区签约患者试行长处方管理"，针对高血压、糖尿病、冠心病、脑血管病四类慢性疾病稳定期治疗的患者且符合五项条件时，社区医生可以按照慢性疾病管理的有关条件，开具最长不超过 2 个月量的常用药品，列出了适于长处方的药品目录[3]。

2017 年 3 月北京市人民政府关于印发《医药分开综合改革实施方案》的通知（京政发〔2017〕11 号），要求北京市行政区域内政府、事业单位及国有企业举办的公立医疗机构和解放军、武警部队在京医疗机构执行。其中"（六）完善分级诊疗制度"中提到：完善家庭医生签约服务，对高血压、糖尿病、冠心病、脑血管病等 4 类慢性疾病稳定期常用药品，统一大医院与基层医疗卫生机构的采购和报销目录，符合条件的患者在基层医疗卫生机构可享受 2 个月的长处方便利，有序分流三级医院门诊量[4]。

关于长期药品处方的模式，我国还没有具体的界定和统一的规范。此前孙雯娟、朱珠等学者陆续概述了英国 Repeat Prescriptions 项目和美国的 Medication Refill 项目，当时根据其字面翻译和专业含义，将其翻译为"可重配处方"，亦称"重配处方"[5-7]。

第一节　何谓慢性病长期用药处方

一、长期用药处方的定义和内涵

长期用药处方是由处方者根据患者病情长期治疗需要而开具的处方，授权患者在一定时间内无需再次就诊，就可以凭借此处方到指定的医院或患者就近的药房数次取药，限定取药间隔和总次数。在此过程中，要有适当的临床观察与基本用药评估来确保药物的使用和疗效，同时还需详细的取药记录并保存在患者定期复查的病历中。

长期用药处方上包括常规处方的信息，如患者姓名、年龄、出生日期、住址、就诊卡号等基本信息，以及开具处方者的信息、签名和日期，还需要注明长期用药处方的使用次数、终止期限及取药间隔（如周、月、季度）[8]。

长期用药处方不仅约定了处方者的医疗责任，及患者的知晓、依从责任，还约定了处方者与患者的合作关系。这种约定关系是有法律效力的，同时也被多国医疗质量组织认可[9]。

对应于长期用药处方的是长期用药品调配（repeat dispensing）的过程，即药师根据长期用药处方进行多次药品调配的过程，使得患者在既定时间段内无需再挂号找医生就可以拿到治疗所需的药品[10]。其基本流程是：收到长期用药处方后，药师核对患者个人信息、疾病情况和用药情况，按照该处方约定的药品品种、用量和间隔，给患者调配和发放药品，收取当次的处方调配费；同时，建立长期用药处方登记卡，由经手药师登记每次取药的日期、品种、数量等信息。这些记录有助于保障患者在用药疗程中的安全有效且不发生漏发、错发等问题。药师还应询问患者的病情是否变化，判断用药方案是否需要调整。末次调配完的原始长期用药处方由药房保存；当所有重配次数用尽或尚未全部取药但处方已到期时，药房会把原始长期用药处方收回并交给相关质量管理组织或保险机构[11]。

在手写处方时代，患者必须拿着纸质长期用药处方在指定的药房取药；现阶段，多个国家均允许患者自由选择一家药房取药，但在长期用药处方有效期内不得变更。一些国家还建立和完善电子处方服务系统（Electronic Prescription Service, EPS），便于患者从联网药店中每次随意选择一家药房就近取药[12]。

长期用药处方适合病情稳定的慢性非传染病，患者可便捷地获取药物、维持长期药物治疗，不必为开药而频繁去门诊挂号和就诊，使门诊的医疗效率提高，使医师主要接待病情变化或复杂、真正需要就诊的患者；同时，其规范的管理体系、严格的操作流程和不断完善的法规，有效利用医务人员的技能和时间，有效保障了患者用药安全，实现了医患双方共赢[13]。

二、不同国家和地区关于长期用药处方所使用的术语

长期用药处方，英国采用的术语为"repeat prescription"，其突出的意义为处方可重复使用；美国则将其称为"prescription refills"或"refill"，强调在医生授权后的一段时间内可对处方再次执行和调配。瑞典、澳大利亚等国家开展长期用药处方项目时，采用的术语也都分别参照了美国或英国的定义和模式。我国台湾地区采用"慢性病连续处方"的术语。国内相关文献对这类处方的翻译和界定也不尽相同，有长程处方，重配处方，可重配处方，长期处方，长期连续处方等不同术语。根据这类处方的内涵，笔者认为表示为长程连续处方是相对比较规范的。为了与《中国防治慢性病中长期规划（2017~2025）》文件保持一定的统一性，也为了方便理解交流，本书暂将此术语统一改为"长期用药处方"，今后在研究和制订规范性文件时需要进一步研讨。部分国家和地区在介绍该项目时使用的常见术语，见表1-1。

表1-1　不同国家和地区对于长期用药处方所使用的术语

术语	国家或地区
medication refill	美国、加拿大、荷兰
prescription refill	美国、加拿大、荷兰、爱尔兰、中国台湾
repeat dispensing	英国
repeat prescribing	英国、爱尔兰、芬兰、荷兰
repeat prescription	英国、西班牙、新加坡、澳大利亚

备注：法语、日语、瑞典语等语言的专业术语，未在此表列出。

第二节　慢性病长期用药处方的起源与发展

早在 1967 年 7 月 29 日，英国 Dr. J. F. K. Stephenson 在写给 "the British Medical Journal" 的信中，描述了一种非常方便使用的卡，即长期用药处方卡，即可以使患者在一段时间内使用而不用再看医生的处方。无独有偶，1968 年 3 月 22 日，新西兰克莱斯特彻奇日报刊登一则消息 "Charges for Repeat Prescriptions"，报道说一些患者付给医生大约 75 美分的费用，就可以不用频繁就诊而凭长期用药处方拿到药物，并且是法律允许的[14]。

1971 年，长期用药处方的探索初见雏形但应用范围较小[15]。慢性非传染病患者需要长期治疗，经常就医可复查病情变化，随访观察治疗效果；其中部分病情稳定的患者无需或无法频繁到医院就诊。长期用药处方的做法最初由全科医生发起和认可[16]。

20 世纪 80 年代后，为了减轻医生的工作压力，全科医生积极推进长期用药处方，处方卡（Prescription cards）、协定处方（drug sheets）、重配记录（repeat registers）、计算机软件系统、信息网络化等简化重配过程的方式应运而生；另一方面，外界舆论从医疗质量和患者安全的角度质疑这一做法的严谨性，他们担心不找医生复查即获得持续治疗用药可能存在诸多隐患，例如：长期用药处方申请程序过于简单，处方权有可能被滥用、医生无法及时掌握病情变化等[17]。

美国的长期用药处方雏形可追溯到 1941 年，并于 1999 年在华盛顿州的 Bremerton 海军医院和 Everett 海军门诊进行的长期用药处方试点[18、19]。这些尝试奠定了长期用药处方的基础，药师可随访患者药物治疗情况，患者凭长期用药处方在一定时间内可多次取药。这个有效期从最初 60 天、6 个月，到如今 12 个月。

欧洲的瑞典、德国、芬兰、荷兰等国家相继也开展了长期用药处方项目[20-25]。据文献统计，荷兰 1997 年就有大约三分之一的患者可从社区全科医生诊所获得长期用药处方[26]。对患者和医生，使用长期用药处方更加方便，但是也有一些弊端，例如处方过多和限制不足。这些弊端可以通过较为完善的记录系统来弥补。患者通过打电话给诊所前台接待员申请长期用药处方，然后接待员负责将长期用药处方准备好，部分诊所要求医生在这些准备好的长期用药处方上签字即可，也有部分诊所要求医生将部分信息手写在处方上。由于时间的限制，授权处方的过程往往在没有患者病历的情况下进行。因此，也并没有固定的对处方指证及必要性的监管过程。为了更深入了解关于长期用药处方的相应问题，研究者对社区全科医生进行了深入的面谈。研究结果显示，不同医生对长期用药处方的用法有差异。部分医生遵循专门的长期用药处方规则，有些医生并不觉得其长期用药处方的处理有什么不妥，然而他们却并没有发觉自己开出的长期用药处方中的差错。有些诊所助理在帮助处理长期用药处方时，缺乏明确的工作流程。并不是所有医生都认可诊所助理在处理长期用药处方过程中的重要性。值得关注的是，部分医生认为药师在处理长期用药处方中没有什么特别的作用，却信任药师管理着长期用药处方是很重要的步骤。芬兰与荷兰情况类似，在芬兰的社区诊所（Primary Care Clinics），老年患者及精神方面、心血管方面的药物使用者经常通过免就诊方式获得长期用药处方。这就意味着这些患者的病情不是由一个医生亲自管理着。同时，诊所前台接待员（部分为注册护士）也往往不会评估患者的用药情况。芬兰可提供 12 个月药量的长期用药处方，这也就意味着，如果患者情况稳定，可能隔几年才会接受一次医生的检查[27]。

　　长期用药处方拓宽了患者取药方式的选择性，充分发挥了药师的职能，给药师发挥其专业知识和专业技能提供了机会和平台，让他们帮助患者恰当地使用药物、减少浪费。研究表明，由药师进行长期用药处方的用药审核既有利于发现用药相关问题，也分担了全科医生的工作负荷。多年临床实践表明，长期用药处方能够减轻医生的工作量，节省医生时间，使医生集中更多的时间和精力为病情紧急或危重的患者进行诊疗服务[25]。

第三节　全球开展慢性病长期用药处方的概况

一、关于慢性病长期用药处方的文献研究概况

以（prescription refill* ［Title］）OR medication refill* ［Title］）OR repeat prescription ［Title］）OR repeat prescribing ［Title］）OR repeat dispensing ［Title］）OR refill clinic ［Title］）OR refill ［Title］）OR refills ［Title］）构建检索式，在PubMed 数据库检索 2016 年 4 月以前发表的、语言为英文的、与长期用药处方相关的文献，共检索到文献 215 篇。在 215 篇文献中，筛出与本研究相关的随机对照、横断面调查等一次文献，综述、荟萃分析等二次文献，报道与评论等有数据文献共 87 篇，具体筛选步骤见图 1-1。

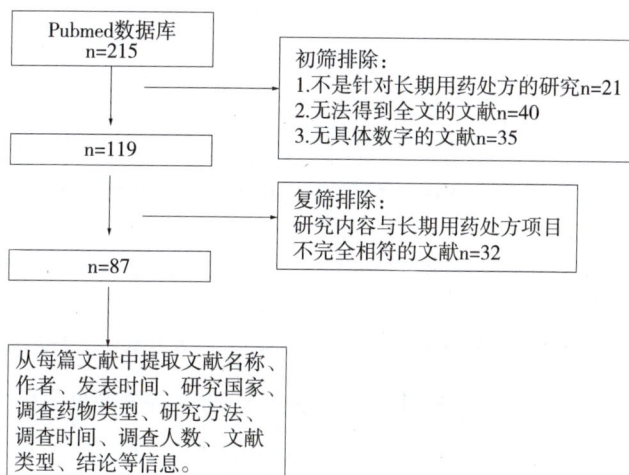

图 1-1　文献检索与筛选步骤

将每篇文献所得信息整理到 Excel 表格，并统计分析后按国家分类整理文献的结果见图 1-2。

由图 1-2 可见，全球已有十多个国家和地区实施长期用药处方项目。文献数量从一个侧面反映全球开展长期用药处方项目的情况，美国、英国、瑞典、荷兰和加拿大的文献列居前五位。其中美国和英国的文献总和超过全部

文献的一半，可见美国和英国是开展长期用药处方后研究较多的国家。

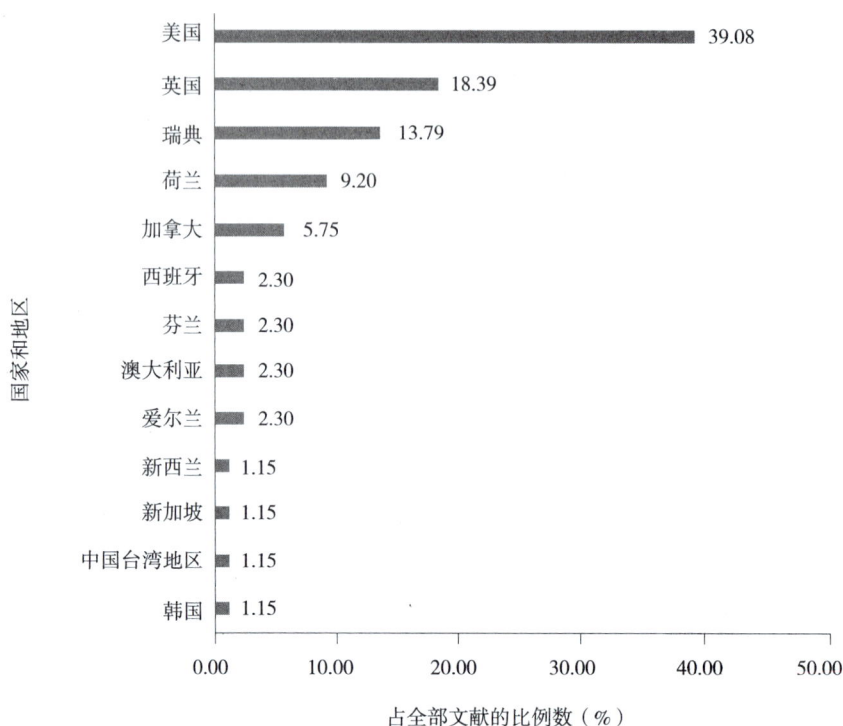

图 1-2 不同国家和地区的长期用药处方文献数量占比

二、不同国家和地区的长期用药处方使用情况概况

英国是最先报道长期用药处方占比的国家，早在 1985 年对英国纽卡斯尔大学附属的 29 所诊所进行调查时报道，长期用药处方占全部处方的 12.5%~33%。同时还测算用仿制药替代原研药的话可以节省 11.4% 的医疗费用[27]。Zermansky AG. 等[28] 1996 年随机挑选英国利兹市 57 个全科诊所的长期用药处方进行调查后发现，长期用药处方占所有处方的三分之二，其费用占所有处方费用的五分之四，大约 24 亿英镑。Petty DR 等[29] 在 2014 年再次对英国长期用药处方的使用率进行调查时发现，当年 NHS 系统中长期用药处方的使用率为 77%。

Lillis S 等[30] 在 2011 年对新西兰电子网络中心提供的 97 个全科诊所

的数据进行总结时发现，长期用药处方占全部处方的 19%~75%。而 De Smet PA 等[31]对 2004 年荷兰的数据分析后发现，长期用药处方的占比为 29%~75%。这也从另一侧面体现英国长期用药处方项目开展的规模在全球属于前列。美国 2005 年处方药物支出为 1600 亿美元，Miller AH 等[33]对公立医院长期用药处方的研究表明，29% 的患者使用了长期用药处方。对中国台湾地区 1005 名 2 型糖尿病患者的调查也发现，使用长期用药处方可以大大节约医疗花费[34]。

从文献中采集的部分国家和地区在不同年代使用长期用药处方的规模，列于表 1-2。

表 1-2　文献研究中部分国家和地区在不同年代的长期用药处方占比

国家	时间	长期用药处方的占比（%）
英国[27]	1986	12.5%~33.0%
英国[28-29]	2014	66.6%~77%
荷兰[32]	2004	29%~75%
美国[33]	2005	29%
芬兰[35]	2009	12%~56%
新西兰[30]	2011	19%~75%
中国台湾地区[34]	2011	30%

备注：长期用药处方占比为长期用药处方数与同期该国家或地区处方总数的比值。

荷兰的文献研究表明，长期用药处方占总处方的 42%；15~25 岁患者中，25% 的处方为长期用药处方，而 75 岁和以上的患者中有 61% 的处方为长期用药处方。长期用药处方药品中最多的为降压药，其次为安眠药、抗焦虑药、避孕药。在一篇基于七个社区诊所的研究中，长期用药处方药品占 75%；换言之，54% 的避孕药物、51% 的精神科药物、47% 的心血管药物使用长期用药处方，比例最低的药物为抗生素（10%）。医生们信任药师管理长期用药处方的审核与调配，医生和药师的合作可以有助于提高长期用药处方系统的运作[26]。

类似于英国、荷兰的慢性病长期用药处方项目，芬兰的长期用药处方也主要基于社区诊所。文献表明，其长期用药处方多用于中枢神经系统、心血管系统、呼吸系统和肌肉骨骼系统的用药。统计显示芬兰 19% 的处方是患者没有经过再次就诊就得到了长期用药处方，而规律地评估患者用药可以避免不必要的就诊，尤其是作用于神经和精神的药物，就更有必要防止相应的对药品的依赖[27]。另一篇芬兰的研究指出，社区药师可以主动介入长期用药处方服务，对患者进行提问，并将相关用药信息提供给处方医生。通过药师的主动介入，医生可以更好的发现并解决患者的用药相关问题，从而提高处方的质量[36]。

三、部分国家和地区长期用药处方项目可处方的药物类别

对 87 篇文献中不同国家和地区纳入长期用药处方中的药品及其类别、不宜纳入的药品进行梳理，结果见表 1–3。

表 1–3　文献研究中不同国家和地区长期用药处方涉及的药物种类一览表

国家和地区	文献中纳入的药品	所属药物类别	不得纳入的药品
爱尔兰	他汀类药物	调节血脂类药物	
北爱尔兰	非甾体抗炎药	非甾体抗炎药	
芬兰	所有药物	所有药物	
荷兰	口服降糖药、降压药、调节血脂类药物、吸入皮质类固醇、吸入糖皮质激素	降糖药、降压药、调节血脂类药物、平喘药	
加拿大	降低眼压的药物、口服降糖药物、吸入皮质类固醇、心血管药物	降低眼压的药物、降糖药、平喘药、心血管药物	
美国	血管紧张素转化酶抑制剂、血管紧张素受体阻断剂、β受体阻滞剂、钙通道阻滞剂、利尿剂、口服降糖药、他汀类药物、甲状腺激素替代药物、抗抑郁药、选择性 5-羟色胺再摄取抑制剂、抗惊厥药、血清素 - 去甲肾上腺素再摄取抑制剂、补钾药、拟钙剂、双膦酸盐类药物、青光眼用药、平喘药、抗癌药、避孕药（具）	心血管药物、利尿剂、降糖药、降压药、调节血脂类药物、甲状腺激素类药物、抗抑郁症药、抗焦虑药、抗惊厥、镇痛药、电解质平衡调节药、维生素类、眼科用药、激素及其有关药物、平喘药、抗癌药、避孕药（具）	非甾体抗炎药、抗变态反应类药

续 表

国家和地区	文献中纳入的药品	所属药物类别	不得纳入的药品
瑞典	降糖药、降压药、他汀类药物、β受体阻滞剂、选择性不含肝素的血小板聚集抑制剂、血管紧张素转化酶抑制剂、利尿剂、抗癫痫药、抗精神病药、非选择性单胺再摄取抑制剂、选择性血清素再摄取抑制剂、双膦酸盐类药物、甲状腺激素替代药物、雌激素、平喘药、泻药、激素、避孕药（具）	降糖药、降压药、调节血脂类药物、心血管药物、抗癫痫药、抗精神病药、抗抑郁症药、激素及其有关药物、甲状腺激素类药物、平喘药、泻药、避孕药（具）	
中国台湾地区	降糖药		
西班牙	口服内分泌激素	激素及其有关药物	
新西兰	所有药物		急性感染用抗生素、食欲抑制药、减肥药（如奥利司他，利莫那班和西布曲明）、戒烟药（尼古丁、安非他酮、伐尼克兰），急性疼痛用镇痛药、镇咳药、注射用利尿药、注射用安眠药和镇静药、初次使用的抗抑郁药
英国	抗溃疡药、抗酸药、非甾体抗炎药	消化性溃疡病药物、催眠药、抗焦虑药、非甾体抗炎药、避孕药	较为昂贵的药物，皮质激素类药物，其余同新西兰

对所有长期用药处方相关文献中所研究的药品种类进行统计后发现，对高血压、糖尿病、高血脂等慢病治疗药物是被研究最多的，远远高于其他类的药物，其次有抗病毒药物、精神科药品等，这些药物在文献中出现的频次见图1-3。由于慢性病的患患者数众多、用药疗程长，在定期随访条件下可以长期使用等特点，是长期用药处方最适合的药物类型[30]。艾滋病治疗用抗病毒药物、精神科药物等的服用依从性较差时，可以通过长期用药处方的模式

和每次取药时的复核与督促来提高其依从性。

并非所有的药物都适合长期用药处方。如图 1-3 所示，一些病程短、病情变化大的疾病用药，包括治疗急性感染的抗生素、食欲抑制药、减肥药、戒烟药，治疗急性疼痛的镇痛药、镇咳药、注射用利尿药、注射用安眠药和镇静药、初次使用的抗抑郁药等[30]均不适合长期用药处方。就避孕药而言，英国和美国把它列入了可以长期用药处方使用的范围。根据每个国家的管理法规和支付方式不同，纳入长期用药处方项目的药物类型也不同，有些国家和地区允许医生来判断和决定。

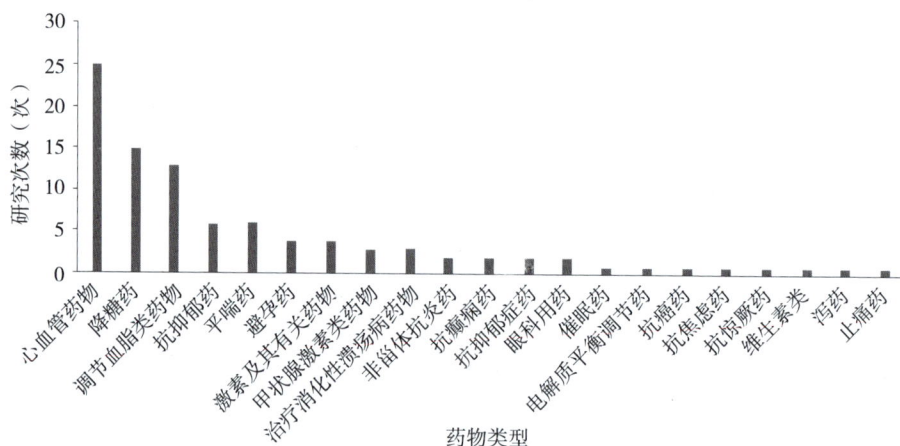

图 1-3 **87 篇文献中涉及药物种类及其相关研究数量**

针对癌痛患者的长期止痛需求和老年患者长期失眠的需求，美国、英国、澳大利亚的特殊管理药品分类、允许长期用药处方的药品管制级别及可处方量等管理方法和实践经验，值得参考和进一步研究。请参看相关章节和附件。

长期用药处方的有效期，根据药物种类或国家的不同而不同。芬兰可提供有效期为 12 个月药量的长期用药处方，这也就意味着，如果患者情况稳定，可能隔几年才会接受一次医生的检查[27]。而每张处方的药物量也有差异，例如美国每次处方量为 1~2 个月量，英国与荷兰每次处方量为 1~3 个月量。

四、长期用药处方与用药依从性

长期用药处方的取药记录可用于回顾性分析患者的服用依从性。文献研究发现，患者用药依从性在 38%~86% 之间，因药物种类、服用次数、国家以及人群基本特征不同而不同。在这些报道中，慢性病药物的依从性较高。Schectman JM 等[32]对美国某大学附属的普通内科医院 340 名患者的慢性病治疗药物长期用药处方的研究中发现，平均处方依从性在 83.9%~86.0% 之间，将患者的信息及时回馈给医生可提高患者的依从性。Morningstar BA 等[35]对加拿大慢性病患者 3 年的长期用药处方依从率调查报道，平均处方依从率为 86%，并且每日服用一次药物的依从性较高。

研究还表明，年龄、文化水平、受教育程度、种族、语言、药物类型等等都是影响患者依从性的因素。美国的 Bailey JE 等[19]对 1395 个患者的依从性影响因素调查表明，不同药物、剂量、年龄、治疗方案等都是其影响因素。Delgado J 等[22]对加拿大 886 个使用长期用药处方的艾滋病患者的依从性研究显示，依从性与年龄、明确诊断艾滋病、性别、医生的经验有关。美国 Gazmararian JA 等[37]发现健康认知力较低也是长期用药处方依从性差的原因之一。英国 Kunutsor S 等[38]对一家医院 332 位抗病毒药物使用者的依从性调查发现，外出旅游、收入紧缩、遗忘等都是影响依从性的原因。

对长期用药处方的取药记录进行回顾性分析发现，提高患者依从性的方法如下：

（1）信息化系统完善：Moreno G 等[39]对美国华盛顿医疗保健合作系统中 509 位患者使用长期用药处方的途径进行研究时发现：33.1% 的患者使用电话来操作，31.6% 的患者使用网络来操作。完善这些系统可以大大提高患者的依从性。Ascione FJ[18]在对美国 102 位社区患者的长期用药处方依从率影响因素的调查研究中表述，使用提醒系统使得没有及时来取药的延迟时间从 19.15 天降到了 6.6 天。

（2）较多的患者教育：Gazmararian J[40]发现自动电话提醒重配处方、图片处方卡、培训药师清晰的健康问题交流可提高患者对疾病的认知，从而提高长期用药处方的依从性。

（3）药品以及剂型的影响：Law A 等[41]在更改避孕药服用方法对长期用药处方模式的影响的研究中发现，大约有三分之一的口服避孕药物处方没有及时重配，改为避孕环或贴剂等方式的延迟重配率达到42%~45%。

（4）更完善的服务和团队来服务患者。Salanitro AH 等[42]对美国3 307 699名慢病患者的调查发现，简化和统一长期用药处方使用模式，加强药师的作用，避免多个医师和药店间的差异，可大大提高依从性。Schectman JM 等[32]发现，加强团队之间的沟通和协作，将患者的信息回馈给医生可提高患者依从性。

五、药师在长期用药处方项目中发挥审核、干预和随访等作用

从事长期用药处方审核与调配的药师，在英国和日本都有专门的培训，考核通过之后方可上岗。参见本书第三章和第五章。

英国 Bond 等[43]在对19个医疗机构、3074个患者、62个社区药师的随机对照干预研究中，考察了社区药师在管理和监测长期用药处方中的作用，结果表明：药师共发现12.4%的患者具有依从性、药物副作用、药物不良反应、药物相互作用等问题。说明了药师在团队中的重要性。

澳大利亚 King 等[45]在2014年发表的对25个成人长期用药处方评估研究中发现，药师在优化用药方案，提高药物的疗效、安全性以及患者依从性方面起到关键作用。通过药师的主动介入，医生可以更好的发现并解决患者的用药相关问题，从而提高处方的质量[36]。

苏格兰 Hamley 等[45]的研究表明，将临床药师整合到初级医疗照护团队，形成药师与其他医务人员合作，是一种合理并有成本－效益的可获益的尝试。

关于药师在长期用药处方项目中的做法和作用，还可参见美国、英国、澳大利亚、新加坡等国家和中国台湾地区的相关章节和附件。

第四节　慢性病长期用药处方项目的独到之处

从长期用药处方的发展历程、操作流程及利弊分析可见：①其不断完善的工作模式，使医疗资源得到更加有效利用，改善了患者诊疗过程。②在药师的指导下，患者便捷地获取长期治疗所需要的药品与用药指导。③促进了

药师与临床医师的联系与沟通，为医生分流了患者，避免了重复开药的无效就医，节约了门诊时间，提高了医疗资源利用效率。

一、长期用药处方项目的社会效益 [3-5, 18, 38, 39]

经过多年的摸索和实践，从医务人员到患者，从政府到民间，对长期用药处方的作用已基本认可，其优点包括：①提高了处方行为的质量；②提高了患者获取所需医疗服务的便捷性；③增强了患者用药安全性；④降低了全科医生的工作负荷，使其有时间为急需治疗的患者服务；⑤更适宜地发挥相关医务人员和服务人员的技能，有效利用时间；⑥优化就医过程的效率；⑦减少患者就诊次数及相关成本；⑧更好地利用各种医疗保健服务资源。

在多个国家，通过成立以药师驻店为主的诊所来突出药师在长期用药处方中的作用，通过药师与医生的合作，从而减轻医师工作量、方便患者长期服药，提高依从性。药师发挥的主要作用包括通过提醒患者定期来监测各项实验室指标，确保患者长期用药的安全性和有效性，以及长期用药处方合理使用的时间等；通过定期随访来审核目前患者服用的所有药物之间是否存在药物相互作用等，来保证患者的用药安全。药师不仅可以看到患者的长期用药处方，还可以通过信息系统看到关于患者就诊、检查和既往用药史的所有信息。通过药师的审核，可尽量避免出现不合理用药和重复用药的现象；甚至是患者已经通过其他的长期用药处方拿到并使用的药物，药师也可以知晓并审核其是否存在重复用药。通过筛选，可以让药师关注和服务那些存在药物相关需求的患者。

社会公共设施也会影响长期用药处方项目的开展情况，例如交通就是影响患者依从性的一个因素。如果在社区间缺少交通工具，如果患者的长期用药处方需求没有及时被受理，这样就得多次来诊所。这样会增加患者的服药成本，以及有可能会出现患者断药的现象。反之，长期用药处方也会促进社会公共事业的发展。因此，与政府多方合作，成为社会体系中的一个环节，长期用药处方的社会效益不容小觑。

二、对国家医疗服务体系的益处 [12, 23-25, 43]

从国家层面来看，长期用药处方项目对医疗服务系统的益处是：①保证以安全、有效和适当的方式用药；通过长期用药处方的项目，可以有效的保证患者定期定量的服用药物，并且通过定期监测来评估用药适宜性。②突出以患者为中心的医疗体系。长期用药处方在各国的开展都符合全球视角下的以患者为中心的医疗服务理念。该项目的开展都是为了给患者提供更便捷、更个性化、更安全有效的医疗服务。从患者申请长期用药处方开始，到预约取药、审核处方、评估监测患者使用长期用药处方的依从性以及适宜性，再到跟踪随访，都旨在全程跟踪服务患者。这也就要求有更完善的体系来支撑。

随着互联网和软件系统的不断发展，以互联网为主的长期用药处方系统应运而生。可以在不同地点共享患者信息，以及评估患者使用长期用药处方的合理性和适应性等等，这使得患者可以在互联网系统内的任意地点持长期用药处方取药。这样可以有效地利用资源，减少浪费。通过互联网，患者能随时随地得到更详尽的用药指导，可准确地了解如何使用和管理药品；甚至有机会与医疗专业人士讨论用药情况，了解治疗过程和重要性。还有利于降低发生药品不良反应和不良事件的可能性。同时患者通过互联网也可参与自身健康护理的决策，有助于自我管理等等。不论是从更全面的服务患者还是鼓励患者参与治疗的积极性，都更有利于开展以患者为中心的医疗服务。

三、对国家医疗保险系统的益处 [12, 23-25, 43]

不同国家对长期用药处方的政府补贴以及保险资助情况不同，但提高报销支付比例以及门槛必然有利于增加患者依从性。通过长期用药处方，可以更全面的了解和监测患者长期的用药情况，可有效避免无适应证等用药问题，避免医疗资源以及费用的浪费和潜在的危险。

第五节　我国引入慢性病长期用药处方项目的可行性和必要性

据 2011 年 4 月 28 日发布的第 6 次全国人口普查结果显示，内地总人口 13.39 亿，比 2000 年增加 7390 万；60 岁以上老年人占全国总人口 13.26%。随着近年来我国经济社会快速发展，人民生活水平和医疗卫生保健事业的巨大改善，生育率保持低水平，而老龄化进程加快[1]。

另据《中国卫生统计年鉴》的记载，2002 年我国高血压的患病率为 18.8%，按照当时的人口计算为近 0.67 亿人患有高血压[46]。2010 我国疾病监测地区数据显示，我国 18 岁及以上居民糖尿病患者的患病率为 9.7%[47]。慢性病的管理已经成为我国公共卫生服务的重大项目之一。

《中国防治慢性病中长期规划（2017-2025 年）》所针对的慢性病，主要包括心脑血管疾病、癌症、慢性呼吸系统疾病、糖尿病和口腔疾病，以及内分泌、肾脏、骨骼、神经等疾病[1]。其防治基本原则，既要坚持统筹协调，统筹各方资源，健全政府主导、部门协作、动员社会、全民参与的慢性病综合防治机制；还要坚持预防为主，加强行为和环境危险因素控制，强化慢性病早期筛查和早期发现，推动由疾病治疗向健康管理转变。加强医防协同，坚持中西医并重，为居民提供公平可及、系统连续的预防、治疗、康复、健康促进等一体化的慢性病防治服务。其规划目标是，2020 年的慢性病防控环境显著改善，降低因慢性病导致的过早死亡率，力争 30~70 岁人群因心脑血管疾病、癌症、慢性呼吸系统疾病和糖尿病导致的过早死亡率较 2015 年降低 10%；到 2025 年，慢性病危险因素得到有效控制，实现全人群全生命周期健康管理。

我国近年来已采取构建和扶持基层和社区医疗机构、多渠道预约挂号等多种便民措施，而涌入医疗机构就诊人次数非但没有下降，依然呈现逐年上升趋势，其中相当一部分就是慢性非传染病患者为定期取药而去挂号开药。通过完善分级诊疗政策体系，健全医疗机构分工协作机制，逐步实现基层首诊、双向转诊、急慢分治、上下联动，并引导大医院医生和返聘专家到基层工作，可提高基层医疗服务供给能力和水平；通过完善家庭医生签约服务，并授权签约的家庭医生使用长期用药处方，可方便那些符合条件且病情稳定的患者维持长期药物治疗[4]。换言之，我国引入长期用药处方项目，是解决这部分患者的取药需求和长期药物治疗需求的良策。

在从药品供应型向专业化药学服务的转型中，我国药师的专业知识和药学服务作用尚未发挥。慢性病患者的长期防治工作中，在"强化规范诊疗、提高治疗效果"方面，长期用药处方项目有助于慢性病诊疗服务实时管理与控制，持续改进医疗质量和医疗安全。在"促进医防协同、实现全流程健康管理"方面，没有药师参与的疾病诊疗疗程和健康管理流程并不完整。实现全人群全生命周期健康管理，需要越来越多的专业人员参与，多维度、多领域、多渠道、多创新地服务于慢性病防治。

（朱珠，尚楠，陆浩）

参考文献

［1］中华人民共和国国家卫生和计划生育委员会.中国防治慢性病中长期规划（2017–2025 年）［EB/OL］.http://www.gov.cn/zhengce/content/2017–02/14/content_5167886.htm.

［2］浙江省人力资源和社会保障厅.浙江省人力资源和社会保障厅等 3 部门关于开展慢性病长期用药处方试点的通知［EB/OL］.http://www.zjhrss.gov.cn/art/2015/06/08/art_2341_2067717.html.

［3］北京市卫生和计划生育委员会.北京市分级诊疗制度建设 2016–2017 年度的重点任务［EB/OL］.http://www.bjchfp.gov.cn/xwzx/xwfb/201608/t20160818_157660.htm.

［4］北京市人民政府.北京市人民政府关于印发《医药分开综合改革实施方案》的通知［EB/OL］.http://zhengce.beijing.gov.cn/library/192/33/50/42/438653/154581/index.html.

［5］孙雯娟,Helen Zhang, 朱珠.英国的可重配处方项目及其借鉴意义［J］.中国药师,2013,（07）:1075–1078.

［6］孙雯娟,陈浩,Helen Zhang 等.英国重配处方项目运作中的安全隐患及防范概述

［J］. 中国药师 ,2014,（08）：1388–1393.

［7］孙雯娟 , 陈浩 , 朱珠 . 美国针对慢性病患者取药的方便措施与各州的实践情况［J］. 中国药师 ,2016,（05）：974–976+1018.

［8］National Prescribing Centre. Saving time, helping patients: A goodpractice guide to quality repeat prescribing［EB/OL］.http: // www.npc.nhs.uk/repeat_prescribing/···/library_good_practice_guide_repeatprescribingguide_2004.pdf,2004–01/2012–02–07.

［9］Centre for pharmacy postgraduate education.NHS REPEAT DISPENSING（Book 1）［EB/OL］.http://www.cppe.au.uk.2009–10/2012–6–3.

［10］Board of pharmacy. 2014 law book for pharmacy［EB/OL］. http:// www.gfsoso.net/scholar?q=2014%20LAW BOOK%20FOR%20PHARMACY, 2014–04–01/2014–12–01.

［11］Riege VJ.A Patient Safety Program ＆ Research Evaluation of U.S. Navy Pharmacy Refill Clinics［J］.Advances in Patient Safety,2005,5（1）：215– 218.

［12］National Prescribing Centre. Dispensing with Repeats：A practical guide to repeat dispensing（2nded）［EB/OL］.http://www.npc.co.uk, 2008–09/2012–4–11.

［13］Walker K.Repeat prescription recording in general practice［J］. J R Coll Gen Pract, 1971, 21（113）：748–751.

［14］Balint M. Repeat prescription patients: are they an identifiable group?［J］. The International Journal of Psychiatry in Medicine, 1970, 1（1）：3–14.

［15］Grant G B, Gregory D A, Van Zwanenberg T D. Repeat prescribing: a study prior to the imposition of the limited list［J］. JR Coll Gen Pract, 1986, 36（285）：148–150.

［16］Whitelaw F G, Nevin S L, Milne R M, et al. Completeness and accuracy of morbidity and repeat prescribing records held on general practice computers in Scotland［J］. Br J Gen Pract, 1996, 46（404）：181–186.

［17］Goudie B M, McKenzie P E, Cipriano J, et al. Repeat prescribing of ulcer healing drugs in general practice—prevalence and underlying diagnosis［J］. Alimentary pharmacology & therapeutics, 1996, 10（2）：147–150.

［18］Ascione F J, Brown G H, Kirking D M. Evaluation of a medication refill reminder system for a community pharmacy［J］. Patient education and counseling, 1985, 7（2）：157–165.

［19］Bailey J E, Lee M D, Somes G W, et al. Risk factors for antihypertensive medication refill failure by patients under Medicaid managed care［J］. Clinical therapeutics, 1996, 18（6）: 1252–1262.

［20］Spoelstra J A, Stolk R P, Heerdink E R, et al. Refill compliance in type 2 diabetes mellitus: a predictor of switching to insulin therapy?［J］. Pharmacoepidemiology and drug safety, 2003, 12（2）: 121–127.

［21］De Smet P A G M, Dautzenberg M. Repeat Prescribing［J］. Drugs, 2004, 64（16）: 1779–1800.

［22］Delgado J, Heath K V, Yip B, et al. Highly active antiretroviral therapy: physician experience and enhanced adherence to prescription refill［J］. Antiviral therapy, 2003, 8（5）: 471–478.

［23］Van Wijk B L G, Klungel O H, Heerdink E R, et al. Refill persistence with chronic medication assessed from a pharmacy database was influenced by method of calculation［J］. Journal of clinical epidemiology, 2006, 59（1）: 11–17.

［24］Krigsman K, Nilsson J L G, Ring L. Refill adherence for patients with asthma and COPD: comparison of a pharmacy record database with manually collected repeat prescriptions［J］. Pharmacoepidemiology and drug safety, 2007, 16（4）: 441–448.

［25］Cox S, Wilcock P, Young J. Improving the repeat prescribing process in a busy general practice. A study using continuous quality improvement methodology［J］. Quality in Health Care, 1999, 8（2）: 119–125.

［26］Dijkers, F. W.. Repeat prescriptions. A study in general practice in the Netherlands. s.n.,1997.

［27］Saastamoinen L, Enlund H, Klaukka T. Repeat prescribing in primary care: a prescription study［J］. Pharm World Sci, 2008,30（6）: 605–609.

［28］Zermansky A G. Who controls repeats?［J］. Br J Gen Pract, 1996, 46（412）: 643–647.

［29］Petty D R, Zermansky A G, Alldred D P. The scale of repeat prescribing–time for an update［J］. BMC health services research, 2014, 14（1）: 76.

［30］Lillis S, Lord H. Repeat prescribing–reducing errors［J］. Journal of primary health care, 2011, 3（2）：153-158.

［31］De Smet P A G M, Dautzenberg M. Repeat Prescribing［J］. Drugs, 2004, 64（16）：1779-1800.

［32］Schectman J M, Schorling J B, Nadkarni M M, et al. Can prescription refill feedback to physicians improve patient adherence?［J］. The American journal of the medical sciences, 2004, 327（1）：19-24.

［33］Miller A H, Larkin G L, Jimenez C H. Predictors of medication refill-seeking behavior in the ED［J］. The American journal of emergency medicine, 2005, 23（4）：423-428.

［34］Wang J Y, Lee S H, Lee I T, et al. Effect of prescription refill on quality of care among patients with type 2 diabetes: an exploratory study［J］. Diabetes research and clinical practice, 2014, 105（1）：110-118.

［35］Morningstar B A, Sketris I S, Kephart G C, et al. Variation in pharmacy prescription refill adherence measures by type of oral antihyperglycaemic drug therapy in seniors in Nova Scotia, Canada［J］. Journal of clinical pharmacy and therapeutics, 2002, 27（3）：213-220.

［36］Saastamoinen L, Klaukka T, IlomakiJ.An intervention to develop repeat prescribing incommunitypharmacy［J］. Journal of Clinical Pharmacy and Therapeutics, 2009, 34（3）, 261-265

［37］Gazmararian J A, Kripalani S, Miller M J, et al. Factors associated with medication refill adherence in cardiovascular-related diseases: A focus on health literacy［J］. Journal of general internal medicine, 2006, 21（12）：1215-1221.

［38］Kunutsor S, Walley J, Katabira E, et al. Clinic attendance for medication refills and medication adherence amongst an antiretroviral treatment cohort in Uganda: a prospective study［J］. AIDS research and treatment, 2010, 2010.

［39］Moreno G, Lin E H, Chang E, et al. Disparities in the use of Internet and telephone medication refills among linguistically diverse patients［J］. Journal of general internal medicine, 2016, 31（3）：282-288.

［40］Gazmararian J, Jacobson K L, Pan Y, et al. Effect of a pharmacy-based health literacy intervention and patient characteristics on medication refill adherence in an urban health system［J］.

Annals of Pharmacotherapy, 2010, 44（1）：80–87.

［41］Law A, Lee Y C, Gorritz M, et al. Does switching contraceptive from oral to a patch or vaginal ring change the likelihood of timely prescription refill?［J］. Contraception, 2014, 90（2）：188–194.

［42］Salanitro A H, Kripalani S. Prescription refill management and its effect on adherence: comment on "the implications of therapeutic complexity on adherence to cardiovascular medications"［J］. Archives of Internal Medicine, 2011, 171（9）：822–823.

［43］Bond C, Matheson C, Williams S, et al. Repeat prescribing: a role for community pharmacists in controlling and monitoring repeat prescriptions［J］. Br J Gen Pract, 2000, 50（453）：271–275.

［44］King MA, Pryce RL. Evidence for compliance with long–term medication: a systematic review of randomised controlled trials［J］. International journal of clinical pharmacy, 2014, 36（1）：128–135.

［45］Hamley JH, MacGregor SH, Dunbar JA, et al. Integrating clinical pharmacists into the primary health care team: A framework for rational and cost–effective prescribing［J］. Scottish Medical Journal, 1997, 42（1）：4–7.

［46］中华人民共和国国家卫生和计划生育委员会.《2013 中国卫生统计年鉴》［EB/OL］. http://www.nhfpc.gov.cn/htmlfiles/zwgkzt/ptjnj/year2013/index2013.html.

［47］中华人民共和国国家卫生和计划生育委员会.国家卫生计生委在线发布［EB/OL］. http://www.nhfpc.gov.cn/zhuz/zxfb1/201411/3e8074f217f24dfc9d6d1e58a4ef04de.s html.

第一章 美国慢性病长期用药处方项目的研究与借鉴

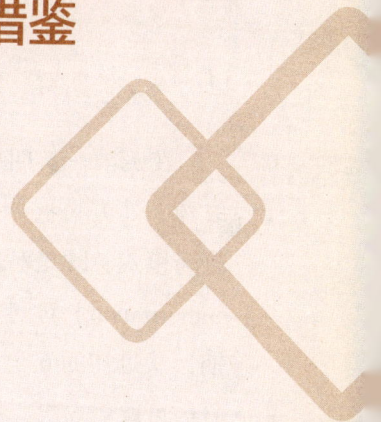

随着全球老龄化社会的到来，慢性非传染疾病给社会养老与医疗服务带来巨大压力。针对病情稳定、以药物治疗维持身体状况的慢性病患者，美国采用长期用药处方取药模式来避免患者频繁就诊，受到患者和医生的欢迎[1-3]。

第一节　美国的慢性病长期用药处方取药模式

一、长期用药处方的界定

在美国，长期用药处方的英文术语为 medication refill，字面意思是再次取药、处方再次调配，表达的是维持长期药物治疗所使用的长期用药处方取药模式，既是对用完了的药品进行再次调配和发放，也是医生授权（refill authorization）对同一处方医嘱的再次执行和调配。这种长期用药处方的有效期，从最初的 6 个月内可取药 5 次、每次取 30 天的药量，到近年来的 12 个月内可取药 6 次、每次可取 60 天的药量[3, 4]。据凯撒家庭医疗保险公司 2010 年公布的数据显示，过去 10 年里全美的处方总金额由 28 亿增长到 39 亿，其中 2/3 以上的处方在医嘱中注明为可多次重配的长期用药处方而非单次有效的处方[5]。

二、长期用药处方的调配流程

美国最早有文献记载的长期用药处方，是 1941 年底特律会议上有关长期用药处方潜在危险性介绍的文章。早期的长期用药处方多是患者个人提出的要求，没有统一的调配流程、用药范围、操作流程，主要决定者和实施者是临床医生，药师职责仅是调配长期用药处方并据此发药，实践中用药风险多[6]。1999 年在华盛顿州的 Bremerton 海军医院和 Everett 海军门诊进行了长期用药处方试点[7]。该试点及后续的实践奠定了长期用药处方的基础，实现了有药师随访患者药物治疗情况、允许患者凭长期用药处方在一定时间内多次取药的便捷流程；药师的作用从最初的调配逐渐深入到各个环节，如审核处方、处理长期用药处方申请、记录和随访患者用药情况等[7, 8]。

长期用药处方可用于如下疾病或科室：心血管疾病，呼吸系统疾病，免疫系统疾病，泌尿系统疾病，过敏症，神经病，精神病，眼科，皮科，妇科等。以慢性病高血压患者的常用药（氯沙坦、缬沙坦）为例，针对单一品种，药师在审核长期用药处方时的操作流程与细节，如图 2-1 所示[7]。

Ⅰ. 收到长期用药处方的重配申请后，根据如下条件，进行处方合理性判断：

（1）用药指征

（2）药品剂量、适应证

（3）计算取药日期

（4）确认预约时间

（5）如果是上一年度的临时（PRN）处方，应该保证开具药品数量可以用到下次预约或者 12 个月

（6）合并用药情况

（7）用药前后的生化检验值，如血清钾、尿素氮、肌酐值等

Ⅱ. 如果上述信息均符合规定，按如下步骤执行：

（1）准许重配

（2）致电处方者进行咨询

（3）电话记录存档

Ⅲ. 如果Ⅰ的结果为不合理，与患者联系并附加如下检查：

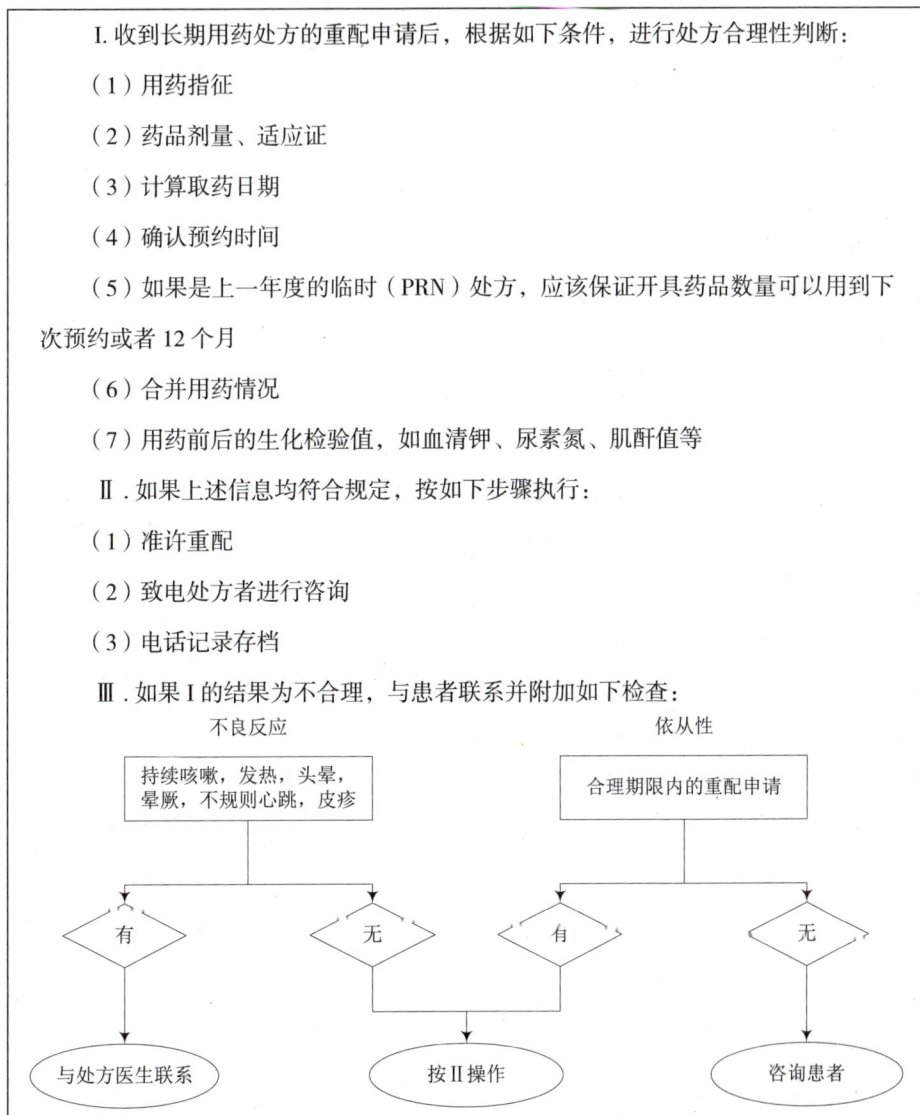

图 2-1　血管紧张素Ⅱ受体拮抗药（如氯沙坦、缬沙坦）的长期用药处方处理流程示意图

第二节　美国慢性病长期用药处方取药模式的技术支撑

随着信息科技的发展，新技术与新方法逐渐融入到医疗领域，对慢性病长期用药处方模式发挥了较大推动作用。早期长期用药处方是由医生手写处方、患者亲自预约、药房手工调配。随着技术支持的开发与深入，长期用药处方自动提醒系统、长期用药处方在线申请系统应运而生；现阶段电子处方广泛应用，与长期用药处方自动提醒系统和在线申请系统连接、融合，并在长期用药处方的运营系统中实现一体化协同作业，使得慢性病长期用药处方运作系统更加人性化、智能化。

一、自动化的长期用药处方取药提醒系统

（一）自动化的长期用药处方取药电话提醒系统[9]

自动化的长期用药处方取药电话提醒语音系统，即药师和药房联合开发的用于自动联系长期用药处方患者的特殊硬件和软件，于 1988 年在美国申请专利。该系统主要原理为通过检索数据库中存储的长期用药处方患者信息和其电话号码，自动联系患者并语音提醒其再次取药时间。患者信息指患者个人信息和处方信息。其中的处方信息包括长期用药处方日期、处方药品、用药疗程等，并以计划表的形式按时间顺序保存。整合装置主要由计算机、电话拨号、语音模拟系统组成。具体流程如下：

（1）再次取药日期临近，电脑控制的拨号系统自动拨叫患者电话。

（2）顺利接通后，语音整合系统通过姓名、开具药品种类以及处方号识别患者。

（3）如果预计已开具的药品即将用完，语音整合系统会自动提醒患者及时取药。

电话语音提醒系统存在局限性，可能存在电话占线或无人应答情况，需要再次拨通，并且受工作时间限制，发送语音提醒一般是早 10 点到晚 8 点。

（二）自动化的长期用药处方取药短信提醒系统[10]

2015 年凯撒家庭医疗保险公司为了给其所属 14 个诊所和 200 家药房的 370 万患者提供更加便捷的取药措施，研发了短信提醒系统。该系统克服了电话语音提醒系统的局限性，以短信形式直接向患者发送再次取药的时间、地点等提醒信息。

1. 短信提醒系统的组成

（1）数据库：包括患者基本信息，生化检验值结果，药房信息管理等数据信息。

（2）定期更新和管理数据库中患者的相关信息，计算患者下一次取药间隔时间的运算方法。

（3）短信自动发送系统。

（4）维护系统的工作团队。

2. 患者接收到的短信内容格式

患者接收到的短信内容格式如下："尊敬的［XXX］，这是来自凯萨家庭医疗保险公司的医疗短信。药房记录显示，您处方号为［XXXXX］的处方药品即将用尽。此信息是提醒您尽快去取药。如果您的医生已对处方做了修改和调整，请忽略此条信息；如果您准备去取药，请致电药瓶上的电话或在凯萨官网填写再次取药申请（官网网址：www. kp. org）。您可亲自来取药或者等待邮寄，邮寄时间约需 7~10 天。谢谢。"

二、自动化长期用药处方申请系统

（一）手写处方时代的长期用药处方再次取药在线申请自动化系统

长期用药处方再次取药申请自动化系统于 1999 年申请了专利[11]，它利用电话和计算机接收患者的长期用药处方再次取约申请，将患者信息数据存入数据库并对长期用药处方信息进行分析判定，如处方类型、药品管控级别等。此系统的优势在于有离线配置功能，患者可不受时间和空间限制进行长期用药处方再次取药在线申请。长期用药处方数据库可按规程分析该长期用药处方再次取药申请的有效性。如果显示申请无效，则系统会自动确认并提示患者的长期用药处方取药申请未通过。

（二）电子处方时代的长期用药处方自动提醒系统[12]

长期用药处方自动提醒系统与手写处方时代提醒系统相比，免去患者亲自到药房或电话申请再次取药，由药师和药房工作人员依靠信息系统自动生成重配申请列表，在预定的再次取药日之前，以短信形式自动发送到患者手机，提醒患者再次取药。所以，电子处方时代极大降低了长期用药处方再次取药的在线申请数量。

每个药房的处理长期用药处方的流程在细节上略有差别，但都是基于长期用药处方的再调配处理原则[12]。以南部某零售药店的长期用药处方再调配为例，其在线申请流程如下：

（1）信息接收：药房信息系统接收电子长期用药处方。

（2）审核长期用药处方是否合格：系统在慢性病用药的患者处方上进行标记，根据预定标准审核判断长期用药处方是否合格。

患者资格判断：除外美国医疗补助计划的参保患者。

药品是否合规：除外短期治疗药品（如，抗生素或其他临时用药）或有其他限制条件的药品。

（3）短信通知患者：当患者新开具的长期用药处方为合格药品，或长期用药处方再调配申请通过审核后，系统自动给患者发送短信通知，并征求患者意愿：取所有药品、仅取某个药或所有的药品都不取。

（4）患者信息反馈：收到再次取药提醒后，如果患者选择等间隔多次取药，还可以回复短信选择适合的取药提醒方式，如电话语音提醒、邮件提醒或者短信提醒。

美国大部分药房都应用自动化电子长期用药处方系统，用以提高患者用药便捷性和满意度。自动化程序节省药房员工在长期用药处方再调配流程中的时间，其节省时间的环节包括长期用药处方再次取药的电话提醒申请和电话语音通知、接收患者的再调配申请等[8, 10, 12]。

三、电子处方支持下的长期用药处方系统

电子处方是医疗信息产业的重要组成，对于加强医疗行为与药房通讯、完善长期用药处方再调配流程有积极作用。在美国，电子处方在降低错误率方面发挥极大作用，也是近年来提高长期用药处方质量与效率最为重要的技术支持内容。

电子处方实现了医生、诊所和药房之间通过计算机网络进行处方传输的过程，将大部分手写处方时代的技术整合，如电子处方系统将长期取药提醒、再次取药提醒系统融合为电子处方系统中的具体环节，管理和应用一体化；为医生提供患者长期用药处方取药历史信息的系统追踪，方便管理患者用药记录、审核药物之间相互作用或配伍禁忌，并在药房与医生沟通中搭建便捷的桥梁。截至 2008 年，全美约 12% 的诊所已应用电子处方[13]。

（一）电子处方支持下长期用药处方功能的提升[12, 13]

（1）电子处方信息系统可以检查和监测长期用药处方的处方日期和用药时长，及时为患者提供再次取药提醒。

（2）电子处方附加功能包括处理长期用药处方在线申请，提供连续、完整的患者用药信息跟踪。

（3）在电子处方支持下，医生登录长期用药处方系统不受时间、地点限制。

（4）在电子处方实施过程中，相关管理部门改变了长期用药处方工作流程，允许患者选择不止一家药房进行长期用药处方申请和调配。

（二）电子处方的积极作用[10, 12, 13]

（1）电子处方简化长期用药处方流程，其节省时间的关键环节包括接打电话、部分工作流程、报告图表等。

（2）降低电话或邮件申请长期用药处方的数量，减少医生与药房电话沟通长期用药处方事宜的发生率。

（3）电子处方在降低慢性病患者用药错误方面作用显著。包括用药剂量、用药监控、提高患者用药依从性、减少药物相互作用等。

（三）电子处方效果评价

美国在实施电子处方后，就电子处方对于长期用药处方流程的作用做了相关的调研[13]。

1. 调查背景

（1）调查样本地域分布：佛罗里达州、马塞诸塞州、内华达州、新泽西州、罗德岛州、田纳西州。

（2）样本数量：64 组临床实践组，共 276 名长期用药处方参与者。

（3）调查对象：64% 是医生，其余为办公室工作人员。

（4）操作标准：如果处方有 3/4 未调配，药房系统自动发送短信提醒患者重配；如果患者仍坚持不继续重配处方，药房应告知患者可能产生的后果或影响。

2. 调查结果

（1）患者用药：45% 是内科用药。

（2）处方类型：39% 是家庭医生处方，24% 是私人医生处方，40% 是专科操作（如口腔科、眼科）。

（3）电子处方应用比例：23% 的医生应用电子处方。

（4）长期用药处方申请方式：33% 的发起者应用药房专线，每周接 3~175 个电话和 35~375 封邮件不等。

（5）满意度：47% 的调查对象表明药房自动提醒系统十分有用。

（6）长期用药处方应用比例：54% 经常使用长期用药处方功能，17% 为有时应用，22% 为偶尔应用，8% 为从未使用。

（四）电子处方对于长期用药处方的局限性[12, 13]

电子处方支持下的慢性病长期用药处方功能并非完美，重配错误风险可产生于长期用药处方的各个环节，概括如下：

1. 信息审核有误：

（1）电脑屏幕大小的限制，导致信息查看不全；

（2）长期用药处方的条目漏看或看错；

（3）电子处方信息出现错误，但是由于药师对于系统过于信任或其他心理，忽视错误信息或者假定错误信息为正确。

2. 系统故障导致的药品信息错误。

3. 审核电子处方时未做好电子标记。

4. 患者放弃重配申请或者信息传输失败，而药房未按时收到电子处方申请（建议做电子申请信息回执），因沟通不畅而影响药品调配和长期用药治疗。

5. 长期用药处方软件技术支持方面，如长期用药处方系统出现小故障不能及时处理、软件更新迟缓等原因。

（五）长期用药处方信息系统的优化方向[12, 13]

1. 收集和核查全部错误数据，防止错误数据再次传播和再次发生；在此基础上改进流程，在实施过程中强化制度落实。

2. 不同地域实施电子化长期用药处方有各自特点，因此各地区应根据自身地域特点开发相应的电子处方软件。

3. 管理长期用药处方的电子处方软件并不完善，为了降低工作流程障碍和药品错误，软件公司需要不断完善电子处方系统，开发错误报告系统等。

4. 目前，许多政府部门、非盈利机构、私人组织已经发布了相关操作标准，强化医院和药房的人员沟通和信息连接。

第三节 美国慢性病长期用药处方的意义与管理评价

一、长期用药处方对提高慢性病患者用药依从性的意义

慢性病患者不连续用药是普遍的公共卫生问题，可导致治疗无效、疾病复发率和再入院率升高、治疗成本增加等风险。近半数的美国成年人患有慢性病并开具慢性病长期用药处方。研究数据表明，与依从性差的患者相比，依从药物治疗方案的患者，其医疗结局良好并能减少医疗护理支出[14]。然而，尽管研究者和临床医生付出诸多努力来提高慢性病患者用药连续性，仍有较高比例患者常常擅自中断药物治疗。

用药依从性差由多种因素导致，目前主要通过个人护理管理、药学服务

项目、咨询服务和长期用药处方再次取药自动提醒等干预措施加以应对。有研究表明[10]，综合管理策略较单一干预措施效果显著，但是多种方法的结合难度高且耗资大。其中，长期用药处方针对的主要目标人群为慢性病患者，其优势在于保证连续用药和便利性，降低取药频率，提高用药安全，它是提高患者依从性的有效策略之一。

以抑郁症治疗为例，试验数据结果表明，药物治疗的患者中，用药3个月后中断给药的比例约为76%。用药不连续不仅有极高复发风险，同时自残和自杀风险也急剧升高[15]。

慢性病之一的高血压同样存在不连续用药问题，不连续使用降压药可直接造成疾病复发，增加医疗管理机构的成本[16]。因此，长期用药处方程序中的用药量监测和再次取药自动提醒环节十分必要。同时，各种疾病的疗程间隔不同，因此长期用药处方自动提醒时间间隔及用药量测算的计算公式需要进一步研究[14, 15]。

2015年凯撒家庭医疗保险公司在南加利福尼亚州，针对高血压和心脑血管疾病患者应用长期用药处方自动提醒系统接受药物重配的效果展开深入探究[10]。长期用药处方自动提醒方式包括信件、电子邮件和电话。研究内容包括：与普通护理组相比，两周内长期用药处方重配率；长期用药处方间隔时长；低密度脂蛋白等生化指标值的变化和血压三项指标对比情况。其研究结果见表2-1。

表 2-1　试验组与普通护理组应用长期用药处方自动提醒系统的成效对比[10]

	他汀组	降压药组
两周内长期用药处方重配率	30.3% 比 24.9%	30.7% 比 24.2%
长期用药处方间隔时长	29 天比 36 天	24 天比 31 天
生化指标值的变化	无显著差异	无显著差异

结果表明，长期用药处方自动提醒系统对于应用他汀类调脂药和普利类降压药的患者，在两周内的长期用药处方重配方面有显著作用。此外，对于首次重配他汀类药物或普利类降压药的患者，研究组相比对照组可提前一周进行重配；对于二次重配的患者，研究组相比对照组无显著差异，且在生化

指标值变化方面无显著差异[10]。

二、简化就医流程，医药护技多方共赢

在美国，随着个人医疗护理项目的增加，医生时间被占用的越来越多。由于时间有限、家庭医生增多等因素，许多医生认为其在患者问诊和治疗过程中并不顺畅。如，在面对面的问诊中，全科医师（primary care physician PCP）需要审核和答复长期用药处方申请的电话和邮件、检查生化指标值、记录咨询报告等。患者护理和慢性病管理中通过采用多学科合作，如药师和医生合作，由药师管理长期用药处方门诊，在节省医生时间、保障患者用药安全、提高患者满意度方面非常成功[3，7，8，10]。

（一）长期用药处方对医务人员工作的积极作用

Riege 等在美国海军医院进行的长期用药处方研究，针对药师参与的长期用药处方工作对减轻医务人员工作量方面开展调研[7]。结果表明：

1. 节省处方者时间，分担其工作压力。

2. 药师有机会研究不同药物的治疗情况。

3. 增加处方者与患者的交流时间，为急需医生诊治的患者提供诊疗机会。

4. 减少护士查阅患者用药记录及化验结果的重配操作、节省更多的时间为患者提供护理与指导。

5. 药师获得医生口头医嘱后可开具长期用药处方，缩短护士等待医嘱的时间。

（二）临床药师开展长期用药处方门诊独立授权重配

贝城医疗中心（Baytown Health Center，BHC）是社区医疗护理中心，主要服务贝城社区居民、东休斯顿和附近的社区。贝城医疗中心收集了 2008 年到 2010 年的数据，针对临床药师获得长期用药处方授权后患者用药情况，评估临床药师管理长期用药处方对减轻医生工作量的影响[17]。

为了监测生化检验值、用药依从性并方便医生问诊，临床药师需审核患者病历和电子处方。如果审核不合格，需短信提醒患者或直接电话联系患者。该研究结果表明，临床药师每天审核长期用药处方申请的工作时长为 2 小时。

由临床药师参与审核后，医生处理长期用药处方申请量下降约 60%，给医生的长期用药处方申请量从每天的 10 次降到 4 次。在全部长期用药处方申请中，85% 审核通过，15% 被拒回。在所有长期用药处方申请中，42% 需要干预，有些干预超过 1 次。最常见的干预措施为，提醒患者复查生化检验项目、直接咨询医生或者拒回处方。重配授权被拒回的原因包括患者申请药品错误、患者没有提交重配申请，最多的拒回原因是医生新开具了处方或在原有基础上更新了处方。有 33% 的拒绝原因是在审核患者病历和处方后，认为没有继续治疗的必要。终止重配原因还包括患者不再接受医生治疗、生化指标结果异常需要停止用药、剂量调整而需要新开具处方、需要长期用药处方申请副本、生化值检查过期、没有及时看医生门诊等。

该研究认为，药师与医生合作可以审核患者用药记录，及时监督依从性差的患者，识别错误药物申请或重复用药。药师与家庭医生的合作，可提高药师管理长期用药处方药品重配门诊的质量，减少医生工作量，提高患者护理质量[17]。

关于授权药师独立审核长期用药处方和用药情况，参见本章第六节。

三、长期用药处方的管理评价

2006 年美国俄克拉荷马州开展长期用药处方管理在基层医疗中的作用研究[8]，描述基层医疗过程中管理长期用药处方的有效方法。部分地区的长期用药处方管理是基层医疗机构医生的日常工作，该研究试图挖掘医务人员工作潜能来评价其工作效率，将现场实践解决方案、部分解决方案结合到统一分类法中，开展了一些用于增加肺炎球菌免疫率、管理生化结果、提高对糖尿病患者管理质量的有效评价方法。

这是首次评价长期用药处方管理综合系统对于基层医疗工作的意义。调查显示，较多的医务人员并不满意目前长期用药处方的管理模式，且每天执行长期用药处方管理耗时多，花费大并且错误率较高。实验结果显示，长期用药处方操作最佳步骤为 5 步法，见表 2-2 所示。通过该方法将有效改善长期用药处方工作管理模式，降低管理费用，节省医生时间。此研究也被称为最佳实践研究[8]。

表 2-2　长期用药处方调配的最佳步骤

长期用药处方操作步骤	最佳方法
1. 患者进入重配系统	填写重配需求，以邮件或其他方式传输到药房
2. 联系药房	药房以传真形式发起重配申请
3. 做出决策	最有效、便捷的方式为药师或护士作出重配决策，必要时与医生沟通
4. 通知患者	药师将重配决策反馈给患者，通知患者使用长期用药处方
5. 备份重配记录	由最终决策者及时做相关记录

该研究对第一、二步的改进结果：邮件申请内容清晰，可以减少患者或药房电话申请中易出现的口误（如错报剂量或数量），节省患者联系时间，保证患者用药安全，患者对药房满意度较高。对第五步重配记录的改进结果：由决策者记录并执行，可以明显减少处方转配过程中的错误率。对于紧急重配处方（EMR），便捷、准确、有效地备份记录在重配过程中可加快重配进程[17]。

第四节　美国实施慢性病长期用药处方的多样性

准确和有效地调配长期用药处方是药师提供药学服务的重要工作，并且是开展患者用药教育的重要途径。2012 年美国华盛顿大学开展了电话采访调查家庭医师执行长期用药处方程序上的异同，以华盛顿州、怀俄明州、阿拉斯加州、蒙大拿州、爱达荷州等 5 个州的 11 个临床实践基地为研究点，考察长期用药处方草案和规程的多样性[18]，主要内容包括长期用药处方草案、临床药师的角色价值、临床表现评定、激励措施、用药安全教育以及住院医师在各基地实习情况。其研究结果如下：

（1）实施长期用药处方单位的性质（$n=11$）：独立诊所（18.2%），大学附属医院（36.4%），私人医疗护理中心（18.2%），社区医疗中心（1%），联邦政府下属医院（18.2%）。

（2）各州长期用药处方患者投保类型为（$n=9$）：美国医疗补助计划（31%），美国国家老年人医疗保险制度（20%），个人投保（29%），自费（10%）以及其他（10%）。

（3）实施长期用药处方单位的药师配备情况（n=11）：配备临床药师占90.9%，临床药师有长期用药处方权的占72.7%，临床药师已通过规范培训的占72.7%。

（4）临床药师的职责：不是所有医疗机构都配备临床药师，各机构临床药师的岗位各异。部分诊所、社区医疗中心和医疗护理中心的临床药师，被授权允许开具部分药品使用长期用药处方；其中，部分医疗机构的临床药师职责包括：审核患者用药错误、是否有漏检的生化检查，出现严重问题时与医生联系。

（5）各研究点都有各自的长期用药处方程序，且操作环节不尽相同（详见表2-3）。例如，仅有约36.4%（4/11）的研究点具备正式的、经权威专家认定的书面协议（formal written protocol）。有正式协议的实践，都会在授权之前按规定审核用药记录；没有正式协议的机构不到一半；81.8%（9/11）的基层全科医生有授权长期用药处方的权利；有正规长期用药处方程序的诊所，比没有正规程序的诊所切换授权重配药房的频率更高。

表2-3　各研究点的长期用药处方流程各环节异同一览表

研究点	有无正式重配流程	是否可以转配处方	长期用药处方申请接收者	首次授权长期用药处方者	首次审核未通过，二次授权者	是否进行复审	复审内容
1	有	是	药师或PCP	PCP	药师	是	生化值，末次重配
2	有	否	药师	药师	PCP	是	生化值，血压，末次重配
3	有	是	药师	PCP	其他处方者	是	生化值，末次重配
4	有	是	护士	PCP	其他处方者	是	记录，末次重配
5	无	否	药师	药师	其他处方者	否	无
6	无	是	药师或护士	PCP	其他处方者	是	生化值，血压，末次重配
7	无	是	药师	PCP	其他处方者	是	无提及
8	无	否	PCP	PCP	其他处方者	是	生化值，末次重配

续　表

研究点	有无正式重配流程	是否可以转配处方	长期用药处方申请接收者	首次授权长期用药处方者	首次审核未通过,是否进行二次授权者	复审	复审内容
9	无	否	PCP	PCP	其他处方者	否	无
10	有	是	护士	PCP	其他处方者	否	无
11	有	是	护士	PCP	其他处方者	否	无

综合以上调查研究，以及医疗保健和患者安全研究中心对 31 家美国基层医疗诊所的调查表明，美国长期用药处方的操作环节存在缺陷及安全隐患[18]。安全隐患包括禁忌证的常规筛查、门诊处方多样性、使用药品多样性等。多数慢性病长期用药处方由药师或者患者发起申请，通过电话、短信、邮件等方式将具体重配信息告知护士或其他工作人员进行分析、处理，处理分析结果再传输到患者记录中以备长期用药处方的调配，这些信息传递环节均易产生差错。有研究表明，转配流程的人数从 1 个增加至 4 个或更多，差错率从 25% 增加至 100%[19]。增加长期用药处方工作人员可以提高复核频率并且平衡误差，但也会是误差根源，因此合理的环节设置和人员配备是未来研究重点。

第五节　美国部分地区慢性病长期用药处方的药品分类

适用于慢性病长期用药处方的药品类别在不断完善，哪些药品可以纳入长期用药处方使用，并保证患者应用的安全性，在联邦和各州药房管理法中有明确规定。各地医院或药房也在此基础上有各自的长期用药处方药品名录。

一、长期用药处方药品目录的筛选原则

北卡罗拉那州药房法[20]中长期用药处方的药品遴选原则：针对治疗窗窄的药品进行重配时，根据上次发放的药品，选择同一生产厂家的相同规格药品。除非药师事先通知处方者优先选择另一品规的药品并且经处方者及患者同意，方可选用其他品种。另外，refill 这个术语包含了新的内容，即对应用治疗窗窄的药物的患者，在其原处方即将过期时，需开具新处方的提示建议。

二、长期用药处方的药品重配原则

1. 美国华盛顿大学医学中心发布的药品重配协议，将长期用药处方的药品按药理作用分 12 类，具体针对每类药物特点制定重配标准，并详细介绍了重配流程和注意事项[21]。

2. 北亚特兰大初级医疗长期用药处方政策对可重配药品规定如下：除另有规定，可提供患者三个月剂量的维持用药，如降压药、降脂药、降糖药、甲状腺素；需要每 3 个月定期预约复查的药物包括：麻醉药、管制药品❶、助睡眠药[22]。

3. 2014 年加利福尼亚州药房法对透析药品有如下重配规定：经处方者授权，患者可得到 6 个月量的重配药品，此重配记录应由药房保管 3 年[4]。

4. 贝城医疗中心下属的社区药房规定：允许临床药师重配药物包括降糖药、降脂药、降压药、抗凝药，及慢性心衰、哮喘、慢性阻塞性肺疾病、甲状腺功能异常、慢性过敏、胃食管反流、慢性炎症性疼痛（NSAIDs 类药物）等病症的维持治疗用药。其他类药物的重配审核需转发给患者指定医生进行。临床药师在审核长期用药处方申请时，还应查看生化指标值[17]。服用不同药物时所需监测生化指标的间隔时间见表 2-4。

表 2-4　服用不同药品所需生化指标复查的间隔时间表[17]

药品名称	化验值	检测周期
胰岛素	HbA1c	6 个月
二甲双胍	HbA1c, SCr	6 个月
磺脲类药物	HbA1c, SCr	6 个月
噻唑烷二酮类降糖药（TZDs）	HbA1c	6 个月
	LFTs	第一年 2 月/次，之后 6 个月/次
甲状腺类药物	TSH	12 个月
ACEI,ARB	SCr,K	6~12 个月
利尿剂	SCr, 电解质	6~12 个月
他汀类药物	Lipid panel	6~12 个月
	LFTs	初次应用 3 月/次，之后 6~12 个月/次
依折麦布	Lipid panel	6~12 个月
	LFTs	6~12 个月

---

❶　管制药品，相当于我国的特殊管理药品。

续　表

药品名称	化验值	检测周期
烟酸	Lipid panel LFTs	6~12 个月 初次应用 3 月 / 次，之后 6~12 个月 / 次
贝特类药物	Lipidpanel, SCr, LFTs	6~12 个月
茶碱	茶碱血药浓度	6~12 个月
地高辛	BMP 地高辛血药浓度	12 个月 12 个月
NSAIDs	Hgb/Hct, SCr	12 个月
沙丁胺醇		用量不超过 1 吸入器 /30 天

第六节　美国慢性病长期用药处方相关法规

一、美国药房法规简介

《美国联邦法规》（Code of Federal Regulations，简称 CFR）是总指导原则[24]，是美国联邦政府执行机构和部门在"联邦公报"中发表与公布的一般性和永久性规则的集成，具有普遍适用性和法律效应。其中第 21 章是美国食品药品管理局（Food and Drug Administration，FDA）、美国缉毒局（Drug Enforcement Administration，DEA）和国家麻醉品控制政策办公室（Office of National Drug Control Policy，ONDCP）对药品和食品的相关规定。

经国会授权，各州行政部门以联邦管理法规为依据，制定有各州特色的管理法案[20~23]；经国会准许，各州行政部门根据联邦行政程序法案（Administrative Procedure Act）颁布管理细则并在联邦公报（Federal Register，FR）[25] 上发布，随后准许实施。根据美国药房理事会全国联合会颁布的《标准州药房法》（Model State Pharmacy Act and Model Regulation of the National Association of Boards）[26]，各州可以颁布本州的药房法。

《标准州药房法》强调对各州颁布的药房法进行管理约束，对突发公共卫生事件的长期用药处方以及药房日常工作有详细的规定与要求[27]。

二、长期用药处方的法律规定

（一）2016 年修订的《美国联邦法规》

2016 年修订的《美国联邦法规》中 Section 1306.22，对慢性病长期用药处方的相关规定如下，详见附件一[24]：

1. 自开具之日起，Ⅲ、Ⅳ类管制药品（Schedule Ⅲ or Ⅳ）的长期用药处方重配时长不能超过 6 个月，重配次数不超过 5 次。

2. 每次重配取药时，都应该在处方背面或电子处方记录中做出标记。若记录在其他文件项下，如用药记录、电子处方记录中，需保证文件内容与处方内容一致。

3. 以下信息可通过处方号检索到：调配或重配的药品名称、剂型、数量，调配或重配日期，执行人姓名。

4. 如果药师在处方背面签字或在电子处方记录上进行注解，即视为处方已再次调配完成。

5. 处方医生可以通过口头重配授权药师对Ⅲ或Ⅳ类管制药品进行重配。

6. 电脑程序可以用于存储和检索原始处方中Ⅲ或Ⅳ类管制药品重配信息依据条件，以及重配具体要求和限制。

7. 长期口服避孕药，可给予重配六次的长期用药处方。

8. 对于慢性病用药，现有处方量用完 75% 或以上时，可以申办下一个长期用药处方。

9. 对于患者准备境外旅游、应急等特殊情况，药师审核后可允许提前重配[22]。

（二）Ⅱ类管制药品的长期用药处方

1961 颁布的《美国管制药品法案》（Controlled Substances Act，CSA）麻醉品单一公约（Single Convention on Narcotic Drugs），是最早确定管制药品分级的法案[28]。根据管制药品成瘾性将药品分为五个等级，即Ⅰ、Ⅱ、Ⅲ、Ⅳ、Ⅴ类管制药品。Ⅰ类管制药品没有临床应用合理性并且滥用危害严重的药品；Ⅱ类管制药品有临床应用合理性且滥用危害严重的药品；Ⅲ，Ⅳ，Ⅴ类管制药品有临床应用合理性并且被认为滥用可能性较低的药品[24]。

2013 年修订的《联邦管理法规》1306.12 条规定，Ⅱ类管制药品不适于长期用药处方[28]。但满足如下条件，医生可以授权患者一次性得到 90 天用量的Ⅱ类管制药品，即授权加倍重配处方（multiple prescription）：

1. 每个单独处方都有合理医疗目的并且由医生按专业规程开具。

2. 执业医生提供每张处方的书面指导，用以告知药房最早的可再次调配的日期。

3. 为患者提供加倍重配处方不会增加药品滥用或不合理用药的风险。

4. 开具加倍处方的药品必须经州法允许。

5. 执业医生完全遵从实施办法规定，且这些规定也要符合州法的要求。

管理规定没有批准或支持执业医生为患者开具加倍处方或Ⅱ类管制药品的长期用药处方。执业医生应该根据临床经验和临床背景以及就诊频率，对是否为患者开具加倍处方作出判断。

（三）关注特殊管理药品的管理法规和级别变化

当某些处方药升级为管制药品或管制级别提高时，在长期用药处方的审核和执行中需要及时调整，严格守法。例如，2014 年美国药品缉毒局（DEA）发布将氢化可待因产品（HCPs）归入Ⅱ类管制药品，并于同年 10 月 6 日开始执行；处方医生和药师需及时知晓这一变化，在管制药品的重配、部分调配、转配以及集中调配中，随国家法规、各州法规和医保限制做出相应调整[29]。

三、各州药房法关于长期用药处方的规定

美国有 50 个州，各州根据本州特点制定适合的药房法规。如《北卡罗拉那州药房法》（Pharmacy Laws of North Carolina）[20]由北卡罗拉那州会员大会制定，2017 年 3 月最新修订。涉及长期用药处方的内容主要包括：长期用药处方重配原则、重配药品筛选，以及关于调配、重配、转配、邮寄或普通递送处方申请的一些规定。

关于长期用药处方的限制因素、紧急长期用药处方以及其他等三个方面，比较新罕布什尔州[30]、亚利桑那州[31]、华盛顿州[21]、北卡罗拉那[20]、加利福尼亚州[4]的药房法规定，就长期用药处方的异同点进行汇总，见表 2-5。

表2-5 美国部分州《药房法》关于长期用药处方规定的异同

地区	长期用药处方限制因素	无长期用药处方时的紧急调配	其他
新罕布什尔州	对于标有PRN，或Ad lib*或有类似标注的重配处方，允许药师按患者需求进行重配，但应严格按照订购数量及用药指南进行调配。超过授权重配日期1年的处方不得重配，此后如果需增加药品，原始处方无效，需开具新处方[26]	也称临时药品供应（Interim Supply），在无处方者授权情况下，药师应运用专业药学知识分区分紧急处方，包括Ⅲ、Ⅳ、Ⅴ类管制药品，重配条件如下： a. 如不重配可能导致治疗中断或者增加患者病痛 b. 自然或人为灾害导致发生导致药师与处方者联系中断；药师无法与处方者联系 c. 按原始处方供给未超过72小时药量	助理药师不能直接接收处方者电话授权的重配处方
亚利桑那州	a. 处方授权不能重配情况： (1) 处方者没有授权重配 (2) 授权重配期限超过1年 b. Ⅱ类管制药品不能重配 c. 处方开具之日起重配周期不能超过6个月 d. 长期用药处方授权之日起，超过1年不能重配[27]	如果自然灾害或恐怖事件发生，如同时满足以下两点要求，药师可临时重配最多30天的处方药： a. 药品对患者治疗方案或发生命安全十分重要 b. 药师无法与处方者联系（药师尽力辨认标有紧急处方标写重配的内容，归档留存以备日后作为证据）	重配任何手写、电子转配，口头授权处方、电子转配无论是原始处方还是电子转配处方都需要迅速备份，由药师存档
华盛顿州	a. Ⅱ类管制药品不能重配； b. 包含Ⅲ、Ⅰ、Ⅴ类管制药品的长期用药处方期限6个月内不能超过5次，处方者更新除外； c. 长期用药处方授权之日起，超过1年不能重配，标记有PRN的处方超过1年作废[28]	如果联系不到处方者，并且根据药师的专业判断此处方为紧急处方，药师可以调配足够量的药物（但不能超过72小时用量），并且迅速通知处方者	抗精神病药、抗抑郁药、抗癫痫药、化疗药、抗病毒药、免疫抑制剂等，由疾病治愈疗程决定，此类药品重配时长最少为24周，最多不超过48周
北卡罗来纳州	标记有PRN的长期用药处方限不能超过1年，到期后原处方规定另有许诺续配[23]	紧急情况下，Ⅱ类管制药品可以根据医生的口头授权进行调配，无特殊情况不准许重配	
加利福尼亚州		紧急处方在几类特殊情况下，无需医生授权即可重配，如停止药物可导致患者用药治疗中断对患者健康造成严重伤害[2]	4063和4064部分对危险药品或紧急处方的授权问题有明确指示，除开具方者（prescriber）授权，危险药品及危险装置置不得重配

备注：Ad lib 即适量，主要指临时调配的溶液剂。

备注：A 无长期用药处方时的紧急调配，是指在长期用药处方办好之前或因无法抗拒原因而无法办理的情况下，药师为维持慢性病药物治疗用药而采取的临时补救措施。

四、关于授权药师开具长期用药处方[32]

详见本章附件 2。

第七节　启示与借鉴

美国的慢性病长期用药处方取药模式，有完善的法规保障，有详细、具体的流程，有必要的技术和信息支持系统，符合患者需求、医生需要以及社会效益。它为患者提供了更便捷、优质的取药服务；减轻医生工作负荷，充分发挥医生职责，改善了繁杂的就医环境。

医生的人力成本高、工作时间和精力有限，部分州法规已允许药师独立处理患者的处方重配申请，开具长期用药处方，明确药师在长期用药处方项目实施的责任和义务。

（孙雯娟，朱珠，陆浩）

参考文献

［1］孙雯娟，Helen Zhang，朱珠. 英国的可重配处方项目及其借鉴意义［J］. 中国药师，2013,16（7）：1075-1078.

［2］孙雯娟，陈浩，朱珠. 英国重配处方项目运作中的安全隐患及防范概述［J］. 中国药师，2014 (8): 1388-1393.

［3］孙雯娟，陈浩，朱珠. 美国针对慢性病患者取药的方便措施与各州的实践情况［J］. 中国药师，2016，19（5）：974-976.

［4］Board of pharmacy.2014 law book for pharmacy[EB/OL]. (2014-04-01). http://www.gfsoso.net/scholar?q=2014%20LAWBOOK%20FOR%20PHARMACY.

［5］Kaiser Family Foundation. Prescription Drug Trends Fact sheet–May 2010 Update[EB/OL].http://kff.org/health–costs/fact–sheet/Prescription–drug–trends–fact–sheet–may–2010/

［6］Ralph J. Mill. Journal of the American Pharmaceutical Association. Potential Hazards in the refilling of prescriptions[EB/OL].(1943). http://www.sciencedirect.com.ez.library.latrobe.edu.au/sdfe/pdf/download/pii/S009595611530565X/first–page–pdf

［7］Riege VJ. A Patient Safety Program & Research Evaluation of U.S. Navy Pharmacy Refill Clinics[J]. Advances in Patient Safety, 2005,5(1):215–218.

［8］Ferrel CW, Aspy CB, Mold JW. Management of Prescription Refills in Primary Care: An Oklahoma Physicians Resource/Research Network (OKPRN) Study[J].J Am Board Family Medcine,2006,19(1):31–38.

［9］Pilarczyk.United States Patent[P]. U.S.Patent:4.766, 542, 1988–08.

［10］Harrison T N, Green K R, Liu I L A, et al. Automated Outreach for Cardiovascular–Related Medication Refill Reminders[J].The Journal of Clinical Hypertension, 2015,18(7):641–646.

［11］Reichert RR. On–line pharmacy automated refill system[P]. U.S.Patent:5970462,1999

［12］Grimm M, Ford H, Grubbs K, et al. Patient perceptions regarding enrollment in automatic prescription refill programs[J]. Journal of Pharmacy Technology, 2013, 29(5): 231–239.

［13]Goldman R E, Dub é C, Lapane K L. Beyond the basics: refills by electronic prescribing[J]. International journal of medical informatics, 2010, 79(7): 507–514.

［14］Matlin O S, Kymes S M, Averbukh A, et al. Community pharmacy automatic refill program improves adherence to maintenance therapy and reduces wasted medication[J]. Am J Manag Care, 2015, 21(11): 785–791.

［15］Hansen RA,Dusetzina SB. Prescription Refill Records as a Screening Tool to Identify Antidepressant Non–Adherence[J]. 2010,19(1):33–37.

［16］Bailey JE, Lee MD, et al. Risk factors for antihypertensive medication refill failure by patients under Medicaid managed care[J]. Clin Ther,1996,18(6): 52–62.

［17］Nguyen M, Zare M. Impact of a Clinical Pharmacist–Managed Medication Refill Clinic[J]. Journal of primary care & community health, 2015, 6(3): 187–192.

［18］Guirguis–Blake J, Keppel GA, Force RW, et al. Variation in Refill Protocols and

Procedures in a Family Medicine Residency Network[J]. Family Medicine, 2012,44(8):564–568.

［19］Lynch J, Rosen J, Selinger HA, et al. Medication management transactions and errors in family medicine offices: a pilot study[EB/OL]. (2008–08–01). http://www.ncbi.nlm.nih.gov/books/NBK43758/?report=printable

［20］North Carolina Pharmacy. Pharmacy laws of north Carolina,chapter 90[EB/OL]. (2012–03–01)http://www.ncbop.org/LawsRules/Statutes.pdf

［21］University of Washington academic medical centers. Medication Refill Protocol[EB/OL]. (2012–05). http://depts.washington.edu/druginfo/Refills/algorythms.pdf

［22］North Atlanta primary care. Prescription refill policy[EB/OL].(2012–10–01). http://www.nffm.md/client_files/file/Prescription–Refill–Policy–for–Portal.pdf

［23］UNC Internal Medicine Clinic. ADD/ADHD C– Ⅱ Medication Policy & Procedure[EB\OL]. (2012–6).http://www.med.unc.edu

［24］United States, Office of the Federal Register. Code of Federal Regulations[EB/OL]. (2016–03–31). http://www.gpo.gov

［25］Federal Register. The Daily Journal of the United States Government. https://www.federalregister.gov/

［26］National Association of Boards of Pharmacy® (NABP®). The Model State Pharmacy Act and Model Regulation of the National Association of Boards[EB/OL]. nhttps://www.nabp.pharmacy/

［27］NABP (National Association of Boards of Pharmacy). National Association of Boards of Pharmacy Model State Pharmacy Act [EB\OL]. (2012).www.nabp.net/news/assets/06–07LEL.pd

［28］United States, Office of the Federal Register .Controlled Substances Act [EB/OL].(2017–01–24).http://www.fda.gov/regulatoryinformation/legislation/ucm148726.htm#cntlsbb

［29］Pharmacy Quality Assurance Commission. Patient care laws and rules for pharmacy[[EB/OL].(2014 10–01).http://www.doh.wa.gov/portals/1/Documents/Pubs/690214.pdf

［30］State of New Hampshire Board of Pharmacy .Laws and Rules governing the State of New Hampshire Board of Pharmacy[EB/OL].(2012–06–01).www.nh.gov/pharmacy/ laws/pharmacists.htm

［31］Arizona State. Board of Pharmacy [EB/OL]. (2013–09)www.azpharmacy.gov

［32］MultiCare Health System. Pharmacist Refill Authorization[EB/OL]. https://www.multicare.org/file_viewer.php?id=11802&title=PHARMACIST+REFILL+GUIDELINE

附件 1　2016 年修订的《美国联邦法规》中 Section 1306.22

（a）处方自开具之日起Ⅲ或Ⅳ类管制药品（Schedule Ⅲ or Ⅳ）连续重配时长不能超过 6 个月，重配次数不超过 5 次。

（b）每次重配处方都应该在处方背面或电子处方记录中作出标记。若记录在其他文件项下，如用药记录、电子处方记录中，保证文件内容与处方内容一致。

（c）以下信息可通过处方号检索到：

（1）调配或重配的药品名称。

（2）调配或重配日期。

（3）调配数量。

（4）药师首次调配药品剂量。

（5）处方调配的总次数。

（d）如果药师在处方背面签字或在电子处方记录上进行注解即视为处方已调配完成。

（e）处方医生可以通过口头重配授权药师对Ⅲ或Ⅳ类管制药品进行重配：

（1）6 个月内处方总重配次数不能超过 5 次（含原始处方调配次数在内）。

（2）药师得到口头授权需要记录在原始处方背面或者在电子处方中记录，记录内容包括日期，重配数量，重配授权号码，原始处方或者电子处方记录需要显示口头授权的医生，以及接收授权的药师。

（3）每次附加重配授权的量需要等同于或者少于原始处方的药品剂量。

（4）对于重配次数大于 5 次，以及超出重配期限的处方需要重新开具并将此类处方单独存放。

（f）作为 a 到 e 的选择，电脑程序可以用于存储和检索原始处方中Ⅲ或Ⅳ

类管制药品重配信息，依据以下条件：

（1）所有的申请需要提供在线检索(通过电脑监控或者纸质记录）原始处方信息，包括但不限于以下信息，原始处方号；处方开具日期；患者名称和地址；医生 DEA 登记号；管制药品名称，疗效，记录，数量，处方重配需由处方医生授权。

（2）所有的申请需要提供在线检索（通过电脑监控或者纸质记录）Ⅲ或Ⅳ类管制药品（长期用药处方重配期限在 6 个月之内的）的长期用药处方重配史，包括但不限于以下信息，处方重配药品名，重配日期，重配数量，识别码，调剂药师的首字母或者名字，全部处方重配的日期。

（3）药师重配原始处方、传真处方或口头授权处方涉及Ⅲ或Ⅳ类管制药品时，其重配信息必须正确记录入电脑，并且记录该事实的文件必须由药师个人独立正确记录。

如果重配处方申请为拷贝内容，并且证实数据真实可靠且有重配处方药师签字，此次调配药师需要核查数据真实性，并且以同样正式格式（格式同签署支票或者法律文件，例如 J.H.Smith 或 John H.Smith）签字，且自调配日起在此药房保存 2 年。重配处方打印后72 小时内，可以在任何一家药房重配。药房可以配备指定用药记录本或备份文件，便于药师对重配过程签字或注释。备份文件作用是证实当日录入电脑的长期用药处方信息审核完成，在药品调配后保存 2 年。

（4）电脑申请可以提供重配数据的打印版，使用的药房有责任在法案和实施条例下维护这种行为。如对于特殊用法用量的管制药品需要进行 refill-by-refill 审计跟踪。重配处方打印结果应包括处方者姓名、重配日期、原始处方申请编号。接收电子重配申请的零售药店，其处方记录中心应有能力将打印文本于 48 小时之内送至指定药房，如果 DEA 特殊代理人或者转让员要求药房提供打印文本，药房需要证实其传输文件的凭证（如，邮戳）。

（5）如果指定药房的计算机申请系统出现故障，药房需要启动备用程序处理Ⅲ或Ⅳ类管制药品的长期用药处方申请。这些辅助程序首先应确保重配申请有原始处方者授权且未超出长期用药处方最高次数。所有的操作数据在电子系统恢复应用时再进行输入。

（g）当归档原始处方、传真处方或口头授权处方涉及Ⅲ或Ⅳ管制药品时，药房需要应用（a）到（e）中的一个方法，或者直接应用（f）。

（h）当归档电子处方重配信息时，药房需要提交满足这章1311符合条件的申请信息。

（孙雯娟　朱珠　陆浩　译）

附件 2　关于药师开具长期用药处方的授权

MultiCare ✚ **BetterConnected**	用药指南 版本 1.7-1

标题： 关于药师开具长期用药处方的授权

　适用范围： 该政策适用于所有 MultiCare 卫生体系内享受 MHS（Multi Care Health System）医疗服务的门诊患者。

　政策概述：

　旨在建立 MHS 指南以授权药师恰当、安全地开具长期用药处方。指南还制定了 MHS 医生和药师之间的合作执业协议，从而为开具长期用药处方以及必要时开具相应的实验室检验提供规范化的权限。

　背景／原理：

　由于患者重新开具药品的需求导致医生和护士工作量增加，从而严重影响了 MHS 诊所的工作。此外，开具长期用药处方的延迟也常常导致患者中断治疗。药师，作为掌握着药学知识的重要专业人员，能够判定药物治疗的适宜性。考虑到药师的专业知识技能，许多综合卫生体系已经成功地授权药师来负责长期用药处方的重新开具。授权药师以合作的方式开具长期用药处方，目的在于加速重新开具药品的流程、减少医生在重复开具药品上花费的时间、通过药师进行药品审核进而促进患者安全以及将患者的院外免疫接种录入病历。授权药师开具长期用药处方旨在为家庭医生服务模式的组织目标提供支持，在医疗团队的密切合作下改善患者健康状况并提高患者满意度。

　特别说明：

　药师长期用药处方权适用的情况：持续用药（疾病和药品见第Ⅳ部分）并有长期用药处方需求的患者。

　药师长期用药处方权不适用的情况：需要开具管制药品、华法林的长期用药处方或需要开具短期治疗处方的患者。曾用药品、家庭医生的口头医嘱或停用药品。当出现上述药师长期用药处方权不适用的情况，患者处方申请会被转送给医生进行处理。

　特殊情况的处理：对于 EPIC（注：美国广泛使用的一种电子病历管理软件）中列为 On-Hand，No script，Sample（注：部分特殊的处方状态，例如在等待处方到达等）的处方，药师需要审查病历并提供文件证明。如有文件证明，处方重配机构将进行重配。如没有文件证明，则会将患者转送给医生。

　程序：确定资格：

　A. 确定患者重新开具药品的需求是否符合药师长期用药处方权适用的情况。

　B. 如果重新开具药品的需求符合适用／不适用的情况，则进入第Ⅱ部分；否则患者的需求将转送给主诊医生进行处理。

　Ⅱ. EPIC 病历审查

　A. 确定最后一次就诊的日期，并审查 MHS 医生的相关医疗记录。

　B. 如果需要开具长期用药处方，应查看实验室检验结果。

　C. 药师通过其专业临床判断来决定是否需要额外信息来评估开具长期用药处方的适宜性，并于病历中记录备案。需要考虑的因素可能包括：

　1. 药物的适应证

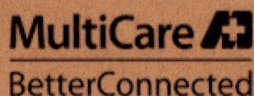

续 表

| **MultiCare** ✛ BetterConnected | 用药指南 版本 1.7-1 |

2. 药物治疗的依从性

3. 患者的并发症

4. 潜在药物相互作用或重复用药

D. 如果合格通过全面审查，则按照第Ⅲ部分开具长期用药处方。如果没有充足的信息能够明确可否恰当重新开具药品，则应根据情况采取以下行动：

1. 若药师认为需要进一步明确情况，则会向医生发送信息。潜在问题可能包括治疗疗程、药物相互作用、重复用药、治疗禁忌证或者可能需要主诊医生进一步评估的其他因素。

2. 根据当前的临床实践标准，若有必要，药师会开具实验室检验。

3. 对于需要到医生处就诊的患者，会以转发此次问诊的方式直接为患者进行预约；药师会视情况为患者开具足够的药品以保证能够使用到与医生见面。

Ⅲ. 授权程序

A. Epic 需要的文件（例如：电话问诊）。需要包含的信息如下：

1. 最后一次就诊的日期

2. 如有需要，最后一次实验室检验结果的日期

3. 对于开具长期用药处方以及开药数量的简短评估和理由 *

B. 更新 Epic 中的药品列表，并使用 Surescript（注：电子处方系统）、传真或电话将医嘱发送至患者取药的药房。* 如果适宜，长期用药处方可允许开具的最长时长为一年（从最后一次就诊 / 实验室检验日期开始计算）。

四、持续用药

药师需要有合作处方权方可对持续用药开具长期用药处方。有以下适应证的持续用药可考虑应用于长期用药处方的开具：

疾病状态或药物类别 *	
痤疮	勃起功能障碍
过敏	胃肠道疾病
阿尔茨海默氏病	痛风、高尿酸血症
贫血	激素疗法
心绞痛	高脂血症
心律失常	
抗凝	高血压
惊厥	偏头痛
精神病	营养补充剂
关节炎	
焦虑症	骨质疏松症
良性前列腺增生	疼痛
长期使用的抗菌药 / 抗病毒药	帕金森病
充血性心力衰竭	戒烟

MultiCare	用药指南
BetterConnected	版本 1.7-1

疾病状态或药物类别 *	
避孕 抑郁症 皮肤病	呼吸（哮喘 / 慢性阻塞性肺病） 甲状腺功能异常 血管疾病 - 抗血小板
糖尿病	

★具备适宜的医疗机构治疗方案相关文件的其他适应证也可以考虑。

Ⅴ.管制药品

管制药品将会被转送给医生进行处理。

Ⅵ.监测指南

根据现行基于证据的实践标准，若有必要，需要审查患者的实验室检验结果。更多常见药品类别的实验室监测指南详见附录 A。

Ⅶ.质量控制

关于药学干预的质量和适宜性，由临床药师或医师通过对药师开具长期用药处方的问诊过程定期进行同行审查，从而确保质量。

相关政策：

MHS P&P：药房：电子处方传输

MHS P&P：关于药师开具长期用药处方的授权指南

相关表单：无

患者教育：此链接提供了药师如何为临床照护提供支持的信息。（注：此连接为美国药师协会发表的题为"扩展药师在社区医疗机构的角色"的文章，链接：http://www.aacp.org/advocacy/engage/casestudies/pages/expandingpharmacistroleinpcmh.aspx）

该附录来自美国 Multicare 医疗系统，链接如下：

https://www.multicare.org/file_viewer.php?id=11802&title=PHARMACIST+REFILL+GUIDELINE。

（范倩倩　陆浩　译）

第三章 英国慢性病长期用药处方项目的研究和借鉴

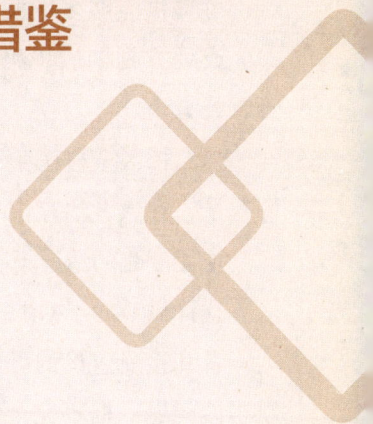

随着人口老龄化程度加重，慢性病的医疗与管理已经成为英国国民医疗保健体系（National Health Service, 以下简称 NHS）的最大问题和挑战。药物治疗作为最方便和最常用的慢性病管理方法，在目前 NHS 的所有支出里位居第二[1]。

慢性病长期用药处方（Repeat prescription）是指在接受固定药物治疗的随访期内，对药物可耐受、药效稳定、病情得到有效控制的患者，医生可提供能够多次使用的取药处方[1]。待长期用药处方的所有重配次数完成或处方到期后，患者需要预约医生进行复查，获取下一时间段的长期用药处方。

社区全科医生（general practitioner，以下简称 GP）需建立和书写治疗记录，在患者治疗记录上设定长期用药处方的复诊时间，在复诊到期之前且病情无变化的情况下，允许其可以重复申请和继续使用自己的长期用药处方药。这样做节约了 GP 的时间和精力，减少了不必要的复诊，增加了 GP 会诊新患者和接受急诊的可用时间；同时也重点解决了患者预约难和等待时间长的就诊问题。据不完全统计，在 2014 年英国 NHS 所有处方药物支出中，慢性病长期用药处方占 80%[1]，可见慢性病长期用药处方应用广泛。

第一节　英国慢性病长期用药处方的取药流程和服务规范

慢性病长期用药处方实施后，患者的取药流程也随之发生了变化。从最初患者自己"申请处方－领取处方－去药店配药"的复杂流程，到现在只需"定时到药店取药"的简单模式，患者取药变得更加方便和安全。目前，英国长期用药处方的取药模式主要分为两大类：药房提供的长期用药处方代理服务（Non-NHS repeat prescription Services）和 NHS 的长期用药处方连续调配服务（NHS Repeat dispensing Services）（见图 3–1）。患者可以根据个人情况，选择适合自己的处方服务[1]。

```
                    ┌─────────────────────┐
                    │   慢性病长期用药处方    │
                    │  Repeat Prescription  │
                    └─────────────────────┘
```

图中结构：

慢性病长期用药处方 Repeat Prescription

药房长期用药处方代理服务 NON-NHS Repeat Prescription Services

国民医疗保健体系内的长期用药处方连续调配服务 NHS Repeat Prescription Services

长期用药处方管理服务 Managed Repeat Services

长期用药处方代理领取服务 Repeat Collection Services

长期用药处方代理申请服务 Repeat Ordering Services

医师最多授权12个月的可连续调配长期用药处方，患者和药剂师在此期间无需重复申请

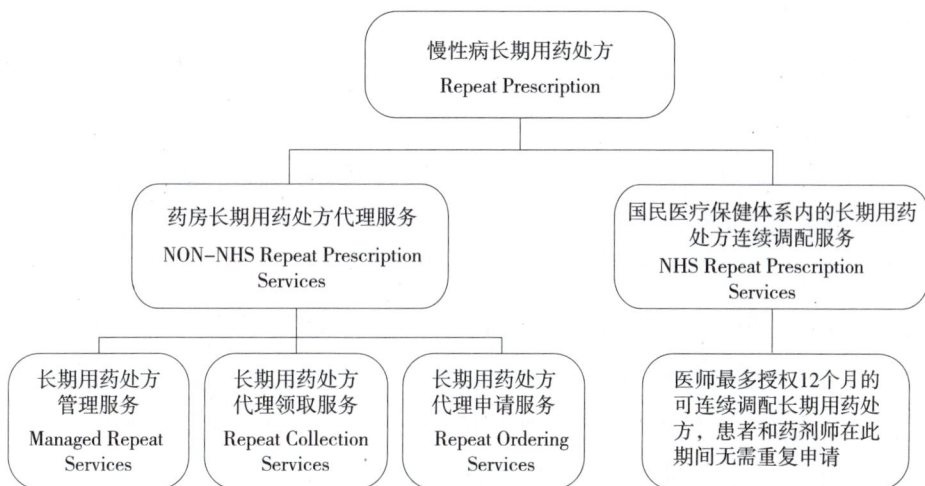

图 3-1　英国慢性病长期用药处方的取药模式

一、慢性病长期用药处方的药房代理服务

为了方便患者，减少患者自己申请和领取处方的繁琐过程，药房在传统的取药模式上，推出了以药房为代理的长期用药处方管理服务。药房代替患者申请和领取慢性病长期用药处方，节省患者往返时间和次数，减轻交通资源压力，提高取药效率。在如今的电子处方（electronic prescription services，以下简称 EPS）时代，GP 可以直接将电子处方发送到患者指定的药房，简化了服务的流程。药房长期用药处方服务建立在患者的需求上，确保患者可以准时和方便地拿药，从而提高患者用药的安全性和依从性，减少药品浪费。药房在提供服务的同时，记录患者完整的用药史，便于及时发现和更正患者的处方问题，减少社区诊所和 GP 的相关工作量。

长期用药处方的药房代理服务对以下患者具有特殊意义：

（1）弱势群体，比如患有精神疾病或者缺乏交流能力的患者，他们对已经熟悉的常用药房的依赖性很大；

（2）时间观念差的患者，药房会帮助他们管理处方的申请和领取事宜，避免因忘记按时取药而导致药品不足的问题；

（3）对行动不便、不能去诊所的患者，除了处方申请和代领，药房还提

供送药上门服务；

（4）没有网络或者不能上网的老年患者，无法完成在线申请和办理长期用药处方[3]。药房代理服务可帮助这些老年患者。

（一）长期用药处方的药房代理服务主要有以下三种方式

1. 长期用药处方管理服务（Managed Repeat Services）

由图 3-1 可见，药房全权代理患者慢性病长期用药处方的申请和领取，并按时调配。患者每次在药房取药后，在处方侧联的"长期药品目录"中提前选择下个月需要的药品，并签字授权药房代理申请。药房根据患者下次取药时间，提前 7 天代表患者在诊所申请所选药品，诊所一般需要 2 个工作日审查和授权处方，药房随后代理领取处方药物并准备调配。在英格兰地区，13% 的患者使用此项服务。

2. 长期用药处方代理领取服务（Repeat Collection Services）

患者直接向诊所或者在线申请长期用药处方，并指定自己常去的药房；社区诊所一般需要 2 个工作日审查和授权，允许患者指定药房代替患者领取处方。患者在约定时间去药房取药，或选择药房的送药上门服务。在英格兰地区，81% 的患者使用此项服务。

3. 长期用药处方代理申请服务（Repeat Ordering Services）

患者联系药房并选择所需药物，药房代表患者在诊所申请和领取长期用药处方。患者在约定时间（至少两个工作日以后）直接去药房取药，或选择药房送药上门服务[3]。

本章附件 3 收录了用于申请长期用药处方的患者信息表。

（二）药房慢性病长期用药处方代理服务的取药流程

慢性病长期用药处方用药处方代理服务的取药流程见图 3-2，可概述为以下几点：

1. 授权长期用药处方

GP 和患者签署治疗协议，确认可以采用长期用药处方的模式和药物，并指导患者知晓并执行长期用药处方的模式。GP 设定患者下次的药物、复诊时间和最多可取药次数 n（即 n 张重复处方）；在复诊到期前，患者在不需要就诊医师的情况下，最多可以申请和获取 n 次处方药，即步骤 2~7 可以重复 n 次。医师应确保患者明白定期复查的重要性，如果遇到药物副作用或者在设定复诊时间前停止了用药，患者需要及时联系医师。医师必须记录每次会诊内容，以及决定使用长期用药处方的原因。

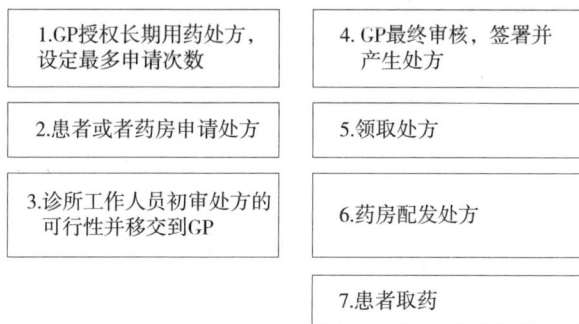

1.GP授权长期用药处方，设定最多申请次数	4.GP最终审核，签署并产生处方
2.患者或者药房申请处方	5.领取处方
3.诊所工作人员初审处方的可行性并移交到GP	6.药房配发处方
	7.患者取药

图 3-2　药房长期用药处方代理服务的取药流程

2. 申请长期用药处方

患者或者药房代理申请长期用药处方，诊所告知患者或者药房处方领取时间。大部分诊所设定的处方领取时间为 48 小时后。

3. 长期用药处方可行性的检查

诊所收到申请后，处方部的工作人员首先确认所申请药品是否在该患者的"长期用药清单"上，检查患者的复诊时间，计算患者长期用药处方的剩余次数。患者上次的处方签署时间也要审查，如果发现申请过早或者过迟，将记录下来并移交 GP 处理。如果没有问题，通过打印处方或者电子处方的形式，把长期用药处方移交给 GP 做最终审核。

4. 产生和签署长期用药处方

GP 收到初审处方后，需要建立和完成患者的治疗记录，记录患者指定的配药药房；需要结合患者的用药记录，检查长期用药处方的安全性和合理性，监督和保障患者安全和合理用药；确定患者使用了正确的药物、剂量和数量，并且不需要复诊。如果一切合理，GP 应在处方上签字，产生具有法律意义的处方。在诊所的处方信息系统里，在患者复诊到期前，长期用药处方的取药次数就会减少一次，即 n-1（重复长期用药处方也就减少一张）。如果患者需要复诊，医师需要提醒患者预约。

5. 领取处方

一般在提交处方申请48小时后，患者可自己去诊所领取处方，或者到自己指定药房领取处方。在当今电子处方信息系统中，GP可以直接把处方发送到患者指定的药房处方系统里。

6. 药品调配及药师的职责

药房获得处方后，药师首先审核处方的合法性，确保处方拥有正确和完整的药物信息；再根据患者在药房的用药记录，检查患者用药的安全性（包括剂量、数量、使用频率、药物与药物之间的相互作用）。

7. 患者取药

根据患者取药记录和处方申请的时间记录，药师可测算患者服药情况，检查其用药依从性，发现用药过量或者用药不足的问题，帮助患者正确和按时用药。

药师还可以通过执行药房高级服务条款中的"药物使用审核（medicine use review，以下简称 MUR）"，发现并分析患者的药物使用相关问题[4]。

（三）药房慢性病长期用药处方代理服务的相关指导和规范

1. 英国皇家药学会发布的《社区药房处方服务管理政策》：

为了完善药房处方管理服务的运行，英国皇家药学会（Royal Pharmaceutical Society of Great Britain，以下简称 RPSGB）指出：药师作为药事服务的一线工作者，在患者慢性病的管理中有着非常重要的作用，药师需要确保患者正确和优化用药，在正确的时间服用正确的药物，在获取最大治疗益处的同时，降低药物危害。具体内容包括：

（1）如果药房提供处方代理服务，药师必须确保服务质量，保证患者的用药安全，并减少药品浪费；

（2）药师应确保患者的用药最优化，可申请患者真正需要的药品；

（3）应提供所有可选择的处方服务项目，由患者选择最适合自己的服务；

（4）支持和鼓励药房和诊所尽可能地使用 NHS"长期用药处方连续调配服务"；

（5）鼓励患者对药物治疗的自主管理，对自己的健康负责；

（6）如果患者决定让药房代理申请处方，药房需要获得患者的"授权同意书"；

（7）药房处方代理服务需要由患者、药房和诊所的三方认可；三方必须了解处方的申请和领取流程；

（8）药师应提供患者用药教育，尽最大职责协同医生和其他医护人员为慢性病患者提供最安全的药物治疗；

（9）药师要最大可能地会诊患者，识别并解决患者的用药相关问题；

（10）通过运用团队合作、信息技术等方法，药房应帮助药师获取更多的时间，充分利用 NHS 的资源，来提高患者的用药安全和医疗成效[2]。

2. 英国皇家药学会发布《药房长期用药处方代理服务的执业参考指导》

为了指导社区药房完善和管理长期用药处方服务，英国皇家药学会在2015年10月联合英国总药房理事会（General Pharmaceutical Council，以下简称 GPhC）推出了《药房长期用药处方代理服务的执业参考指导》[2]，要求每个药房执行，重点概述如表 3-1。

患者服务授权	药房必须向患者全面介绍服务模式，提供相关的参考资料，通过口头、书面或者实际行动来获得患者的授权
高质量的药事服务	药房需要提供高质量的配药和用药服务，确保患者安全和有效的用药，在正确的时间服用正确的药物
审核用药记录	药房必须拥有完整的配药记录和患者用药记录系统，便于用药审核
服务质量改善系统	药房需要拥有服务回馈和服务改善系统，通过定期收集和审核回馈信息，改善服务质量
患者隐私安全	药房需要最大可能的保护患者隐私，不可以泄漏患者任何个人信息和用药信息
综合合作服务模式	建立以患者为中心的"医生—药师—患者—家属"服务系统，通过多方建议来设计和完善服务模式
服务效能	提高患者的用药依从性，减少药品浪费

3. 标准操作规程

根据英国药学理事会的要求，药房提供的所有服务都必须符合标准操作规程（Standard Operation Procedures，以下简称 SOPs）。药学服务协商委员会

（Pharmaceutical Services Negotiating Committee，以下简称 PSNC）在 2015 年发布的《药房长期用药处方管理服务》中介绍了 SOPs 中应该包含的内容，各个药房可以用来参考并编写自己的 SOPs[6-7]。各个诊所根据自己所在地区的长期用药处方操作模式，在《长期用药处方操作政策和实施草案》中规定长期用药处方的操作规范，建议当地合作药房参考并纳入药房 SOPs 中。

本章附件 1 是沃林顿地区（Warrington）的《长期用药处方操作和申请指导原则》，其中详细介绍了长期用药处方在当地诊所的运行方法，同时指导并规范当地合作药房的长期用药处方服务，还涉及对出院患者和养老院的长期用药处方运行[8]。

本章附件 2 介绍了英国坎布里亚郡（Cumbria）的《长期用药处方操作和申请指导原则》[9]。

二、NHS 长期用药处方连续调配服务（简称连续调配）

在社区医疗中，慢性病长期用药处方的使用达到所有处方的三分之二以上，占社区医疗开支的 80%。社区医师每年开出近 4 亿 1 千万张慢性病长期用药处方，其中 80%（3 亿 3 千万）都可适用于连续调配；如果可以实现服务转型，将节省社区医师 270 万小时的工作时间[1]。对比药房的处方代理服务，连续调配在整个取药流程中，完全省去了申请处方的环节（见图 3-3），患者只需定期到药房取药。这减轻了药房申请和管理处方以及诊所处理处方的工作量。

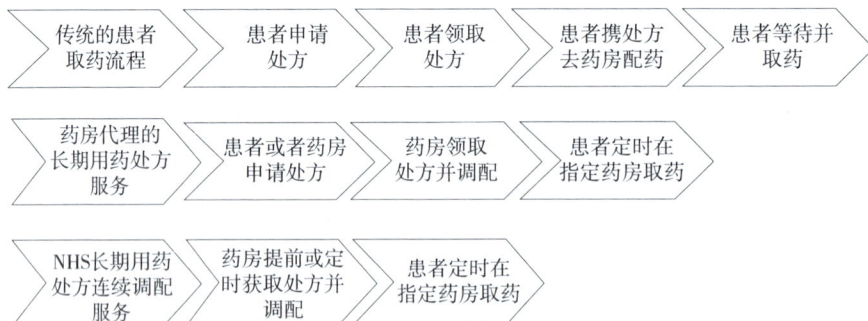

图 3-3　三种长期用药处方服务模式的比较示意图

为了更好的管理慢性病长期用药处方，从 2005 年开始，英国政府将连续调配列为《英国社区药房契约架构（Community Pharmacy Contractual Framework）》中的"基本药事服务"，即所有的社区药房都必须提供此项服务。从 2009 年 7 月开始，连续调配可以在电子处方（Electronic Prescription Services，以下简称 EPS）的平台上使用，称为电子长期用药处方连续调配（Electronic Repeat Dispensing，以下简称 eRD）[1]。电子处方简化方便了连续调配的操作，医生可以省去繁琐的操作和管理，直接在电脑系统上授权、签署、产生长期用药处方，取消或者更改长期用药处方，大大提高了工作效率和患者用药安全[10]。

（一）适用患者

大部分使用慢性病长期用药处方的患者都适用于 eRD 的模式。GP 需要临床确定 eRD 的可行性，并与患者签署知情同意书；GP 还要确定患者指定的药房可以运行 eRD。

NHS 长期用药处方连续调配服务适用患者类型包括：

（1）病情和用药稳定、使用单一药物的患者，比如使用左旋甲状腺素的甲状腺激素缺乏者；

（2）病情稳定、接受多种药物且治疗效果稳定的慢性病患者，比如高血压、糖尿病、哮喘患者；

（3）可以很好的自主治疗季节性疾病的患者，比如每年春夏季使用抗组胺药氯雷他定的过敏患者[1]。

（4）连续调配不可以用于 II 类和 III 类特殊管制药品，及病情不稳定或者需要紧急治疗的患者[10]。服用较多药物或者频繁住院的患者，也不适合使用长期调配服务[8]。

需要"临时用药（When Required Medicines，以下简称 PRN）"的患者，一般另外开具单独的处方，与常用长期用药处方分开，便于处方的管理和调配。"临时用药"的连续调配周期比较灵活，在处方有效期内，患者可以根据自己的需求和药房协商调配，药师需要根据患者的临床需求以及用药史来判断患者是否合理用药[1]。

```
┌─────────────────────┐      ┌─────────────────┐
│ 1.GP授权连续调配处方eRD，  │      │ 4.药房处方       │
│   批量授权最多12个月      │      │                 │
└─────────────────────┘      └─────────────────┘

┌─────────────────────┐      ┌─────────────────┐
│ 2.所有授权处方发送并保存    │      │ 5.患者取药       │
│   到电子处方中控系统中     │      │                 │
└─────────────────────┘      └─────────────────┘

┌─────────────────────┐
│ 3.药房按需或按时下载处方    │
└─────────────────────┘
```

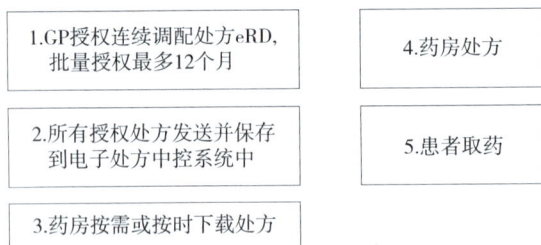

图 3-4　NHS 电子长期用药处方连续调配服务（eRD）的主要流程

（二）eRD 的取药流程可概括为以下步骤

图 3-4 为 NHS 电子长期用药处方连续调配服务（eRD）的主要流程，要点如下：

1. 社区全科医生授权连续调配处方

通过临床诊疗和患者的许可，GP 决定使用连续调配服务；根据患者的病情和下次会诊时间，GP 授权长期用药处方可以连续调配 n 次，比如患者下次会诊时间是 6 个月以后，那么 GP 可以授权 6 张长期用药处方，设定 eRD 处方要求，内容包括长期调配次数（n）和调配周期（一般 28 天）。GP 可授权的长期用药处方有效期最长是 12 个月，每张处方包含相同的处方药；

2. 产生处方

确定患者的指定药房可以运行电子处方系统后，GP 使用电子处方系统产生 n 张连续调配处方，并将处方发送到 NHS 电子处方中控系统；在药房下载处方和调配之前，所有的处方保存在 NHS 电子处方中控系统中；

3. 获取处方

GP 电子签署后，第一张处方（1/n）会及时出现在患者指定的药房电子处方系统中，后续处方（2/n - n/n）将根据 GP 的设置或者患者的要求，在不同时间获取；一般情况下，第二张处方会在下次取药时间的 7 天内自动发送到药房，药房利用 7 天的时间审核处方，联系供货商送药，以及完成配药。患者可以随时变更自己的取药药房，剩余的处方将自动转移到患者新指定的药房；

4. 药房调配和发药

药房收到处方后，按照"标准操作规程（简称 SOPs）"完成调配和发药；药师根据患者在药房的用药记录，检查患者用药的依从性和安全性（包括剂量，数量，使用频率，药物与药物之间的相互作用）。

5. 患者按时和按需在指定药房取药

在药房调配完所有长期用药处方（n）之前，患者和药房不必联系诊所或者 GP[1]。

例如：医师授权给患者 6 个月的长期用药处方，调配间隔周期为 28 天，调配次数是 6 次，即 6 张处方内容一致的长期用药处方。如果第一张处方（1/6）在 1 月 1 日完成调配和取药，药房需要发送"完成调配信号"到电子处方中控服务器，由此证明患者已经完成取药；患者的下次取药时间为 1 月 28 日，药房可以在 1 月 21 日下载第二张处方（2/6），利用 7 天的时间准备和完成药品调配和发药。

药师可以根据患者的特殊需求，按需下载和调配处方。比如患者要出国度假，药师需要根据临床和专业判断，提前手动下载下一张处方。药师必须审核患者用药的依从性和安全性。在患者用药历史记录上明确标明当次拿药时间和下次正确拿药时间。所有处方调配完成后，患者需要预约医生进行药物复查，然后重新获得另一批长期调配处方。

（三）慢性病长期用药处方连续调配的服务规范和指导

1. 英国药学服务协商委员会制定的服务规范

英国药学服务协商委员会（PSNC）在 2005 年将"长期用药处方连续调配服务"列为英国药房必须提供的"基本药事服务"，并发布了全面的服务规定（Service Specification）[10]，主要介绍了连续调配服务的益处、服务大纲和要求，以便于药房参考和执行。

为了更适时和有效管理患者的长期用药处方，英国 NHS 和 PSNC 都大力推广"NHS 连续调配(NHS Repeat Dispensing)"。NHS 在 2005 年开始实施之初，尽管社区药方和诊所都大力推广此项服务，可是使用率较低。在英格兰地区，只有 8.05% 的处方药运用于此项服务。为了确保此项服务可以持续帮助患者和国民医疗保健体系，英国药学服务协商委员会要求所有的药房于 2015 年 3 月 1 日起，根据社区药房契约合作中的最新指示，针对所有适合此项服务的患者进行宣传和教育，加大"NHS 连续调配"的使用。药房需要协助诊所选取符合条件的患者，针对患有慢性疾病且病情稳定、需要长期使用固定药物的患者，尤其是已经在药房使用长期用药处方代理服务的患者，帮助社区诊所提高"连续调配"的使用。与此同时，地方临床医药服务委员组（Clinical Commissioning Groups，以下简称CCGs）应指导和督促其管理范围内的诊所和医师，加大对此项服务的落实[10]。

2. 英国药学继续教育中心的培训科目

英国药学继续教育中心（Centre for Pharmacy Postgraduate Education，以下简称CPPE）为"长期用药处方连续调配服务"提供了完整的在线学习和考核课程，所有药师在实施此项服务前都必须先接受培训。该课程介绍了长期用药处方连续调配服务的实施目的和益处、操作方式，运行中各种常见问题及其解决方法，帮助药师更有信心地与诊所和医师达成共识，共同建立"长期用药处方连续调配服务"[11]。

3. 英国国家医疗服务系统（NHS）联合英国医学会（British Medical Association，以下简称BMA）和药学服务协商委员会（PSNC）在2013年发布《连续调配实施指导方案》

2013年发布的《连续调配实施指导方案》重点介绍了"连续调配"对诊所、医师以及患者的益处，给出了成功实施"连续调配"的十大建议：比如增强诊所和药房的合作；更新和完善处方信息系统，便于长期调配服务的操作；所有医护人员需要完成相应培训，了解服务流程等[12]。

4. 标准作业程序

CPPE为药房提供了SOPs的模版，药房可以根据自己的运行系统完成SOPs的建立[11]。

第二节　英国关于慢性病长期用药处方的指导原则

一、英国总医学理事会发布《优良处方指导原则》

英国总医学理事会（General Medical Council，以下简称GMC）推出的《优良处方指导原则（Good Prescribing Guide）》，其中一章专门介绍了长期用药处方的实用建议，要求每个诊所建立适合自己的《长期用药处方操作政策和实施方案（Repeat Prescribing Policy/Protocol）》。实用建议包括：长期用药处方药的申请；诊所对患者的用药纪录；申请和调配周期；重复授权要求；用药审核；患者转诊；养老院使用指导等。在 GP 和患者建立长期用药处方记录的时候，需要注明病情的管理方案，其中包括使用长期用药处方的原因和复查时间。与此同时，GP 还需指导患者在服药期间的注意事项。

为了确保长期用药处方的合理运用，GP 需确保以下几点：

（1）对适宜的患者对症下药；

（2）正确的剂量和药量，特别是剂量变化的药物，比如高警示药品；

（3）监控患者的病情，确保药物使用的正确性和疗效；

（4）确保只有完成培训的专业人员来准备和授权长期用药处方的申请；

（5）定期审核用药的合理性；

（6）定期审查长期用药处方药的安全性和必要性[8]。

二、英国国家处方中心于 2004 年发布关于长期用药处方的首个实践指导

英国国家处方中心（National Prescribing Centre，以下简称 NPC）在 2004 年 1 月结合医师、药师、护士、患者、诊所管理人以及其他医药专家，共同发布了《节省时间，帮助患者：提供高质量长期用药处方的优良实践指导》，首次详细介绍了该指导原则的用途、使用方法，建立长期用药处方的目的和意义，长期用药处方的完整操作流程，包括长期用药处方授权与申请，长期用药处方的产生和签署，药物审核，患者信息和指导，各方医药人员的作用和职责等[14]。

英国国家处方中心 2011 年被 NICE 取代，但是 2004 年的这份指导原则被视为经典，还是被广泛地运用到英国各个地区《长期用药处方操作政策和实施方案》中。

三、各州郡纷纷制定其《长期用药处方操作和申请指导原则》

根据英国总医学理事会（GMC）推出的《优良处方指导》（Good Prescribing Guidance）和国家处方中心的《节省时间，帮助患者：提供高质量长期用药处方的优良实践指导》，各个诊所结合地方临床医药服务委员组（CCGs）的要求，纷纷制定各自的《长期用药处方操作政策和实施方案（Repeat Prescribing Policy/Protocol）》。帮助患者更方便地取药和更安全地用药，减少了运行错误导致的危害；帮助诊所提高工作效率，减少问题和投诉，更有效的安排员工时间；帮助地方临床医药服务委员组（CCGs）减少药品浪费，减少用药错误及危害，提高用药安全和有效性[15]。

本章选取了流程规范、内容细致的两个地区的长期用药处方操作手册，见附件 1 和附件 2。

四、英国国家医疗与照护卓越研究院与"NICE 质量与持续改进案例分析"

英国 NHS 下属 Walsall 临床委员会发布了《药师主导的慢性病长期用药处方管理：确保处方适宜、减少浪费》的报告，其中英国国家医疗与照护卓越研究院（The National Institute for Health and Care Excellence，以下简称 NICE）于 2014 年 11 月发布的"NICE 质量与持续改进案例分析"，重点介绍了药师在诊所中的作用，尤其是对慢性病长期用药处方的管理。诊所药师和医生及其他护理人员组成权威的医疗团队，在减少药品浪费、降低药物伤害及副作用，提高长期用药处方运用的质量方面发挥了重要作用[16]。NICE 建议诊所和地方临床医药服务委员组（CCGs）在医药团队中增加药师，组建药师团队。

第三节　英国慢性病长期用药处方实施方案

1. 接待和答复慢性病长期用药处方的申请须知

Pharmacy's name and address	Patient's age: Date of Birth:	Patient's Title, Forename & Surname: Patient's Address: Patient's NHS number: xxxxxx	Patient's name and address: Patient's NHS number: Page 1 of 1
	Prescribed Medication　　　　Page 1 of 1 Alendronic Acid 70 mg tablets 4 tablet Take one weekly Lansoprazole 30mg gastro-resistant capsules 28 capsule Take one each morning Paracetamol 500mg tablets 100 tablet Take two when required There is THREE medication on the form.	EPS code:	Prescribed Medication Information Paracetamol 500mg tablets (100 tablet) Pharmacy information: new medicine when required for pain Patient Information Please tick the medicine(s) you require – Please only order what you need, allow 2 full working days before collection. Next review date: Repeat Medication Alendronic Acid 70 mg tablets - Take one weekly, 4 tablet　( ) Lansoprazole 30mg gastro-resistant capsules - Take one each morning, 28 capsule　( ) Paracetamol 500mg tablets – Take two when required, 100 tablet　( )
Prescriber's signature:	Date:		Prescriber's name:
	Prescriber's name and registration number: Practice address and contact number: Type of prescription:　FP10XXXXXX		Prescriber's practice address:

图 3-5　英国长期用药处方和长期用药清单样本

英国的处方分为主联和侧栏，主联是处方（见图 3-5 左侧部分），侧联是该长期用药处方的用药清单（见图 3-5 右侧部分）。当患者取药后，可以选择自己保存侧联，用于下次申请。如果选择药房代理处方服务，药房负责保存侧联和申请药物。患者如果选择自己提交申请或者药房处方管理服务，患者必须亲自在处方侧栏选择需要药品、签字和日期，患者可以自己领取处方或者药房代理领取。患者如果选择药房代理申请服务，药房必须确定患者所需药物，在侧栏盖章（包括药房地址和联系电话），签字和日期[8]。诊所一般需要 48 小时来开出处方。比如患者周五申请处方，需要等到下周二才可以领取。

使用 NHS 长期用药处方连续调配服务的患者无需保留侧联，因为此项服务不需要患者重复申请处方。

诊所收到申请后需审核的项目：①确定申请药物在长期用药处方药品清

67

单上；②检查药物信息，比如药名、规格、剂量等；③检查下次就诊复查时间；④检查申请周期，发现过早或者过迟的申请；⑤移除超过一年没有使用的药品；⑥给予最多28天的发药量[15]。

本章附件6为各种慢性病的复查周期。

2. 如何处理患者手头药品不足的紧急申请

紧急申请需要立即交给处方管理人员，初审后马上交给GP复核；患者如果过早申请长期用药处方，通常意味着药物使用过量，诊所工作人员需要通知GP进行审核和授权。在临床上，应高度重视过量用药，意味着该患者有可能对药物成瘾或者存在浪费药物的现象。如果申请被通过，GP需要记录授权原因[8]。

3. 如何处理胰岛素、甲氨蝶呤、华法林等高警示药品的调配处方

如果患者服用高警示药品，每次申请处方时，建议复印最新的血生化检查结果或者检查记录，连同处方侧联（长期药品清单）一同提交，以便于GP审核[8]。

（1）胰岛素

胰岛素剂量必须写"unit"，不可以缩写成"U"或者"IU"；给患者提供胰岛素治疗护照❶，上面应记载患者用胰岛素的商品名和用药信息；应给患者提供信息告知书，包括如何使用胰岛素治疗护照，以及使用胰岛素的常见问题。

（2）锂剂

教育患者对副作用和毒性症状的认识；提供锂剂治疗书，锂剂的患者版信息告知书，以及锂剂预警卡；根据NICE的指导，提供定期的血液检查，检查锂剂的含量和甲状腺功能并记录，根据血检结果调整锂剂剂量并记录；患者每次申请长期用药处方的时候，医师需要复查血检报告，确定最新的结果和剂量是否合理；药师在每次调配药品的时候，需要审核患者的锂剂治疗书，确定患者是否完成了定期的血检。

---

❶ 治疗护照：即治疗用药登记本。

（3）甲氨蝶呤

在患者使用甲氨蝶呤之前，医生需要向患者解释治疗的益处和危害，安排定期血检并发放患者治疗书，指导如何正确服用药物，确保患者理解所有注意事项并同意使用甲氨蝶呤。医师需要和其他医护人员达成患者合作管理协议，确保处方和药检责任的分工，保证患者理解血检的重要性和流程，指定血检部门必须将血检结果通知医师。长期用药处方的申请需要医师单独审核，医师需要结合患者的治疗和用药记录，根据患者的血检结果授权处方，确保患者服用正确的剂量。处方上必须明确标明每周使用剂量，最长提供四周的药量。每次的血检结果和剂量变化，都需要记录在患者治疗书上。药师在配药过程中也需要检查患者的血检状况。医生、药师和患者必须了解服药后可能出现的不良反应，比如呼吸困难、持续干咳、呕吐或者腹泻。

（4）华法林

使用华法林的患者需要发放一份个人治疗手册，上面记录患者的基本信息，还有血检的时间，INR 数据，剂量和下次血检时间。在收到长期用药处方申请时，医生或者指定的医务人员需要检查患者的用药记录，确定患者已完成了定期的 INR 检查，记录结果并确保患者使用正确和安全的剂量。用药剂量需要以毫克（mg）为单位，不可以其他数量形式出现。如果患者同时使用与华法林有相互作用的其他药物，需要实施额外的 INR 检测，确保剂量适宜[9]。

4. 出院患者和养老院患者的用药申请

（1）出院患者

住院诊疗期间，医生通常使用新药或者改变患者长期用药处方中的药品。为了保证患者使用正确的药物，必须严格审查和管理出院后的用药情况。患者的社区全科医师和药师都必须对"出院用药信息表"做全面检查，结合已有的记录，更新新药品和新剂量，检查药物和药物之间的相互作用，删除不需要的药品，形成一份最新的"药品使用清单"。如有任何问题，需及时联系医院。GP 需要在审核后的"出院用药信息表"上签字和日期，并保存到患者用药档案中。如果诊所在收到医院"出院用药信息表"之前，接到患者对长期用药处方的申请，诊所需要及时联系医院，获取"出院用药信息表"传真件[15]。

（2）养老院患者的用药申请

养老院的医护人员需要根据患者的"服药执行记录（Medicine Administration Record，以下简称 MAR）"或者处方侧栏的"长期用药处方药品清单"，按月申请患者的长期用药处方药。医生最多授权 28 天的用药量，过量申请必须通过医生的审核。如果患者的"服药执行记录"需要改动，比如患者服用新药或者新的剂量，必须得到医师检查并同意更改[8]。

NICE 于 2014 年 3 月发布了《养老院的药物管理指导原则》[18]，重点指导养老院应该如何管理患者的用药申请：

（1）养老院的护理人员或者社会工作者需要接受过相应的专业培训，拥有充足的时间去完成用药申请，检查药房调配给患者的药物；

（2）养老院根据自己的运行模式和患者的个人状况，协同医师和药房选择用药申请模式。NHS 的长期调配适合病情和用药稳定的患者。养老院和患者也可以选择药房提供的处方领取和配送服务；

（3）为患者办理处方申请是养老院的工作和责任，养老院的医护人员需要直接向诊所提交申请，不可以让药房代理申请；

（4）完整记录每个患者的用药申请。药房完成调配和送药，护理人员必须结合申请记录，核对真实药物的正确性。

5. 处方应包含的必要信息

《英国国家处方集（简称 BNF）》指出，处方上必须填写的法定信息包括：处方签名；处方者的执业信息；手写签字；电子处方系统接受处方者的电子签名；处方者的地址；处方签署日期；处方者的执业属性（医师，牙医，独立处方者等）；患者全名、地址；如果患者不足 12 岁，写明患者的具体年龄。

非法定信息包括药物信息：药物全名；规格；药物剂型（片剂，胶囊，液体等）；剂量和使用频率；总药量[19]。

对于 NHS 的长期用药处方，必须明确标明允许重配的次数。若允许重配次数为 6 次，那么第一张处方还必须标明"连续调配第 1/6"。

6. 如何处理特殊管制药品需求和处方书写要点

除了上面介绍的必要处方信息，Ⅱ类和Ⅲ类特殊管制药品需要额外的处方法定信息，包括：①药品剂型：片剂，胶囊，或者缓释剂；②明确的剂量：比如一次一片，一天三次，每次间隔 8 小时；③总药量：书写必须包括文字和数字，如"调配 28（贰拾捌）片"；④如果牙医开具的处方，需要标明"牙科治疗专用"。

第Ⅰ类特殊管制药品不可医用，所以本章不予讨论[20]。

对于长期用药处方的使用，第Ⅱ类和Ⅲ类特殊管制药品需要医师和用药管理团队根据患者的个人情况认真分析，以免造成药品上瘾和滥用。Ⅱ类和Ⅲ类特殊管制药品的处方申请，必须交由授权医师审核，处方生成后只接受医师的手写签字，不可使用电子处方和电子签字授权，每次最多开具 30 天的药量[8]。由于每次处方申请都需要医师特别审核的特殊要求，长期来说不可以使用Ⅱ类和Ⅲ类特殊管制药品不可以重复调配[20]，所以不可以使用 NHS 长期用药处方连续调配服务。

第Ⅳ类特殊管制药品可以用于长期用药处方连续调配，第一次调配（1/n）必须在处方签署日期开始的 28 天内完成，后序的处方（2/n – n/n）有效期为一年[10]。

第Ⅴ类特殊管制药品可以用于长期用药处方连续调配，申请和使用方法与其他处方药品一样，没有特殊要求[10]。

本章列举了英国常用的Ⅱ类，Ⅲ类和Ⅳ类特殊管制药品，参见本章附件 7。

7. 原研药和仿制药的替换原则[21, 22]

理论上，仿制药和原研药的药物成分相同，可以达到相同的治疗效果，可是价格一般要比原研药便宜 80%。由于其价格优势，NHS 鼓励 GP 开具处方时使用仿制药，减少 NHS 的药品开支，把更多的资金投入到其他医疗领域。与此同时，使用仿制药可以让药师更加灵活地为患者配药，减少原研药单一生产厂家、可能供药不足的问题。在药品替换前，医生需要通知患者替换的原因和相关注意事项，并与患者签署药品替换协议。患者如果有任何用药相关问题，可随时咨询自己的签约药师。当然，考虑到患者的用药安全，下列有原研药不宜替换，例：

（1）抗癫痫药：药物在体内的吸收速率可能不同，导致治疗效果不同，比如拉莫三嗪；

（2）缓释药物：在体内的崩解时间和吸收效果可能不同。比如维拉帕米缓释剂；

（3）生物药：生物药由人体特殊的蛋白质合成，合成条件和过程不尽相同；

（4）环孢素：免疫抑制剂，不同厂家的产品在吸收特性上可能存在差异；

（5）治疗窗狭窄的药物：比如锂剂，不同药厂的产品可能产生不同的药理作用强度；

（6）需要物理装置的药品：比如哮喘喷雾剂倍氯米松，用于治疗哮喘，市场上有两种产品，但是药效有差别。

处方中不宜用其仿制药替换的药品，参见本章附件4。

8. 患者依从性审核

（1）诊所和GP的审查：患者申请长期用药处方后，诊所需要进行药物二级审查，指定的医护人员结合患者的治疗和用药记录，确保患者的申请符合用药周期，从而审核患者是否按照医生的要求正确用药；如果发现问题，及时和患者沟通，必要时可安排患者与医生见面。与此同时，移除患者不需要的药物，减少NHS的药品浪费和开支。

（2）药师的作用：每次调配药物时，药师都要审核患者的用药记录，确定患者按时申请处方和按时取药，检查患者的依从性。从2005年4月开始，社区药师可以对其药店的固定患者提供年度"药物使用审核（Medication Use Review MUR）"，从而提高药物治疗的效果，并减少药品浪费。MUR的主要目的就是检查患者的药物依从性，药师用10~20分钟与患者交谈，判断患者对药物的理解情况，发现真实用药情况、副作用、生活习惯等相关问题。英国NHS要求药房75%的MUR要针对全国四大患者群体：服用高警示药品的患者，最近曾住院治疗的患者，患有慢性呼吸道疾病的患者，患有慢性心血管疾病的患者（服用至少4种处方药）[17]。

9. 处方的安全性

（1）英国国家处方中心（NPC）于2010年发布了《处方安全策略》，建议如下：

授权慢性病长期用药处方

有资质的 GP 方可开具长期用药处方；必须设定复诊日期，并结合用药后的常规检查周期；

处理慢性病长期用药处方的申请

患者需要了解诊所的慢性病长期用药处方的申请和使用流程，以及相关规定；申请必须在规定的时间内（一般是 48 小时）得到正确和安全的处理；鼓励患者使用医师建立的"患者长期用药处方药品清单（处方侧栏）"来申请处方，减少电话和口头申请；

审查开具长期用药处方可行性的思考要点

是"长期用药处方药品清单"上的药品吗？药物治疗的复查日期到期了吗？药物的申请提前或者延后了吗？

长期用药处方的产生、签署、以及返还患者

鼓励诊所和 GP 使用电子处方来提高处方的安全性；有资质的 GP 需要检查处方的安全和可行性，然后签字；如果患者需要复查，通知患者预约会诊[23]。

（2）GP 的责任

英国总医学理事会指出，即使最初的慢性病长期用药处方是其他 GP 签署的，复核此时签字的 GP 对其所签署的处方也负有法律责任，所以每次签署处方前一定要审核处方的安全性，并确定下次复诊时间。为了用药安全，尽量安排患者在固定 GP 来签署慢性病长期用药处方。GP 应根据自己的临床知识，开具拥有临床根据支持并适合患者需求的药物。具体说来，GP 应认真地检查患者的治疗记录和复查记录；给患者对症下药；开出正确的剂量（尤其是剂量经常变化的药物）；确保按时检查患者的症状和用药反应；负责慢性病长期用药处方的工作人员必须接受过相关培训；任何药物的改变和副作用都需要及时会诊并记录在案。每次会诊都需要确定患者正确用药，确定药物的有效性，患者的耐受性和依从性[13]。

GP 的用药审核包括以下内容：

①长期用药的必要性和有效性；

②剂型和规格的适当性：比如剂量增加，一片高剂量代替两片低剂量；

③患者对治疗的理解；

④审核检查结果，比如血检、血压等；

⑤检查副作用、药物之间相互作用、禁忌证等；

⑥在长期用药处方药品清单上，移除不需要的药品；

⑦检查处方申请周期和频率；

⑧检查患者自己购买的非处方药；

⑨如果患者的药物治疗稳定，考虑使用NHS长期用药处方连续调配服务[8]。

（3）诊所的责任

建立《长期用药处方操作政策和实施方案（Repeat Prescribing Policy/ Protocol）》；确保诊所工作人员已完成相关培训；指导患者关于慢性病长期用药处方的申请方法，审核时间，领取处方的周期和时间[24]。

（4）药师的责任

在长期用药处方的调配中，药师可直接了解到患者的用药状况，通过每次调配时与患者见面交谈，了解患者的实际用药情况，结合申请和取药时间记录，发现并解决用药问题。药师还可以通过"药物使用审核（MUR）"强化长期用药处方使用的安全性：

①确保药房拥有完善的处方管理系统和SOPs；

②药房提供的任何服务都需要得到患者的"知晓"和"同意"；

③每次调配药品时，都要确认患者的实际用药情况，检查患者的依从性和临床反应。药师可以通过以下询问获取更多信息：您最近会诊医护人员了吗？您最近服用什么新药了吗？您有什么用药问题或者不良反应吗？请检查您的长期用药处方药品清单，您有哪些不需要的药品吗？

④实施完整的患者记录，包括用药记录，副作用记录，以及其他临床反应[3]。

（5）NHS电子长期用药处方连续调配服务（NHS Repeat Dispensing）的安全措施包括：

①每张处方只能调配一次；

②处方者因需要调整患者用药而作废某处方时，需要清楚该处方是否已

经调配；处方者应主动联系药房和患者，记录作废处方和更改用药的原因；

　　③处方者和药房都必须具有完整的患者用药记录，方便审查；

　　④处方者对其签署的所有长期用药处方负有责任；

　　⑤在长期用药处方有效期内，患者可以自由更改取药的药房；

　　⑥医生可以给药师或者患者发送电子留言，提醒患者或者药师取药信息或者药物变化，因此提高了患者的用药安全[1]。

第四节　英国慢性病长期用药处方运作中存在的安全隐患和风险防范措施

　　近几年，英国各部门一直在讨论慢性病长期用药处方的运行模式。地方临床医药服务委员组（CCGs）和社区诊所（GP practice）担心药房的长期用药处方代理服务造成了处方管理不当和药品浪费等问题，建议限制药房对长期用药处方的重复申请和管理权限。部分地区建议推出 Luton Model 或者 Coventry Model 来完善长期用药处方的运行。Luton Model 要求患者自己申请慢性病长期用药处方，第三方（药房）不可以介入。Coventry Model 是一种处方直接申请服务（Prescription Ordering Direct），简称 POD，要求患者通过地方卫生管理中心申请，处方直接发送到患者指定药房。

　　社区药房则担心限制药房处方代理服务会给患者带来不便，尤其是那些弱势群体和已经长期使用药房处方代理服务的患者。以下是 POD 试验区运作后的负面回馈：

　　（1）POD 的服务很有限，它要求患者在上午 9:00 至下午 3:00 之间电话申请处方，而很多患者在上班时间无法完成电话申请；

　　（2）很多弱势群体的身体状况很难申请处方。比如患有听力问题的患者无法正常电话申请；

　　（3）由于处方可达性的减弱，很多患者不能适时获得处方，从而导致用药依从性和安全性降低，最终导致患者病情恶化；

　　（4）限制了患者管理自己处方的选择，违背了 NHS 的核心宗旨；

（5）增多了社区诊所的患者流量和电话咨询，加大了社区诊所和 GP 的工作量和压力；

（6）混淆了患者长期以来的取药方式，给患者带来不适和不便；

（7）加大了药房的负担，药房需要更多的时间帮助患者追踪处方和修改错误申请；

（8）需要强大的 IT 和电话客服团队的支持。

因此，英国药学服务协商委员会（PSNC）和药房之声（Pharmacy Voice）根据国家政策，建议各地卫生管理部门在其管辖范围内，首先推广"国民医疗保健体系的长期调配（NHS Repeat Dispensing）"的运用，减少患者重复申请的需求；在方便患者的同时，减少药房长期用药处方代理服务的使用，最终达到减少药品浪费的目的。与此同时，各个医疗部门需要共同合作，根据患者的个人状况来决定服务方式的运用。患者的自由选择是英国卫生服务系统的基础，因此患者可以选择并随时更换适合自己的处方服务模式。任何医疗部门不能引导或者干涉患者的选择[3]。

第五节　启示与借鉴

英国的慢性病长期用药处方管理与实施，有如下特点：

1. 患者为中心的服务理念

从药房的多种代理服务到 NHS 主导的连续调配服务，目的都是帮助患者更方便的取药，达到安全和有效的用药，减少不必要的药品浪费。患者拥有自由选择处方服务方式和选择药房的权利，任何机构或者个人不得干涉患者的选择。

2. 以社区为中心的医疗服务系统

经过严格培训的社区全科医生通常被称为患者的家庭医生，他们是患者就医的第一站，也是患者迈入医院前的第一道门槛。以 GP 为中心的社区医疗服务，需要尽最大努力帮助患者解决疾病困扰，减少不必要的医院就诊，从而减少国家医疗开支。GP 对于使用长期用药处方的患者，至少要进行年度会诊，确保患者治疗的有效性和安全性，从而减少医院急诊的概率。

3. GP 和社区药师对依从性和安全性的双重审核

患者每次取药时，药师都会审核患者用药的依从性和安全性。患者每次办理长期用药处方申请时，GP 会对患者病情和用药进行评估。

4. 社区药师的作用和价值

在英国，社区药师作为药物专家，工作在医疗服务第一线，直接面对患者，帮助患者安全和有效的用药，减少因疾病或药物不良反应而去医院急诊的发生率。患者可以方便地联络或见到药师，解决小病或不适，从而避开 GP 预约难和等待时间长的问题。

药师通过培训后，可提供 NHS 授权的药学服务，提高公共卫生安全。NHS 授权的药学服务包括患者用药年度审核，新药使用服务，流感疫苗接种，小病诊治服务，紧急避孕药免费调配服务等。药师还可以升级为独立处方者，独立会诊患者，开具药品处方。

5. 有全面的法规指导和规范的操作流程

每个医疗服务环节都有相关的指导法规和 SOPs，避免随意性，减少了人为错误。

6. 快速、简单和安全的全国电子处方操作平台

电子处方简化了长期用药处方服务流程，方便了患者取药，减轻了医疗工作人员的工作量；同时，加强了患者用药的安全性，减少了人为错误。全国电子处方操作平台变为英国长期用药处方的未来，长期用药处方项目使每个使用者受益：

诊所：①减少了来诊所申请和领取慢性病长期用药处方的患者；②减少了手写处方的复杂工作量；③减少了手写处方的丢失，加强了数据和信息管理；④减少了以往手写处方的分类和管理。

处方者：①可以自由设定并控制最短和最长的处方有效期，长期用药处方有效期最多可达 12 个月；②可以协助患者更换取药指定药房；③减少了处理、审核和签字的复杂流程；④有了电子签名，就不必签署每一张处方；⑤处方者责任化，会诊处方者授权长期用药处方后，对其所签署的处方负有

责任，在此期间不需要其他处方者重新签字和授权，因此增强了临床和管理的质量；如果用药有变化，医生需要及时和药房沟通，预防用药错误；⑥电子信息储存减少了处方的丢失；⑦增强了患者的用药安全性和合理化，处方者可以更好地管理处方，随时可以作废并重新授权新的处方，并做电子记录；⑧处方者可以准确地追踪和管理处方，了解处方的调配状况并作出调整；⑨电子系统可以更新患者信息，如果患者死亡，剩余的长期用药处方将会自动作废，这样大大减少了工作量和药品浪费；⑩减少了去急诊申请药品的患者，患者可以去取药药房获取所需药品[1]。

药房和药师：①提前7天自动下载长期用药处方，药房提前预订供货和调配，加强了药房的药品供应和管理；②药房可以预知工作量并作出工作调整，提高工作效率；③每次发药前审核患者实际用药，检查患者的依从性，只发放患者需要和实际服用的药物，减少浪费（参见 eRD Prescriber quick guide）；④减少了药房去诊所取处方的时间；⑤长期给固定的慢性病患者调配处方，增进了医患关系；⑥药房不再需要分类和储存每个患者的手写处方，管理更方便；⑦药房在每次调配完成后就可以同时完成处方偿还金的申请，方便了药房月终向政府领取偿还金；⑧系统自动更新患者信息，比如患者死亡，减少了不必要的调配和药品浪费[25]。

患者和家属：①患者每次取药都得到用药审核，定期见到药师并讨论自己的药物治疗问题；②患者可根据自己的度假等特殊需求提前取药，节省了患者为开药而预约医生的时间；③减少了患者由于药房药品不足引起的往返；④患者可以自由地更换取药药房；⑤患者可以直接去指定的药房拿药，不需要重复在诊所申请和领取处方，节省了时间和精力；⑥如果用药有变化，患者不需要再次去诊所退还旧药或者领取新处方，医生可以在电脑系统上直接废除旧处方，授权新处方并发送到药房；⑦医生最多可以授权12个月的处方，方便了患者获取自己的常用药，减少了患者因为药物不足而排队急诊的问题[1]。

（郑帅，朱珠，孙雯娟）

参考文献

［1］NHS England. Electronic Repeat Dispensing Guidance. May 2015. Available online at https://www.england.nhs.uk/digitaltechnology/wp–content/uploads/sites/31/2015/06/electronic–repeat–dispensing–guidance.pdf.

［2］NHS Sandwell and West Birmingham Clinical Commissioning Group. A good practice guide to repeat prescribing. July 2016. Available online at http://www.sandwellandwestbhamccgformulary.nhs.uk/.

［3］Pharmacy Voice and PSNC. Pharmacy Management of Repeat Medication Requests. August 2016. Available online at http://psnc.org.uk/wp–content/uploads/2016/08/Managed–repeats–FAQs–Aug–2016.pdf.

［4］National Prescribing Centre. Saving time, helping patients – a good practice guide to quality repeat prescribing. January 2004.

［5］Royal Pharmaceutical Society of GB. Policy on Community Pharmacy Managed Repeat Prescription Services. Available online at http://www.rpharms.com/policy–pdfs/rps–policy–community–pharmacy–managed–repeat–prescription–services.pdf.

［6］Royal Pharmaceutical Society of GB. Repeat medicine management, prescription collection and delivery services: a professional reference guide. October 2015. Available online at http://www.rpharms.com/unsecure–support–resources/repeat–medication–management––prescription–collection–and–delivery–services.asp.

［7］Suffolk and Norfolk Local Pharmaceutical Committees. Managed Repeats. May 2015. Accessed 28/07/2015. Available online at http://psnc.org.uk/suffolk–lpc/wp–content/uploads/sites/108/2015/05/Managed–Repeat–Final.pdf.

［8］Becky Birchall. Warrington Clinical Commissioning Group. Repeat Prescribing and Ordering Guidance. Version 1.0. July 2014. Available online at http://www.warringtonccg.nhs.uk/.

［9］NHS Cumbria CCG Medicine Optimisation Team. Repeat Prescribing–A practice Guide. January 2014. Available online at https://www.networks.nhs.uk/nhs–networks/nhs–cumbria–ccg/medicines–management/guidelines–and–other–publications/repeat–prescribing–practice–guide/at_ download/file.

[10] The Pharmaceutical Services Negotiating Committee（PSNC）. Repeat Dispensing. Available online at http://psnc.org.uk/services-commissioning/essential-services/repeat-dispensing/.

[11] The Centre for Pharmacy Postgraduate Education. Repeat Dispensing. December 2014. Available online at: https://www.cppe.ac.uk/services/repeat-dispensing.

[12] NHS Confederation Publications. Guidance for the Implementation of Repeat Dispensing. December 2013. Available online at http://www.nhsemployers.org/~/media/Employers/Publications/repeat-dispensing-guide.pdf.

[13] General Medical Council. Good Prescribing Guide: repeat prescribing and prescribing with repeats（2013）. Available online at http://www.gmc-uk.org/guidance/ethical_guidance/14325.asp.

[14] 孙雯娟，Helen Zhang，朱珠，等. 英国的可重配处方及其借鉴意义。中国药师，2013，16（7）：1075-1078.（引用中文文献）.

[15] K Gough. NHS Dorset Clinical Commissioning Group. Medicines Code Chapter 15: Policy for Repeat Prescribing and Medication Review. Version 2. September 2015. Available online at http://www.dorsetccg.nhs.uk/Downloads/aboutus/Policies/Medicines%20management%20policies/Medicines%20code%20chapter%2015%20-%20Policy%20for%20repeat%20prescribing%20and%20medication%20review.pdf.

[16] Walsall Clinical commissioning group. Pharmacist-led repeat prescription management: ensuring appropriate prescribing and reducing wastage. NICE Quality and Productivity Case Studies. November 2014. Available online at: https://www.evidence.nhs.uk/Search?q=Pharmacist-led+repeat+prescription+management.

[17] Davey. NHS Lancashire Medicines Management Group. Guidelines for good prescribing in primary care（2016）. Available online at http://glendalemedicalcentre.org.uk/doc/Guidelines-for-Good-Prescribing-in-Primary-Care-update-FINAL_（1）_（1）.pdf.

[18] The National Institute for Health and Care Excellence（NICE）. Managing medicines in care homes-Social Care Guideline. March 2014. Available online at https://www.nice.org.uk/

guidance/sc1.

［19］The British National Formulary（BNF）. Edition 71. March–September 2016. Page 4 – 8.

［20］NHS evidence: controlled drugs and drug dependence. Available on: https://www. evidence.nhs.uk/formulary/bnf/current/guidance–on–prescribing/controlled–drugs–and–drug– dependence.

［21］NHS Choices. Medicines information – brand names and generics. Available online at http://www.nhs.uk/conditions/medicinesinfo/pages/brandnamesandgenerics.aspx.

［22］Specialist pharmacy service – Branded prescribing: https://www.sps.nhs.uk/articles/ which–medicines–should–be–considered–for–brand–name–prescribing–in–primary–care/.

［23］Top 10 tips for GPs–Strategies for safer prescribing: available on https://bibliosjd.files. wordpress.com/2010/12/prescription.pdf.

［24］Medical Protection. Repeat prescribing for GPs. Available online at http://www. medicalprotection.org/uk/resources/factsheets/england/england–factsheets/uk–eng–repeat– prescribing–for–gps.

［25］NHS Digital. Electronic Repeat Dispensing（eRD）: Dispenser quick guide. October 2016. Available online at http://psnc.org.uk/wp–content/uploads/2016/11/Dispenser–quick–guide. pdf.

［26］Leighton Road Surgery. Repeat Prescription Order Form. Available download online at http://www.leightonroadsurgery.co.uk/repeat_prescription_order_form_t34261.html?a=0.

［27］Health and Social Care Board. Items Unsuitable for Generic Prescribing. September 2016. Available online at http://www.hscboard.hscni.net/download/PUBLICATIONS/pharmacy_and_ medicines_management/prescribing_guidance/Items–unsuitable–for–generic–prescribing.pdf.

［28］British National Formulary, 71st Edition, March – September 2016. Page 7.

附件 1 长期用药处方的操作和申请指导原则

NHS（英国国民医疗保健体系）

沃灵顿

临床医药服务委员组

版本	1.0
主编	贝基伯彻尔，CMCSU（MM）用药管理协会
参编	帕梅拉秀，CWW 区域协会 梅勒妮卡罗尔，CPCW 地方医药委员会 波林·罗伯茨，CMCSU 用药管理协会（养老院用药管理负责人） 乔安妮·古德温，VR,E & S Cheshire CCG 用药管理协会
责任委员会 / 个人	高级医药管理协会 柴郡和默西塞德郡协作单位
发行日期	28/07/2014
复核日期	28/07/2016
目标机构	社区诊所，社区药房，养老院
协助机构	柴郡和默西塞德郡社区药房，柴郡、沃灵顿以及威勒尔半岛药房网
批准机构	沃灵顿临床协作组织初级护理质量委员会
批准日期	2014 年 5 月 28 日

长期用药处方的操作和申请指导原则

本指南为社区诊所、社区药房及养老院的协同合作提供了良好的实践标准，可方便安全、高效地管理长期用药处方。

前　言

我很高兴能分享这份区域性共识及指导意见，希望能够对养老院、医疗机构及药房中涉及的长期用药提供帮助。

本文将为患者提供长期用药处方服务过程中面临的实际问题并提供相关的共识。患者护理过程中涉及到的相关人员，通过相互合作对药品使用进行优化是一个关键性的策略。此外，希望这份共识能成为社区诊所、药房及养老院最终实现患者用药自行管理的起点。

柴郡、沃灵顿、威勒尔半岛区域基层医疗协会主席：格伦·科尔曼

专用术语表

下列用语在本文档中使用：

BNF	主要参考为英国国家处方集，可以增补地方规定
医疗质量管理委员会（CQC）	CQC 是英国所有健康和社会健康服务机构的监管机构
票根	在适当的时候处方的右侧可以用于申请长期药品。可以称作"用药清单""记号列表"或者"b 联"
Datix	一些地方使用的不良反应报告系统
电子处方服务（EPS）	电子化的处方生成、传输及接受系统
药物	指国民医疗保健体系中可以用于处方的任何药物、敷料、器械或设备
用药管理经理 / 用药管理协调人员	负责药物非临床应用相关问题的社区诊所行政人员
国家患者安全机构（NPSA）	是指从 2012 年 6 月纳入到国民保健服务体系，国民保健服务体系在国家患者安全机构专业知识的基础上，从错误中汲取经验来提高患者安全
患者	整个文档中，所有被提及的"患者"，都是指患者或者监护人
长期用药处方	由处方者开具授权患者常规需求的药品，无需每次取药前再找医师就诊。一般诊所规定患者在申请长期用药处方 48 小时后可以领取处方
长期用药处方连续调配	药师根据长期用药处方连续调配的指导，使得患者在既定时间段内获得持续治疗的药品，无需重复申请或者医师就诊

引　言

● 这份指南主要目的在于为社区诊所、药房及养老机构，同时还包括错误高发区域提供最为规范的实践操作指导。这份文档可用于局部会议讨论及相关协定的发展建立，以更加严格的控制长期用药处方和申请系统为目的。

● 长期用药处方可以使患者在不需要医师就诊的情况下，重复获得常用药品，因此减少了不必要的医师诊疗。这是社区诊所工作的一个重要部分，大约包括全科医生 60%~75% 的处方书写，相当于诊所 80% 的开支。

● 2011 年国家基金高度关注到不适宜处方和不必要处方给患者带来的潜在风险及对英国国民医疗保健体系资源的浪费。将医师处方纳入全科医疗服务的质量管理指标，并公布在 http://www.thekingsfund.org/ 上。

● 有证据表明，处方的差错率在 7.5% 左右，1/5 的医院就诊与用药不当相关，其中 2/3 是可以避免的。

● 英国国家处方中心发布报告总结了初诊医疗系统中存在的用药错误和改进策略。同时在 2011 年公布全科医师安全处方的 10 条有效策略，其中包括"长期用药处方安全性的关键点"。

● 医疗质量管理委员会制定药品的安全管理制度，2013 年 4 月普通医疗机构开始在 CQC 注册，药房目前还没有在 CQC 注册。

● 这份指南以患者为中心，包括三个主要部分，分别是社区诊所、药房及养老院。通过设置标准提高长期用药处方的管理和申请系统，并加强相关部门交流，提高患者治疗效果和最大限度地增加服务效率。

为何改进现有系统？

- 清晰、高效的系统可以加强社区诊所、药房和养老院相互合作并提高患者用药安全性。

- 提高了患者安全和处方质量。

- 从减少失误和避免差错方面提高风险管理。

- 在改进现有系统的同时，提高患者对治疗参与性以及药物依从性。

- 提高患者对所需药物的可及性及方便性。

- 确定所涉及相关人员的标准、角色及责任，从而减少查询，节约时间。

- 更准确地发挥专业人员和行政人员的技能。

- 社区全科医生通过使用高效的系统，提高员工对初级问题的鉴别和管理来节约时间。

- 通过控制过度申请不必要的药品和更好地使用 NHS 的资源来减少药品浪费。

- 规避处方错误带来的风险。

- 服从标准，例如：来自专业机构和医疗质量管理委员会的规章制度。

长期用药处方指导原则的操作

第一部分

患者和护理人员

对患者和护理人员的益处

快速有效的长期用药处方的使用和申请流程对于患者和护理人员来说是最重要的。他们可以方便快捷的获得可以信赖和避免伤害的服务。不好的系统或管理不当的系统，将会造成患者的沮丧、时间的浪费以及失误率增加的可能性，从而给患者的健康管理带来风险。

对患者和陪护者的益处：

- 方便快捷的获得他们需要的药品。

- 患者清楚地了解长期用药处方系统的运行，明白什么时候、如何去申请长期用药处方，同时清楚何时、何地可以获得处方。长期用药处方系统需要一个可以复查的审核记录。

- 患者通过这个途径获得具有质量保证、适宜使用的药品，同时满足个体化用药需求。

- 获得详细说明的完整处方，理解如何正确用药。

- 拥有和医疗专业人员交流的机会。

- 减少了用药错误和不良反应的发生。

- 通过增强患者对治疗和用药的决策权，协助自我管理，有助于提高医患诊疗方案的一致性，从而提高健康产出、降低入院率、缩短住院天数及医院的就诊人数。

患者和护理人员的责任

患者和他们的护理人员是使用长期用药处方系统的重要角色，在他们能力范围内，可以承担的责任包括：

● 患者明白长期用药处方的申请系统，了解可以帮助他们安全和及时获得药品的方法。

● 确保患者参与医师的用药复诊，讨论实际用药，以及使用长期用药处方的问题。

● 患者在申请长期用药处方之前应当检查哪些药品是需要的，仅需申请所需药品，然后按照处方说明正确使用。

● 患者应当使用最新的长期用药处方用药清单（处方侧栏）来申请所需药品。

● 患者如果对药品的使用有任何疑惑，应该及时咨询自己的 GP 或者药师，如何时使用药品或者怎么使用药品。

● 确保患者领取的药品是自己申请的所需药品，特别是住院后的药品通常会改变。

● 患者告知医师和药师相关药品的过量储备，从而减少过量药品的申请。

● 患者应当为处方的审核、调配及发放留有充足的时间，尤其是在节假日，业务量增多将会给长期药系统带来额外的压力。

长期用药处方的操作指导原则

第二部分

社区诊所

索引—社区诊所长期用药处方操作指导原则

部分	描述
	标准
1	开始长期用药处方:
1.1	授权长期用药处方
1.2	药物选择推荐和通用名的运用
1.3	药品供应天数或药量
1.4	剂量说明
1.5	授权长期用药处方的使用次数
1.6	新患者的长期用药处方授权
1.7	在医院和其他机构开始的药物治疗
1.8	医师家访和手写处方
1.9	长期用药处方的代理授权
2	长期用药处方的申请
2.1	患者申请长期用药处方
2.2	长期用药处方药房代理服务
2.3	第三方申请
2.4	特殊管制药品的申请
2.5	养老院的处方申请
3	长期用药处方生成
3.1	处方申请和领取期限
3.2	处理长期用药处方的申请
3.3	"高警示"药物请求
4	长期用药处方再授权和用药复诊

续　表

部分	描述
4.1	再授权的临床责任
4.2	用药复诊
5	处方的领取和管理
5.1	完成签署的处方
5.2	领取处方
5.3	传真处方
5.4	邮寄处方
5.5	无人领取或者退还的处方
6	质量保证
6.1	长期用药处方操作和申请草案
6.2	改进长期用药处方操作和申请系统
6.3	错误处理
6.4	审核
6.5	处方安全
6.6	硬件故障的应急计划
7	NHS 长期用药处方连续调配服务
8	电子处方服务

社区诊所长期用药处方的操作和申请标准

这项标准将作为最佳实践标准在某些地区运用

标准	描述
1	只有医师可以授权长期用药处方。如果处方者以外的人员进行授权，那么必须增加一项操作协定，满足长期用药处方操作政策和草案的要求
2	长期用药处方用药清单都将记录在电子病历中并且与适应证相关联
3	不适宜用于长期用药处方的药品
4	所有药物必需提供适当的用法而且必需体现适宜之处
5	按照规定大多数长期用药处方应当满足 28 天的药物供应，养老院的长期用药处方药品供应不可以超过 28 天
6	每位患者的所有药品发药量应当是统一的，也就是说所有药品的供应总量是一致的
7	如果药品在住院和门诊期间更换，出院后应该由处方者输入到社区系统中
8	处方者应当及时更新患者的用药电子记录，记录相关咨询，包括手写处方的详细情况
9	长期用药处方的申请通过使用诊所提供的患者用药清单或网络在线申请，不接受任何形式的电话申请
10	医师仅仅授权患者在用药清单上选择的药品，而不是在清单上的所有药品
11	每个诊所都需要配备与患者的通信系统，通知患者如何申请处方
12	相关的操作协定用来处理特殊管制类药品的申请
13	诊所需在患者申请处方后 48 个小时内产生处方
14	诊所需要建立清晰的长期药用药处方操作方案，指导长期用药处方的使用，并且每年进行审核
15	长期用药处方应当由接受培训的特定员工处理且不受干扰
16	诊所建立相关的医师提示系统和处理流程，比如需要药品复查、监测逾期以及长期用药处方授权过期的患者
17	对于高警示药品的申请，诊所必须建立特殊的操作程序来确保完成必要的血生化检查

续　表

标准	描述
18	当患者所有授权的长期用药处方使用结束前，诊所处方系统需要作出提示，并移交医师重新授权新的长期用药处方
19	所有的年龄超过 75 岁的患者至少每年进行一次药物复诊，同时服用 4 种或更多药品的患者每六个月进行一次药物复诊，药物复诊中还应包括用药一致性的审查
20	应当有简洁的程序用于确保将正确的处方给予正确的患者或陪护者，并予以记录

社区诊所长期用药处方操作流程

1. 开始长期用药处方

1.1 授权长期用药处方

长期用药处方药品应当建立在患者对于药品的有效性、耐受性均是确定的情况下：

- NHS 长期用药处方连续调配服务应当首先考虑。

- 只有医师可以授权长期用药处方。如果诊所允许其他指定成员授权，长期用药处方操作政策和实施方案中必须明确包含相关的特殊协议，例如，在一些诊所中，诊所主管或协助者可以在获得用药处方者授权的情况下添加长期用药处方药品。

- 患者的用药应当与适应证相关联，如果药品用于不适宜的症状，必须记录在患者用药档案中，同时告知患者这种使用方法的不适宜性和特殊性。

- 有些药品不适宜用于长期用药处方的使用。（见附表 1）

1.2 药物选择推荐和通用名的运用

- 在大多数情况下，医师处方药品的选择应当根据当地政策规范和处方集，符合当地卫生经济规划，从而提高处方的质量和效用。

- 在药典允许的情况下，开具的药品条目应当书写通用名。以下除外：

ⅰ）英国国家处方集中不适合使用通用名的药品，诊所临床系统或决策支持软件提醒医师对此类药品的使用；英国药品信息出版了适合使用商品名处方的药品目录。

ⅱ）如果已证实患者对于某种通用名的药物不耐受，那么使用适合患者的商品名药品。

ⅲ）商品名书写在某些地方得到推荐，以达到优化节约成本的目的。

ⅳ）对于使用通用名调配存在高风险的药物，处方者应当采纳用药管理部门的建议或意见使用商品名开具处方。

1.3 药品供应天数

大多数长期用药处方是 28 天的供应，因为这个时间间隔最好的实现了患者的方便程度，良好的医疗实践和最小的药物浪费。医师可以在处方上明确指出供应天数或总药量。

全科医师可以决定不采用默认 28 天药量的建议，但是对个别有风险的患者、经常变化治疗方案的、或药物浪费的患者还是应该减少供应的时间间隔。56 天的间隔可能更适合一些考虑取药方便或减少频繁支付处方费的患者，然而这只能在药物治疗改变风险较低时才能同意使用。

- 药量适合 28 天或更小时间间隔的情况：

  ⅰ）有滥用倾向的药物；

  ⅱ）被认为是有风险的情况。例如：药物在家中的储存要求；

  ⅲ）开具复杂治疗方案的或频繁住院或多变疗法的弱势群体；

  ⅳ）终末期患者接受缓和治疗的；

  ⅴ）进食不方便；

  ⅵ）短期使用的包扎用品；

  ⅶ）高成本的药物

  ⅷ）必要时才服用的"临时用药"。

- 药量大于 28 天的情况：

  ⅰ）口服避孕药和激素替代疗法（3 个月包装）；

  ⅱ）特殊包装；

  ⅲ）28 天不等于特殊包装中的药量，例如 200 个剂量的吸入器为一个包装。

这些患者的其他药物应以更频繁的间隔发放。

- 急症处方应作为一次性使用的处方，直到治疗稳定，特别是对于具有不良反应发生率高的药物。

- 在很少的情况下，例如医师预知到治疗方案可能会有风险或治疗药物会频繁变化的，7 天量处方可能更适合。医师决定需要每周分发的药品，社区药房得到 7 天量的处方后，不能一次发出超过 7 天量的药品。如果社区药房使用监测药物剂量系统来提供药品，一般不需要 7 天量的处方，除非医师希望这些药物以 7 天的间隔调配并发给患者。

● 2006 年药物滥用法规强烈建议对所有 Ⅱ，Ⅲ 和 Ⅳ 特殊管制类药品实施 30 天间隔调配。较短的间隔也可能是适当的。这是用药管理团队的监测参数之一。

● 养老院长期用药处方的供药量不得超过 28 天。

● 那些规律、稳定的药物，应该在每月同一时间，使用同一处方。这个方法可以减少药品量和工作人员在每月几次处理同一患者用药申请的时间。

1.4 剂量说明

● 添加到计算机系统中的所有新药都必须有明确的剂量说明。这包括液体，霜剂，敷剂，鼻喷雾剂，滴剂和所有其他外用产品。没有剂量说明或使用方法不明确的标示不能确保患者准确使用药物，同时对护理者会产生一定的困扰。

● 指定药物以外的包括无麸质食品，浴液润肤剂，气管插口和失禁用品，以及需要定期剂量调整的药物，特别是华法林。对于这些，建议使用标准措辞说明。

1.5 授权长期用药处方的使用次数

● 授权的使用次数是临床决定以及长期用药处方过程的重要部分。患者病情稳定，并且愿意遵医嘱，定期遵守监测要求和慢性疾病检查，才可以开始使用长期用药处方。

● 应尽可能在临床系统上设置最大天数的供应，因为这可以监测早期请求和过度使用。

● 有些药物是不适合长期使用的，只能在短期内实行长期用药处方。例如激素类药物。必须有程序避免过度使用药品的发生。

1.6 首诊患者的长期用药处方授权

● 在第一次处方发出之前，确保获得患者先前的用药信息，例如，向患者询问来自先前全科医师的用药清单，了解患者先前长期用药处方的具体情况，请患者来会诊。一次性处方的使用更适合首诊患者。

1.7 在医院和其他机构开始的药物治疗

● 应该有一个系统来处理从其他机构开始药物治疗的请求，例如出院通知，门诊患者预约。

● 所有此类通知都应由医师添加，在添加到系统之前医师要查看患者临床记录。管理系统里应该确保有一个医师在线并处理这些问题。医师还应确保任何停用的药物已从屏幕上移除，并且在患者病历中记录原因。如果不遵循此指导，就会存在发生错误的重大风险。

● 在某些情况下，处方的责任应该继续纳入二级医疗护理。三色警示列表定义了属于红色和琥珀色的药物，其中处方应该保持二级医疗护理（红色）或责任共享（琥珀色）。

● 如果处方是二级医疗护理，这些药物的处方信息应该仍然保留在社区（一级）系统中，使医师意识到他们所开的药物可能与其他药物之间的任何相互作用。社区用药管理团队可以建议如何做到这一点。

● 根据地方医疗协议，患者出院时至少得到14天的药量，以便社区全科医师接收和处理必要的用药信息。

1.8 医师家访和手写处方

● 医师家访后应该更新患者在诊所的电子医疗记录。如果可以使用远程系统操作，应确保医师能够读取患者详细信息，并且可以将家访内容添加到系统中。

● 如果发出手写处方，药品应当作为"紧急"项目进行添加并作为"手写"处方提交。如果有需要长期用药处方，系统应确保转移到位。任何剂量的改变或停用的药物都应加入记录。

1.9 长期用药处方的代理授权

● 代理授权必须有书面政策的支持；条款包含了诊所负责人/协调员的责任和授权要求。

● 在书面政策的支持下，用药管理药师和药学技术员可以添加新的药物或中止药物；修改剂量说明和药量；重新授权药物，设置用药复诊日期和监测要求。

● 药师或护士增补处方者可以根据商定的临床管理计划授权和开具处方。

● 非医疗的独立处方者可以在其专业领域和能力范围内开具处方。具有专科领域知识的护士，如果涉及到他们专业知识以外的其他慢性疾病状态的患者，则无权为这些条件开具处方。在专科领域开处方前，需要考虑所有疾病和药物的副作用、疾病和药物相互作用。护士不确定的应向全科医师或药剂师寻求建议。护士必须在 2008 年护理助产委员会"药品管理标准"的执业范围内工作。

● 非医疗处方者如果在指定诊所从事处方授权，必须通过 CCG 内的指定人员在 NHS 商业服务管理局注册。当他们离开诊所时也必须注销。

2. 长期用药处方的申请

2.1 患者申请长期用药处方

● 患者应使用"长期用药处方用药清单"来申请药品，并逐一勾选所有选项。勿假定所有药品为患者所需。在申请药品不清楚的情况下，须联系患者并在确认之后再处理申请。

● 患者亲自交付用药清单时，应适时与患者讨论所需药品，以减少浪费、解决患者的用药问题。

● 如果患者没有亲自交付，应通过邮寄、传真或互联网发送用药清单，或者使用置于接待处的处方申请盒中。申请方法应由诊所根据当地实施方案决定，并计入到患者信息。不接受电话请求。医生应确保任何患者的敏感信息受到保护。

● 药房也可保管患者用药清单、完成勾选，并提交申请（参考药房部分）。药房通常提供较长的营业时间，以方便患者提交用药清单。

● 每个诊所都应建立系统方法告知患者如何完成长期用药处方的申请。这些方法既可通过发布诊所信息传单和诊所网站宣传，也可通过在候诊室张贴海报、使用电子留言板和在答复机 / 电话上记录消息提供更多的信息提醒。若患者须额外帮助，需做出额外安排。

● 诊所应该制定如何处理紧急申请的政策。如果患者一直不能按时申请处方，导致用药不足，诊所负责人必须作出相应措施。医生不得指导患者到社区药房获取紧急供应，药剂师可据法拒绝供应。

2.2 长期用药处方的药房代理服务

● 如果患者能够自己申请处方，应鼓励其使用用药清单来申请。药房代理服务对于患者申请的可达性很有帮助，方便出门的老年患者。

● 本指南包括对社区药房代理服务的定义。避免全科医生和药房描述本系统时产生的混淆不清：

　ⅰ.药房接收患者完成勾选的用药清单。

　ⅱ.长期用药处方代理申请服务过程中，申请处方时药房完成用药清单的勾选。

　ⅲ.长期用药处方管理服务，患者在药房处提前勾选用药清单，用于下次申请。

　ⅳ.长期用药处方代理领取服务过程中，药房从诊所获得处方。该过程不一定包含向患者送药的过程。

　ⅴ.药品送达服务。

● 全科医生不得为患者指定某家药房。

● 药房要求应与社区药房申请部分所述的指南保持一致。

● 医生应提倡药房工作人员代表患者填完用药清单时（例如，电话沟通完成勾选），在清单上盖章并留有药房联系方式，签名和日期。因为药房工作人员负责检查是否每个项目必需。

● 患者填完，但药房代理领取处方时，药房需要在清单上盖章，但无需药房工作人员签名/注明日期。理想情况下，患者应该签署/注明日期。或者，另一种识别这些的方法应该是药房和全科医生之间达成一致。医师应确保药房提供一份代理领取处方的患者名单。

● 提倡药房获得患者的书面许可，允许药房代理患者管理和申请处方。全科医生应记录提交第三方的处方。

● 根据 NPSA 指南，对需要密切监测的药物，例如华法林，甲氨蝶呤或锂剂，理想情况是患者将用药记录册或最新监测结果的副本附上用药清单。

● 药房应该及时向诊所和医师反馈关于患者药物终止或清单中不常使用药物。医生应该制定制度确保就反馈信息采取措施，解决关切问题并更新用药清单。

● 全科医生应熟悉药房部分有关处方申请的规定。为实现最大程度的安全并减少药物浪费，进一步了解处方申请的操作细节。

● 经严格管理的药房在长期用药处方的申请中存在不少优良做法。这些做法受益于药房和诊所之间的良好关系和持续沟通，以确保双方和患者都可以接受该做法。

2.3 第三方申请

● 本指南中，第三方被定义为除药房之外的其他供应商，通常是指分配设备承包商（DAC）或器具制造商或补充肠内营养品制造商。

● 患者应按照与申请药品相同的方式申请所需的医用物品和器具，但建议允许诊所的处理超过 48 小时，因为处方通常需要邮寄到承包商处。

● 医用器具或肠内营养品的处方应始终采用单独处方，和其他药品分开。

● 不应定期开具相同处方。新物品的申请应转交医师进行决定，并由参与患者护理的专科临床医生确认和审核。

2.4 特殊管制药品的申请

● 诊所对特殊管制药品的申请应作出特别规定和实施方案。应仔细斟酌决定特殊管制药品的长期使用。

● 医师可以通过计算机生成的所有特殊管制药品的处方。除签名之外的所有细节可以由计算机生成。第Ⅱ、Ⅲ和Ⅳ类特殊管制药品处方只适用于 28 天。供应数量不应超过 30 天，合适情况下可以更短。

2.5 养老院的处方申请

● 根据全科医师、养老院和药房达成的一致意见，养老院应每月使用"服药执行记录（以下简称 MAR）"表或患者长期用药处方用药清单申请处方。

● 申请应通过社区诊所，而非药房。

● 只提供 28 天的药品供应。如要求增加剂量，应向全科医师反馈。

● 应明确说明该月所需药品，且只对其给予处理。如可能出现过两份申请，应提醒全科医师。

● 如果需要改变 MAR 上的用药（例如新药，停药，新剂量），首先应由医师审查，并作出更改决定。

● 用于伤口护理的敷料申请，需要由医师授权，记录在患者的用药记录上。通常不需要重复处方。因非处方选择要求，全科医生应该做出安排以便护理院据此申请敷料，并将此反馈给开处方者检查。

3. 长期用药处方生成

3.1 处方申请和领取期限

● 医生应在 48 小时内完成长期用药处方的处理。如果星期五申请的处方将在星期二准备好。

● 患者或者药房代理申请申请处方时，应告知处方领取时间。通知渠道有诊所处方信息传单，诊所网站，或诊所处方箱上的提醒通知。

3.2 处理长期用药处方的申请

所有长期用药处方必须由经过培训的指定人员通过计算机生成。诊所应制定处理长期用药处方的操作政策和实施方案，并每年至少审查一次，以确保协定和操作实践之间保持一致。协定应确保：

● 处理长期用药处方时不得受干扰；不得同时执行其他职责。

● 不得使用自动处方开具功能。合适情况下可在医疗系统上禁用此功能。

● 用于申请的用药清单应标记诊所开始处理的日期。

● 需检查药物名称，形式，规格和剂量说明，以识别患者申请清单和医师备份长期用药处方用药清单之间的任何差异。

● 处方工作人员须了解如何处理处方疑问，并将疑问和处理结果录入患者记录中，包括非重配药物请求，或重新开具过去药物；应建立处方申请沟通的审计跟踪，因此随后可利用临床制度建立电子跟踪。用药管理团队可以为各临床系统提供具体咨询。

● 医生想向患者传达信息时应尽可能以电子方式完成并打印在处方上。可使用牢固粘贴的单独注释，并记录在患者的临床记录中。

● 药物复诊或监测要求逾期或没有剩余已授权处方时，应告知授权处方的医师。

● 提前或延迟的申请可能表明药物的过量使用或不足，应将其通知医师。抗精神病药，哮喘预防吸入器等使用不足时，需就危急患者或其他人的风险进行评估。过度使用会产生重要的临床影响，例如某些具有成瘾潜力的药物，或造成药物浪费。处理提前申请时，原因应记录在备注中。

● 超过 12 个月没有申请的药品需要停用，但不包括不经常或季节性需要的药物，例如 GTN 喷雾，葡萄糖口服凝胶，花粉过敏用药。

● 须建立明确政策以处理私人处方，确保其不作为 NHS 药物发放。

● 须建立明确制度将处方传至处方者签名。初始处方者若离开，系统应识别负责签署者。临床记录的审查对于处方的签署至关重要。

3.3 高警示药物的申注

高警示药物包括有毒且剂量异常的药物，以及需要根据共享护理协议进行监控的药物。全科医生须建立在开具处方前进行必要检测的程序。高警示药物包括甲氨蝶呤，华法林，锂剂，胰岛素等。

4. 长期用药处方再授权和药物复诊

4.1 再授权的临床责任

● 只有医师可以再授权长期用药处方。长期用药处方再授权时，医师有责任确保药品的持续需求和长期用药处方的持续适当，且确认监测和药物复诊已经按时完成。

● 需重新授权的所有处方都需传至负责医师。处方系统在最后一张长期用药处方开具前完成需要重新授权处方的提醒。

● 不推荐使用延期处方，因为此举会让某些系统取消再授权。

● 重新授权是调整药品用量和时间的良机，使患者可以同一时间完成所有药品的使用。这将避免药物和工作人员精力浪费，因为工作人员不再需要每月处理患者对不同药品的申请。

● 重新授权是评估患者是否受益于 NHS 长期用药处方连续调配服务的

良机。

4.2 药物复查

● 重复用药的患者应根据临床需要定期复查。患者的用药清单上必须明确提醒患者复查日期。

● 建议全科医生对所有 75 岁以上的患者至少每年复查一次，而服用四种或更多药物的患者应该每六个月复查一次，包括依从性的检查。

● 药物复查必须确保所有药物同时完成复查，例如一护士可能对患者的哮喘要进行了复查，但没有复查其他药物。药房的药物使用审核（MUR）是一种针对患者用药一致性和合规性检查，但是这不应被看作等同于医师的药物复查。

药物复查应包括：

ⅰ 每种药物的持续有效性和需要；

ⅱ 剂量和呈现的适当性，如剂量已经被向上滴定，则可以给予更高规格的制剂；

ⅲ 患者对治疗的了解；

ⅳ 监测，试验，检查和跟进；

ⅴ 副作用，药物相互作用及药物禁忌检查；

ⅵ 不必要药物的停用；

ⅶ 适当的处方申请频率；

ⅷ 相同药量的所有处方药；

ⅸ 非处方药的使用；

ⅹ 稳定用药时考虑是否使用 NHS 长期用药处方连续调配服务。

5. 处方领取和管理

5.1 完成签署的处方

患者可通过在接待处或邮寄的方式获得处方，也可由社区药房代理领取或通过 NHS 电子传送直接发送到患者指定的药房。

5.2 领取处方

- 患者明确了解领取处方的时间。

- 建立完善的处方领取流程，确保正确的患者领取正确的处方。接待人员应该检查患者的身份和地址。如接待人员不认识的患者亲戚或朋友领取，他们必须出具身份证明，并在处方领取记录上签字。

- 代表患者领取处方时，身份确认必须严格检查，特别是特殊管制药品处方的领取，领取者必须签字。

- 未成年人领取处方将由诊所负责人或医师斟酌决定，并需得到父母或监护人为其领取处方的许可。

- 建立并记录处方领取记录书。

- 有少数患者必须亲自领取处方。这些患者的电子记录上必须显示有明显的屏幕警示。该警示应清楚标记在用药申请清单上并转移到已开具处方上。员工应确保这些处方只由患者领取。

5.3 传真处方

- 处方可以传真到社区药房，但只限于特殊情况。长久记录传真的发送时间和地点，以及后期领取原始处方的时间。

- 根据医师要求传真的处方须在合理时间内送达至社区药房。全科医生有责任就传真处方一事电话通知药房。

- 如果社区药房要求传真处方，则其有责任稍后领取原始处方。

5.4 邮寄处方

- 患者的姓名和地址应与邮寄地址的信封进行核对，以确保处方送达至正确的患者或机构。

- 姓名、地址和处方中的药物名称应记录在处方日志中，包括发送日期和邮寄人的姓名。

5.5 无人领取或者退还的处方

- 从处方签署起一个月后未领取的任何处方须经由医师再次审查。从计算机处方系统中删除处方时，需要有证明人的参与和监视，在保密的情况下进行粉碎和废物处理，并做记录。

- 如无法取消最后一次开具的处方，序列号应录在患者记录上，并且标明处方未领取。然后处方应粉碎处理。
- 诊所需要建立和药房的沟通程序，通知药房没有领取的处方。

6. 质量保证

6.1 长期用药处方操作和申请草案

- 草案中须有一个清晰的书面协议来描述在长期用药处方中涉及到的每个人的职责和作用。
- 每个诊所应该根据实践编写，每两年评估一次。
- 指定专人负责草案的管理，并且确保所有员工都经过充分的培训。
- 所有的员工包括临时代理处方者，都需要经过培训，熟悉长期用药处方系统如何工作，并且知道个人职责所在。
- 保证所有员工都阅读过此草案，并建立记录和复查系统。长期用药处方的使用也应该包括在新员工的入职培训计划中。

6.2 改进长期用药处方的操作和申请系统

- 用药管理协会的药师通过在各个诊所的考察和工作，总结好的操作草案并传播到其他诊所。

6.3 差错处理

- 应该建立一个系统负责调查并且总结错误。由于医师需要对所开具的药品处方负最终责任，因此需要确保系统健全。任何形式的过失都应报告和记录，并在定期的诊所会议上讨论和学习。
- 如果由于处方错误造成严重医疗实践，比如导致一个或更多患者在治疗过程中发生可以避免或不可预估的死亡或严重伤害。必须在战略执行信息系统（StEIS）中报告，CCG 可以进入此系统中并作进行调查。所有此类事件都必须向相关的研究中心作报告，并就此事件的情况进行调查分析。

6.4 审核

- 为确保患者及医护人员通过安全使用系统保证用药安全，长期用药处方系统需每年进行一次审核。

● 诊所负责人将确保审核顺利实施，并负责学习和更新操作草案，完成相关员工培训。

6.5 处方安全

● 所有空白和已完成签署的处方必须以安全可靠的方式储存。这项操作必须在服从国家指南的情况下，建立标准操作规程（SOP），确保所有工作人员完成培训。

● 所有工作人员必须知道如何处理处方丢失以及处方被偷的情况；并且将其在标准操作规程中进行详细说明。

● 应该定期对处方安全进行风险评估以确保系统安全运行。

6.6 硬件故障的应急计划

● 此操作规程应制定应急计划来应对停电故障或系统故障，从而确保打印及手写处方是清晰的。

● 一旦问题得到解决，临床系统信息应该录入此过程所包含的条款。

7. NHS 长期用药处方连续调配服务

● 为病情稳定并长期需要使用药品的患者提供了另一种方式，患者可以在不需要联系诊所和申请处方的情况下，在药房直接领取处方药。

● 严格管理的连续调配服务可以减少医师和诊所操作规程的工作量，提高患者服务质量，减少药品浪费和加强社区药房的作用。

● 患者会被授权长期用药处方主副本，副本最多 11 个，也就是提前授权最多 12 张处方。这样可以允许在重复调剂的周期内直接调剂药品，而不需要每次再回到诊所申请处方。

● 连续调配服务并非适合所有患者。它适合慢病患者，因为在批量重复调配处方期间，慢病患者很大程度上在用药方面可能相对稳定。使用大量药品的患者或需要频繁住院治疗的患者不适合纳入长期用药处方的连续调配服务。

● 开始使用连续调配服务钱，医师必须得到患者的同意。

● 这项服务的运行模式必须建立到诊所长期用药处方操作草案中，例如

SOPs、处方申请协议和员工培训。

- 连续调配处方必须与标准长期用药处方分开处理。

- 在分发主副本之前，诊所接待员必须检查医师在主本上签字。

- 患者的用药记录上必须被明确注释连续调配服务的使用，在此期间，标准长期用药处方不可以继续授权。

- Ⅱ类和Ⅲ类特殊管制药品不能使用连续调配服务。Ⅳ类特殊管制药品的连续调配处方，首次调配必须在 28 天内完成。第一次调配后，后续长期用药处方在正常有效期内是合法有效的（一般是一年）。

- 在每次调配时，药师负责检查患者的依从性和其他临床因素来判断是否适合连续调配。药师如有任何问题，都可以和诊所医师及时沟通。

8. 电子处方服务（EPS）

电子处方服务（EPS）目前正在逐步实践。EPS 可以使医师通过计算机系统生成和传输电子处方。药房可以将处方下载到自己的处方操作系统中。这使得处方的生成和调配更加简单和快速，方便了患者，提高了医护人员的工作效率。

对于患者和医护人员，EPS 将带来更高效和安全处方服务：

- 电子处方服务提高患者安全，降低由于不清楚或字迹模糊的处方导致调剂错误的可能性。

- 允许及时取消不适宜的处方。

- 防止处方的丢失。

- 减少虚假处方的数量。

- 药房可以在患者取药之前提前准备好处方，节约患者在药房的等待时间，使药师更易于管理工作流程和库存。

- 缓解患者去诊所领取处方的不便。

- 消除药师在处方调剂系统中重新输入处方信息的必要，从而节省时间和提高调剂的精准度。

- 对于 NHS 的连续调配处方，可以更方便地完成电子化保存，因此降低了处方丢失的风险，并且改善了处方开具和调配的问责制。药房不再需要保留和存储长期用药处方，因此减少工作量和存储空间。

当使用处方电子传送，要注意以下要点：

● 处方必须由医师以电子签名方式授权，并发送到电子处方中控系统，由药房下载和调剂。

● 除了授权医师，其他任何人不得使用电子签名。

● 涉及电子处方的问题，诊所必须建立相应的临床管理和风险管理草案，从而确保安全性和患者隐私的保护。草案必须遵照 NHS 最新的信息技术标准。

长期用药处方的申请指导原则

第三部分

药房环节

目录一　药房的长期用药处方指导原则

章节	说明
	药房长期用药处方的操作和申请服务标准
	概述
1	患者沟通
2	药房与全科医师的交流
3	药房工作流程
4	药房接受患者用药清单
5	药房代理处方申请服务
6	药房长期用药处方管理服务
7	长期用药处方的药房代理领取服务
8	药品送达服务
9	电子处方服务
10	NHS 长期用药处方连续调配服务

药房长期用药处方的操作和申请服务标准

所有药房须根据标准操作规程（SOP）提供具体的长期用药处方服务。SOP 应最大程度涵盖以下内容。

此为最佳的行业标准，并具有示范作用：

标准	说明
1	患者应主动参与药房服务
2	患者应签署协议；协议细节需保留，且通告全科医师
3	患者应尽力提醒药房任何关于药物的变更或停用，例如住院后的药物变化
4	须建立全科医师通告用药清单向患者无误传达信息的流程
5	出于风险考量，SOPs 应详细规定口头处方的申请和其相关培训内容
6	取药时，需要与患者确认是否需要所有申请的药物，尤其是按需服用的药物
7	经患者同意后药房向其提供服务，尤其是代理申请和处方管理服务
8	须仔细监控（如华法林、甲氨蝶呤、锂剂等）高警示药品，最新检查结果和日期应向医师提供，附上相关记录
9	把没有调配的处方退回医师，并附上简明原因
10	通告诊所患者要停用的药品；同时通告全科医师
11	药房应为长期用药处方的每次申请和供应建立跟踪追索制度
12	根据临床管理要求记录每起服务事故、失误或错误，适当时应通告患者的全科医师
13	处方开具完成应通知患者；用时不少于 2 个工作日
14	用药清单如果未能完全体现患者需要的药物，由受正规培训的服务人员联系患者并确认
15	药房代理领取处方，须对用药清单盖戳
16	通过重复申请系统申请药物，由于潜在的用药变动，患者或看护人员不应提前大于 10 天申请药物
17	患者通过电话申请的，药房经手人员应在用药清单上签名，签署日期并盖戳以通晓全科医师
18	手写处方风险高，无法避免的情况下应力图准确和易认
19	作为药房处方管理的关键一环，在向患者分配药物时须询问是否仍需全部药物
20	从诊所取回处方后应与药房的记录审核。任何药物缺失或多余情况应及时与医师沟通处理

药房长期用药处方的操作和申请指导原则

概述

药房向患者提供一系列服务，增加了患者急需情况下获得处方的渠道，同时其加长营业时间为患者提供了便利；此类服务同时有助药房减少药物调配量，从而降低风险。但该服务必须永远将患者的利益放在首位。

由于药房长期用药处方调配系统促进药房和全科医师群体之间的沟通，改善两者关系，出现了诸多成功的管理案例，保证了两者的互惠合作。

社区药师可通过多种途径参与长期用药处方项目。参与度的理解不清可导致概念混淆，因此下文详细介绍此类服务，以促进理解，减少对长期用药处方使用的困扰。

ⅰ.药房接受由患者填写的用药清单。

ⅱ.药房代理申请服务，该系统下药房代理患者勾选用药清单。

ⅲ.药房处方管理服务，该管理模式下患者提前在药房申请下次的药品。

ⅳ.药房代理领取服务，药房代理提交用药清单和领取处方，该服务不一定包含将药物送达至患者处。

ⅴ.药品送达服务

ⅵ.NHS 长期用药处方连续调配服务

1.患者沟通

● 药房提供的此类服务应由患者要求，而非药房强制。患者应签署协议，患者可随时更改协议。患者签署协议后药房方可代表患者提供服务，协议内容需保留。

● 应向患者或患者护理人员告知其责任范围。药物变更的风险是最大隐患，因此从一开始就应告知患者，任何情境下的药物停用或变更都需要及时通知药房，尤其是住院后的药物变化。

● 药房应确认要求方是否为患者本人；若不是患者本身，应确认要求方有权代表患者。该点在电话沟通中尤为重要。

● 药房保存用药清单时须确保其万无一失，确保患者信息不泄露。若患者习惯性将用药清单留给药房保管，应确保向患者提供最新版本的用药清单复印件；没有复印件的，可向其提供影印件。患者可能需要向住院医师或牙医提供用药清单信息；全科医师需要根据用药清单信息决定是否替患者安排体检，是否预约流感疫苗注射。在此情况下药房须无误地提供此类信息。

● 口头代理申请处方具有额外风险。为控制风险，用药清单上须写下同一药物的不同剂量和剂型：

i. 口头申请的过程中，药房人员应获得患者用药的电子记录或用药清单。

ii. 详细记录申请方（患者或照料患者人员）和经手申请药房方人员通话记录。为日后店内审计之用，应记录申请日期和具体申请药品。

iii. 电话沟通时应确保患者的个人信息不被旁人听到，做好保密工作。

iv. 药房 SOPs 应详细规定由谁处理口头请求，并规定店员培训，以确保店员人手足、资历硬，向患者提供安全高效服务。

v. 应规定何种情况可接受电话请求。例如，在和患者事前讨论后可向其提供处方管理服务。

● 建议使用剂量监测系统（Monitored Dosage System，以下简称 MDS）用药，患者在每次申请时尤其注意非罩板包装药物（例如药膏或吸入器），以避免重复申请造成积压或浪费。

● 每次调配药品后，与患者确认下次是否需要所有长期用药处方药品，尤其是按需使用的药物。

2. 药房与全科医师的交流

● 鼓励药房增进与当地社区诊所的讨论交流，建立安全、高效、浪费低、可供患者自由选择的互惠制度。为达到最佳效果，鼓励全科医师参与讨论，确保过程有序高效进行。

● 与社区全科医师的合作在处方管理服务和处方代理申请中尤其重要。

药房在向患者提供服务之前，须与全科医师就服务内容达成一致意见。全科医师指导原则也鼓励与药房积极沟通，以消除长期用药处方操作中的误解。

● 须仔细监控（如华法林、甲氨蝶呤、锂剂等）方可开药的高警示药品，最新检查结果和检测数据应向医师提供，最好在申请处方时将记录附到用药清单上。

● 担心患者能力不足，无法重新申请药品的情况下，须与全科医师协商解决，找出重新申请的合适方法。此点适用患有学习障碍、老年痴呆、头脑不清晰的患者，以及使用剂量监测系统用药或罩板包装用药辅助的患者。在患者同意的情况下须记录协商内容、日期、参与其中的药师和全科医师以及合适的审查日期。

● 将所有"未调配"处方送回全科医师处并附上简短说明（如，重复用药、患者不需要、药物中断、患者未申请等），便于全科医师根据患者未接收的处方药修改记录。

● 患者在取药之际表示不再服用某种药物的情况下，药房须提醒诊所，该情况同时也须向全科医师汇报，以便医师审查患者依从性和更新长期用药处方用药清单。在合适情况下也须与患者和全科医师交流潜在的用药不足或用药过度问题。如有需要，须进行药房高级服务"药物使用审核（MUR）"。相关信息记录到患者的个人医疗档案中。

3. 药房工作流程

● 本指导原则汇聚了优良的行业经验，旨在增进与社区诊所的工作交流。英国总药房理事会（GPhC）制定的行为准则和职业操守为本指导原则奠定了基础。药房必须根据标准操作规程提供服务，并且符合 GPhC 标准。

● 确保通过审计跟踪识别每个处方申请和供应。所有干预载入患者医疗记录中，以便能够处理任何可能出现的潜在风险查询。

● 根据临床管理要求记录并报告每起服务事故、失误或错误，并以适当方式通告患者的全科医师。

4. 药房接受患者用药清单

● 药房实际上充当了患者投放用药清单的"邮箱"。许多药房延长了开放时间，为患者提供便利。药房完成药品调配，患者几日后即可取药，或者选择药品配送服务。患者应被告知处方何时调配完成。诊所和全科医师至少需要 2 个工作日处理和产生处方，所以患者在药房的取药时间一般在申请处方的两天后。

● 药房标准操作规程应包含以下几点：

ⅰ 若用药清单上并未注明患者的要求，经正规培训的药房人员应询问患者需要申请哪些药物。药房在任何情况下不提倡"地毯式"申请，尤其是须根据具体情况选用的药物，必须确保患者申请真正需要的药品。

ⅱ 药房如果代替患者领取处方，需在用药清单上盖章，方便诊所处理处方后根据药房分别处理。

5. 药房代理的处方申请服务

● 通常情况下，患者在下次提药之前将用药清单存于药房。在断药前几天由患者电话联系药房，或特殊情况下药房联系患者来申请药物。该服务不同于"重复管理服务"，后者通常是患者在上次取药之际直接申请下次需要药品。前者在申请和开具处方期间的药物变更风险相对较低。

● 患者如果来药房申请处方，药房须要求患者勾选用药清单。若药房工作人员通过患者的电话申请处方，所需药物直接记录到患者最新的用药清单上。该制度规避了患者使用过期用药清单定药带来的风险。

● 药房标准操作规程应包括以下几点：

ⅰ 确定患者或护理者认为是必需的药物，并确保在可能的情况下排除不必要的"地毯式"用药请求，以避免药品浪费或药品过量储存。应特别注意非每月需要的药物，例如，根据具体情况使用的药物，吸入器，药膏等。

ⅱ 考虑到日常起居变化或患者状态的变化（如临时需住院），患者/护理人员应早于断药前 10 天申请药物。应记录特殊情况并传达给全科医师。全科医师和药房达成一致的处方处理天数有利各方的实际操作。

　　iii 如果患者电话联系药房，药房人员确认患者所需药物后，应在用药清单上签名、签署日期并盖上药房邮章以向全科医师确认药房代理申请或领取。没有药房信息的用药清单表示药房仅帮助患者投送申请表，并没有参与到患者的实际申请过程中。

　　iv 确保患者 / 护理人员发起申请。可使用处方提醒系统，但获得患者 / 护理者同意之前药房不可申请处方。

　　v 从诊所领取处方时应对照药房的用药清单记录进行检查。处方中出现的任何缺失或多余药品应由全科医师处理。

　　vi 药房没有患者用药清单的情况可能出现，但应尽量减少该情况，并提醒患者通过用药清单申请以降低风险的重要性。在无法避免的特殊情况下，申请须包含和用药清单内容一致的信息。药品必须按照患者的真实需求，而非复制此前分配的药品重复申请。药房须根据患者用药记录提高申请准确性，即使该记录未能和全科医师记录同步。患者用药记录打印后，若申请药品与全科医师处不同，并可能包括一次性或停用药物时，则需谨慎处理。手写请求极具风险，在无法避免的情况下应力求准确、易认。字迹模糊、拼写错误会对药房产生不利影响，增加患者风险，并最终累及与社区诊所和医师的关系。

　　vii 为预防患者不按照用药清单申请药物，社区诊所应有一套独立的风险管控系统。应鼓励药房与诊所及时沟通，以保持申请内容一致。

　　viii 患者申请非长期用药处方药品时，应由患者本人与社区诊所直接联系申请。

C. 药房长期用药处方管理服务

　　● 在药房提供的长期用药处方管理服务中，患者通常在上一次收到药物时预购下次药物。这其中管理药物变更和药物浪费带来的风险一直是全科诊所和医师的工作隐患。应敦促药房与全科医师商议解决方案。

　　● 患者来取药时，须在用药清单上勾选下月所需药物。建议患者在用药清单上签名，因为患者提前近一个月申请，使得处方打印之前的药物变更风险更大。

- 药房标准操作规程应考虑加入以下几点：

ⅰ 患者选择该服务时，必须向其强调，中途出现药物变更或住院时有义务联系药房。如果患者经常变更药物时，应该考虑此项服务是否适合。

ⅱ 确定患者必需的药物，并确保在可能的情况下排除不必要的"地毯式"用药申请，以避免可能造成的药品浪费或过量储存。应特别注意非每月需要的药物，例如，根据具体情况使用的药物，吸入器，药膏等。

ⅲ 向患者留言，告知其取药时间。

ⅳ 药房领取处方时应对照用药清单记录进行检查。处方中出现的任何缺失或多余药品应由全科医师处理。

ⅴ 作为该服务的重要一环，向患者调配药物时应询问是否仍需所有药物。SOP 须详细规定如何就"未调配"药物反馈给医师。PSNC 指导原则规定，处方须明确指明"未调配"，并就整张处方和单条内容向全科医师提供反馈。

ⅵ 在同时使用处方管理服务和送药上门服务时应特别注意，因为送达药物时患者唯能和快递人员沟通。药房应建立药物调配时对药物必要性进行二次核查的制度。

ⅶ 药物浪费随着处方时间增长而加大；如果处方时间超过 56 天，则不适合处方管理服务。

ⅷ 在严格按照清晰的标准流程管理此类服务的情况下，药房得以在申请时和患者取药时逐一检查每种药物是否是患者所需。患者有机会就自身疑问和药房沟通，从而整体增进患者意识，助力疾病治疗。

7. 长期用药处方的药房代理领取服务

- 代理领取服务须取得并记录患者的服务协议。须向患者解释服务详情，包括处方领取时间和配药时间。

- 药房呈给社区诊所的用药清单上须药房盖章，表示药房将代理患者在诊所领取处方。

- 患者将用药清单提交给诊所后，药房须记载此患者姓名，向诊所领取处方时需要核实。
- 药房领取处方时，须核查药房是否有权代患者取处方和配药。若不具权限，处方应交还医师，或直接转给有此权限的药房。

8. 药品送达服务

- 药房须确保送药员执行与药房接待处同等的标准，以顺利将患者的担忧传达给药房。为此药房应该建立跟踪审计制度。
- 此项服务的最大隐忧在于处方的下次申请。药房须考虑如何就仍需药物进行二次核查。若患者在药品送达之后意识到此点，药品已无法重返库存，造成处方成本浪费。

9. 电子处方服务（EPS）

电子处方服务（EPS）目前正在向全科医师推广。该服务允许全科医师使用他们的计算机系统生成和传输电子处方。借助 EPS 平台，全科医师将电子处方发送至患者选择的药房，之后药房下载处方。该平台提高了处方和配药效率，为患者和药房带来便利。

处方申请仍需按照社区诊所、药房和患者之间达成的协议进行。

对患者和医疗人员来说，EPS 既提高效率，又增进安全：

- 降低处方字迹模糊带来的配药失误可能性，提高患者的安全。
- 允许立刻停用临床上不适用的处方。
- 预防处方丢失，降低二次处方的风险。
- 减少欺诈性处方的数量。
- 实现取药前备好处方，节省配药时患者的等药时间，便于药房管理工作量和库存。
- 省略患者或药房去诊所领取处方的步骤。
- 省略药房重新录入处方信息的步骤，节省时间的同时提高配药准确性。

NHS 长期用药处方连续调配服务允许医师对处方的批量授权，也使得药师能在患者到店之前进行配药准备。处方的电子存储简化了连续调配服务的流程。

- 降低了成批处方丢失的风险。
- 处方修改后无需再将纸质版送还至医师签字。
- 药物、临床状况或个人情况发生变动的，可以取消尚未完成的连续调配处方。
- 通过对处方开具和药房配药实行问责，药师负责检查患者是否坚持用药，或是否出现其他影响持续供药的临床因素。
- 长期用药处方的持续时间可根据患者用药审查，监测流程或社区诊所的其他临床和行政职能进行调整。
- 处方重复授权的工作量大大降低。

发送电子处方时，须注意：

- 医师将电子处方发送到 NHS 电子处方中控系统，药房随后可以下载处方，处方须由医师授权，并以电子签名为确据。
- 除授权者之外，其他人不得使用其签名。
- 社区诊所须建立有关电子处方的临床管理和风险管理问题的议定书。该议定书须符合最新版的 NHS 信息技术标准。

10. NHS 长期用药处方连续调配服务

- 在此服务中，患有慢性病且病情稳定的患者需要新处方时，无需联系诊所或者医师，可直接在药房取药。
- 患者会被授权长期用药处方主副本，副本最多 11 个，也就是提前授权最多 12 张处方。这样可以允许在重复调剂的周期内直接调剂药品，而不需要每次再回到诊所申请处方。
- 处方主本包含授权信息，药房须妥善安全保管；经患者要求，可开具原件复印件。
- 每次配药时，药师负责检查患者是否坚持服药，以及是否存在其他影响持续供药的临床因素，诸如，患者服药是否遇到任何问题，患者最近是否住院，或患者药方是否出现变动。如有任何问题值得警惕，药师须通知诊所。

● 药品、临床状况或患者状况出现变动的情况下，处方中的剩余配药可取消，并将剩余的处方复印件销毁，或经医师要求将其归还医师。

● 当诊所配备电子处方系统后，全科医师可以使用电子版本的长期用药处方，从而简化操作，加强安全。

长期用药处方指导原则

第四部分

养老院

　　本节主要介绍养老院申请长期用药处方的操作指导。社区药房和诊所需要建立处理养老院长期用药处方的申请草案；社区药房和全科医师应该协助养老院共同制定养老院的操作草案。社区药房、诊所和养老院保持良好沟通十分重要。

目录一　养老院长期用药处方指导原则

章节	简介
	养老院长期用药处方的操作和申请标准
	法律问题和全国性指导方针
	指导原则
1	患者自理用药
2	社区诊所或医师与药房的关系
3	给药系统
4	培训和教育
5	咽食障碍患者
6	长期用药处方的申请
7	可以不服从 28 日供药周期的例外情况
8	检查现有库存
9	处方
10	药物送达与检查
11	记录系统

养老院长期用药处方的操作和申请标准

以下标准汇聚行业内优良经验，一定情况下具有示范作用。

标准	简介
1	为实现有效的药物申请与供应，养老院宜固定使用一家药房
2	养老院须经正规培训员工负责所有申请环节
3	养老院尽可能指定一名常用药师和医师解答任何疑问
4	诸如磨粉服用在内的未经许可的服药方式须经全科医师授权，并登记在患者的服药执行纪录（MAR）上
5	处方申请系统须突出一个月以内的用药变化
6	药膏和口服液须标注开瓶日期，除非另有说明，一旦开口须在六个月内服完
7	药膏和口服液开口超过三个月仍未用完的，须咨询医师是否可减少药量，以免浪费
8	保质期内未服用的按需时（临时）使用的药物无需扔掉，可在下月继续服用，以减少浪费
9	按需时使用的药物在用量说明上须注明用法、用量、间隔和每日最多用量。带有"谨遵医嘱"说明的药品服用须询问药师
10	养老院须确保通知药房任何药物的停用，以及患者用药记录/用药清单不符的情况
11	处方申请周期为28日
12	养老院应为医师和药房开具处方和供药预留足够时间。建议最低两周
13	药房不能代表养老院申请处方
14	应由养老院保管处方申请记录
15	28日期间如需添加新药，新药用量须和当下药品同步，而且确保满足下个28日疗程的处方要求，并录入患者服药执行记录里
16	养老院工作人员可养成记录所有疑问的良好习惯，以促进跟踪审计便利化
17	养老院工作人员不得将药品装入其他瓶中；这属于二次配药和非法行为
18	如连续六月及以上没有申请某种药品，应通知全科医师是否可停用该药
19	养老院工作人员须根据MAR表和所需用药清单检查医师开具的处方，随后才可将其送至药房。需检查处方是否包含所有申请药物，是否有异常情况，及是否有患者未要求的药品
20	社区药房应在疗程开始前至少两天，送达下一28日疗程的所有药物和MAR表
21	养老院工作人员须根据申请记录检查药物，发现问题，并就问题与药师/医师妥当交流
22	药房须提供可供患者查阅的所有药物的信息介绍
23	MAR作为一份法律文件，养老院在最后一次记录后须保管至少三年

法律问题和全国性指导方针

养老院药物管理须按照 2008 年《健康与社会护理法》的规定进行。其中第 13 条规章表示：

"注册者须保护用户不受药物不善使用和管理带来的危险。为此，注册者在药物获取、记录、分发、使用、保管、配药、给药和处置方面做出妥当安排，符合法律规定。"

该法同时规定，护理质量委员会是监管单位。该委员会颁布的文件《质量服从指导；质量与安全的基本标准》为养老院提供了守法指导。该文件第 9 章适用于药品管理。

第 9 章规定，养老院应该：

"建立制度，确保其行为符合 1968 年《药品法》和 1971 年《反药品滥用法》及其属法规，2006 年《特殊管制药品安全管理法》，以及英国皇家药师协会和其他相关职业机构制定的专业指导意见。"

因此，任何针对养老院制定的指导方针必须注意遵守这些限制性规定。我们建议除养老院工作人员外，与养老院有工作往来的社区药房和社区诊所的全体员工应对相关法律和指导有基本了解。英国皇家药师协会制定了社会护理服务指导原则，其颁布的《社会护理服务中的药物问题》可在官网上查询。

指导原则

1. 患者自理用药

应积极鼓励养老院居民尽可能地进行用药自理。在某些情况下，这意味着他们将负责申请自己的药品。不过在大多数情况下，养老院负责处方的申请。以下政策适用于养老院接管为居民申请处方的行为责任。

2. 社区诊所或医师与药房的关系

• 护理质量理事会（CQC）的质量标准强调了建立以人为本的护理制度，并且向居民提供全方面的护理咨询，确定治疗方案时要考虑居民本人的观点。这些观点须被纳入药物治疗协议的每个方面。

• 养老院通常与多家不同的社区诊所合作。例如，一家 40 张床位的养老院可与 10~12 家社区诊所合作。这种情况下，居民须决定在哪家注册（前提是社区诊所和医师无异议）。在某些地区，地方临床医药服务委员组为养老院打造了本地化的医疗加强服务。该情况下，一家指定的社区诊所负责整个养老院，该养老院大部分居民会选择此家注册。居民也可按照自己意愿到别家注册。

• 为实现有效申请和供药，一致认可的做法是一家养老院应与一家药房合作。

• 养老院工作人员可能与多家社区诊所合作，但合作药房只有一个。应尽可能保证该家药房既能处理急性疾病的处方，又能处理长期用药处方。

3. 给药系统

• 多数养老院采用的用药制度是用药监测系统（MDS）。目前有多种不同的用药检测制度，Nomad 制度（塑料盘包装，7 天用药）和 Venalink 或 Manrex 制度通常指的是罩板包装。很多养老院认为这些包装比传统的药箱更为安全。然而实际上，由于液体药物和某些固体药物不适合罩板包装，所以养老院不得不同时使用药瓶和药盒用药。

● CQC 的检查标准中不要求养老院必须使用 MDS 的给药系统。MDS 的使用和融资由养老院和药房共同安排。社区药师应遵守 MDS 的专业指导。当作出此决定时，双方应考虑以下几点：

ⅰ 没有法律要求对 MDS 的使用。

ⅱ 只有某些药品可以放入 MDS 中，所以一些药品仍然需要在其他系统中分配。

ⅲ 养老院将需要建立程序来处理剂量变化，因为 MDS 的使用可导致剂量改变延迟和额外浪费。在某些情况下，例如，频临死亡患者的药品，MDS 可能不适用。

ⅳ 只有正常的药品可通过 MDS 分配。所需的药品应该单独分配以实现用量灵活性并减少浪费。

ⅴ 如果使用 MDS，给药的人仍需负责确保正确的药品给予正确的患者，并且知道副作用、特殊的剂量要求，如进食前用药等。

ⅵ 应提供药品信息给患者。

4. 培训和教育

● 为促使长期用药处方的申请平稳运行，员工必须接受培训并胜任操作流程中的每个环节。经过适当训练的养老院工作人员应该负责处方申请过程中的每个环节，该人员应是护士（在疗养院中）或高级护理人员（在住宅中）。

● 养老院负责人应保留一份完成正规培训的员工名单，并确保培训与时俱进。其中需要指定一到两名处方负责人，有助于药房和社区诊所就处方疑问和养老院顺利沟通。然而，养老院负责人应该确保假期仍有足够人手，并且系统不依赖于某一个工作人员。养老院应尽可能在药房和诊所中指定使用固定人员，以方便处方问题的处理。

5. 咽食障碍患者

如果患者不能按规定形式服用药品，应通知医师，以便进行用药审查。这可能涉及简化药方，开具替代药物或替代制剂。虽然提倡按照许可方式服药，但有时需要以未经许可的方式服用（例如粉碎药物，开口胶囊）或在罕见的情况下处方中使用未经许可的产品（特殊制剂药品）。而且有些药物不能粉碎。社区药师或用药管理团队能够建议药物是否可以被粉碎或溶解在水中，但是执行前医师必须授权。如果不按规定形式用药，MAR 表上必须做出适当标注。

6. 长期用药处方的申请

- 社区药房和养老院需要共同开发处方申请系统，确保考虑以下几点：
- 重点检查居民的上个月药品是否有任何更改。
- 除非标签/信息表上另有说明，霜剂、软膏和口服液体通常开口后可以最多使用 6 个月。
- 应该标明开口日期。如果药品包装开口超过 3 个月，请咨询医师是否可减少下次的处方药量。
- 紧需药品、膏霜和软膏等如果仍在保质期内可保留用于下个月。丢弃为浪费之举。
- 任何"谨遵医嘱"的说明应该由医师解释。谨遵医嘱说明书必须包括用法说明，剂量，间隔和最大日剂量。避免用药错误。
- 养老院和社区诊所应该对申请方式达成协议，用药清单或 MAR 表的复印件都可以用来申请。无论使用哪种申请方式，养老院都应该确保社区药房知晓药物停用情况，并且告知诊所 MAR 表和用药清单之间的任何差异。
- 如果停用药物仍在长期用药处方上，通知全科医师该药物已停用，可将其从处方上去掉。
- 药物应以 28 日为一申请疗程（请参照第 7 部分的例外）。
- 允许医师和药房有足够的时间开具处方和供药，这通常需要至少两周。

● 药房不能代表养老院申请药物，这样会承担较高的错误风险，因为药房可能不知道此前一个月患者用药变更。

● 所需药品的申请记录应由养老院保存，便于收到药品后核对。

● 28 日期间如需添加新药，新药用量须和当下药品同步，而且确保满足下个 28 日疗程的处方要求，并录入患者服药执行纪录里。

● 提倡养老院工作人员保留所有查询的书面记录，例如电话交谈等。应建立明确的跟踪审计制度。

7. 可以不服从 28 日供药周期的例外情况

● 养老院供药疗程应为 28 日，但存在一些例外情况：

● 如果某药物在疗程期间加入处方，医师最好在下一疗程开始之前开具当前用药周期内所需的药量，方便用药同步，并避免浪费。

● 需估计治疗或疾病晚期的患者通常频繁更换药物，特别是缓解疼痛和恶心的药物。在患者护理阶段，养老院应该与医师和社区药师将药物定为 7 日一疗程（包括周末），并由社区药房通过药瓶或纸盒配药，以体现频繁换药的灵活性。

● 在其他时间，养老院可申请 28 日以外的药量以应对居民度假这一状况。养老院应向医师做出书面申请。如果居民经常出院，养老院应该与处方者讨论应对措施。可改变用药时间或单独开方。

● 护理人员不得将药物转移到其他容器；此举称为二次分配，属非法行为。

8. 检查现有库存

● 申请药物之前，须确定前一疗期剩下的药物数量。

● 按照患者需求申请药物，如果患者不需要，不申请。

● 须特别注意敷料，外用产品（霜剂，软膏和头皮用洗浴 / 淋浴产品）和失禁产品用量。尽量使用敷料订单。一些临时使用药品可以保存几个月，因此须注意储存，特别是可单独供用的敷料。

- 霜剂，软膏和口服液体必须标明开口日期。除非标签/说明书上另有说明，通常最多可用6个月。

- 应检查是否需要临时药物。如果未申请时间达到6个月及以上，应通知全科医师查看此药物是否可停用。

- 如果居民经常拒绝服用药品，须通知全科医师。

- 申请药物时应考虑最近的送药时间。

9. 处方

- 所有按处方发放的药品必须包括清楚的用量说明，包括液体肠内营养品，霜剂，敷料，鼻喷雾剂，滴剂和所有其他外用产品。如"遵医嘱"的说明不足以使患者恰当用药，则为护理人员带来难题。

- 一旦开具处方，应送到养老院。经正规培训的工作人员应根据MAR表和所需用药清单检查每位居民的处方，然后送到药房。应建立一套确保处方包含所有申请药品的流程。

- 医师应纠正本阶段出现的任何异常或失误。

- 建立确保向社区药师反馈上月的药物变更情况的制度。

- 任何印在处方上，但实际上不需要的药物，应清楚标明"不需要"。 养老院应将所有审查完的处方送至社区药房配药。

- 出现任何不需要的药物须通知医师，以便更新患者用药记录。如某处方药停用，应反馈给医师，以便从长期用药处方中删除，避免将来的混乱。

- 本阶段费时找出差异有利于促进长期进程平稳运行，并节省将来时间。

- 所有处方均按照28日一疗程开量。超出该剂量会给养老院带来实际安全问题。必要时联系医师，请求医师减量。

10. 药物送达和检查

- 社区药房应最少在下一疗程开始前两天提供所有药物和服药执行纪录（MAR表）。

- 经培训的护理人员需要根据他们的药品申请记录，检查药品，并酌情与医师或者药师讨论任何不符之处。

● 检查接收药物的剂量、标签的准确性和 MAR 图表记录信息的准确性。任何药物上如有"谨遵医嘱"或"按照指示"的字样，应由药师解释。

● 所有送到养老院的药物都应带有书面信息。检查所有新药以确保有可用的产品信息介绍。若无，则向药剂师跟进。

● 提倡养老院工作人员保留所有查询的书面记录，例如电话交谈和养老院居民在用药管理过程中的各种措施。应建立明确的跟踪审计制度。

11. 记录系统

● 社区药师通常向养老院提供印刷 MAR 表。该项额外服务没有 NHS 的补偿。只有社区诊所，养老院和药房之间存充分的沟通，才能制出准确的最新图表。

● 提倡向药师告知药物停用情况，以便将停用药物从 MAR 图表上删除。

● 提供 MAR 表的社区药剂师应遵守相关的指导文件，比如《关于社区药师提供健康和社会护理所使用的打印版 MAR 的说明》。

● MAR 表为法律文件。护理质量委员会文件《关于合规的指导：质量和安全的基本标准》指出最后一次记录后的 MAR 表继续保存至少 3 年的时间。

● 如果处方在疗程期间加入新药物，社区药师应该提供新的 MAR 图表。然而，如果无法完成，护理人员有必要在 MAR 图上手写录入新药物。社区药剂师应提供空白的 MAR 图表，以便当现有居民图表上没有足够的空间时，或为新居民手写药物时能够应对。

● MAR 表的任何添加/修改都需签署，注明日期和清楚的说明变化的原因。提倡工作人员向 MAR 图表添加信息以对其进行签名和注明日期，并且随后的核查人员也应签署和注明日期。提倡复印原始处方，将其附到 MAR 图表上，以证明详细的手写记录。

● 由于 MAR 的法律属性，对 MAR 表的任何变更应建立清晰的跟踪审计制度。

附录 1　以下药物不适合做长期用药处方的药物：

药物种类	具体药物或药物种类
抗菌 / 真菌类	口服抗生素 / 抗真菌剂 外用抗生素 / 抗真菌剂
皮质类固醇	口服皮质类固醇 强效的局部类固醇
易被滥用药物	催眠药和抗焦虑药 管制药物 抗吐剂 伪麻黄碱
限用一个疗程药物	伐尼克林
减肥药	奥利司他

此表格并不包含所有该类药物，请就有关特定药物 / 制剂咨询处方预览表或 BNF。

参考文献

［1］节省时间就是拯救患者 . 提高长期用药处方流程质量的实践指导，NHS 全国处方中心 . 2004 年 1 月 http://www.npc.nhs.uk/repeat_medication/repeat_prescribing/resources/library_good_practice_guide_repeatprescribingguide_2004.pdf.

［2］医师处方质量—关于英国全科医师治疗质量的调查 . 国王基金会，2011 年 .http://www.kingsfund.org.uk/publications/improving–quality–care–general–practice.

［3］Garfield et al. 初级护理中的药物使用质量 – 映射问题，致力于解决方案：系统文献概述 . BMC 医学，2009 年 9 月 .

［4］全科医师的安全处方策略 . 全国处方中心，2011 年 http://www.npc.nhs.uk/evidence/resources/10_top_tips_for_gps.pdf.

［5］质量和安全的基本标准.护理质量委员会.2010年3月 http://www.cqc.org.uk/sites/default/files/media/documents/gac_-_dec_2011_update.pdf.

［6］UKMI医学问答"哪些药物可用于初级护理处方？".2013年7月 http://www.evidence.nhs.uk/search?q=%22Which+medicines+should+be+considered+ for +brand%22.

［7］2001年药物滥用规定修正版.www.gov.hk https://www.gov.uk/government/publications/amendments-to-the-misuse-of-drugs-regulations-2001-the-2001-regulations-to-implement-key-elements-of-the-action-programme-published-in-safer-management-of-controlled-drugs-december-2004.

［8］长期用药处方的执行指导.NHS联合会出版社，2013年12月 Http.//psnc.org.uk/wp-content/updates/2013/07/Repeat-dispensing-guide-Dec-2013.pdf.

［9］2008年医疗与社会护理法案第781号 http://www.legislation.gov.uk/uksi/2010/781/contents/made.

［10］皇家药学网站/社会护理制药服务 http://www.rpharms.com/commis sioning/pharmaceutical-services-to-social-care-Settings.asp.

［11］皇家药学网站/社会护理医药处理 http://www.rpharms.com/social-care-settings-pdfs/the-handling-of-medicines-in-social-care.pdf.

［12］皇家药学网站/药物管理图表安全适当生产原则 www.rpharms.com/support-pdfs/marchartsguid.pdf.

初始任务完成小组成员

安迪·唐巴文德医师，处方领导全科医师，西柴郡 CCG

简·赖特医师，全科医师，威勒尔 CCG

简·皮戈特医师，全科医师，威勒尔 CCG

凯瑟琳·道儿医师，沃灵顿 CCG

朱利安·西蒙，药物管理主管，柴郡和默西塞德郡任务扶助部

安娜·英格兰，药学技术员，药物管理小组（沃灵顿），柴郡和默西塞德郡任务扶助部

保罗·罗伯特，处方顾问，药物管理小组（西柴郡），柴郡和默西塞德郡

任务扶助部

格兰达·得柏，高级药学技术员，药物管理小组（威勒尔），柴郡和默西塞德郡任务扶助部

迁安那·古德温，药物管理小组，Vale Royal，东部和南部 CCG

德比·罗威，药物合同小组，CWW 区小组

梅兰·卡洛，威勒尔药物委员会（代表威勒尔和柴郡 LPC）

2013/2014 年文件更新

贝基·波查，处方顾问，药物管理小组（西柴郡），柴郡和默西塞德郡任务扶助部

保罗·罗伯特，处方顾问，药物管理小组（西柴郡），柴郡和默西塞德郡任务扶助部

朱迪斯·格林，高级药学技术员，药物管理小组（威勒尔），柴郡和默西塞德郡任务扶助部

巴布拉·佩林，高级药学技术员，药物管理小组（西柴郡），柴郡和默西塞德郡任务扶助部

杰宁·鲁恩，高级药学技术员，药物管理小组（沃灵顿），柴郡和默西塞德郡任务扶助部

CWW 本地化专业网络

CPCW 区域药物委员会

（尚楠　译；郑帅，Helen Zhang　审校）

附件 2 英国坎布里亚郡长期用药处方实践指南

备注 / 提要：此附件详细总结了长期用药处方的取药流程[9]

2014 年 1 月

长期用药处方系统

前言

在社区医疗中，慢性病长期用药处方是患者获得药品的主要渠道，其使用达到所有处方的三分之二，这部分药费约占到药品总费用的 80%。据估计，在英国，每天约开具 240 万张处方，其中约 192 万张处方是长期用药处方[1]。因此，对社区诊所工作人员和患者来说，制定高效和有效的长期用药处方系统很重要。

设计不当或管理不善的系统，可能会使患者、实际操作人员和其他医护专业人员蒙受损失。它会浪费宝贵的时间，增加犯错的几率，从而给患者健康带来风险。

新的社区医疗服务（简称 nGMS）合约体现了拥有有效和高效长期用药处方系统的重要性，其中包含了药品管理的多种质量考核标准 2。一个管理良好的系统将从以下方面获益：

- 提高处方质量
- 患者更方便地获得他们所需要的药品
- 提高患者用药安全性
- 更好、更恰当地使用相关专业医疗人员和诊所工作人员的技能和时间
- 减小社区医师（简称 GP）和诊所的工作量
- 优化相关工作流程，提高效率
- 增进患者 / 患者家属对治疗的参与性和责任
- 更好地利用英国国民医疗保健体系（简称 NHS）资源

为了满足人口结构的变化和 NHS 的长期发展，长期用药处方系统需要不断的调整和进化，从而减少社区诊所工作中产生的不必要负担。此外，需要

考虑辅助处方者和独立处方者的影响，以及新 IT 系统的实施和社区药店的服务扩展。

什么是长期用药处方系统?

长期用药处方为患者和处方者的一种合作关系，允许处方者授权一个处方，它可以在约定的时间间隔多次取药，而不需要在每次申请处方时找全科医生诊疗。

这个过程中的一个重要组成部分是，处方者确保患者同意并签署治疗协议，包括对药物使用情况和效果进行必要的监测，并定期评估是否不断需要长期用药处方——这应该考虑患者临床审查的具体情况。

下图是一个长期用药处方示意图。

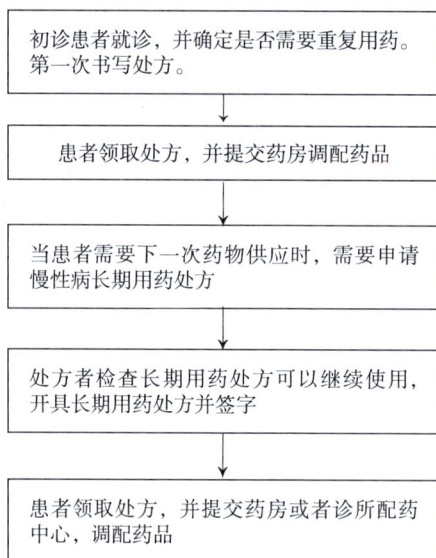

初诊患者就诊，并确定是否需要重复用药。
第一次书写处方。

↓

患者领取处方，并提交药房调配药品

↓

当患者需要下一次药物供应时，需要申请
慢性病长期用药处方

↓

处方者检查长期用药处方可以继续使用，
开具长期用药处方并签字

↓

患者领取处方，并提交药房或者诊所配药
中心，调配药品

图 1　长期用药处方用药处方简化系统

长期用药处方的申请方式可以多种多样，并且可以包括电子（网络）申请、使用处方侧联申请，电话或书面申请，或经由电子处方服务（EPS）的方式。

长期用药处方的领取方式也有很多种，例如患者自己领取，或者直接以电子方式发送到社区药房。事实上，每个社区诊所对长期用药处方系统的使用都有所不同，他们拥有各自的实践模式和创意，所以为了适应当地的实践情况，长期用药处方系统运行的可行性极为重要。

运行良好的系统使患者和患者家属获益

● 更加便捷地获得所需药物；

● 准确地理解和更好地掌握长期用药处方的使用流程，知道何时以及如何申请长期用药处方，并知道什么时间从何处领取长期用药处方；

● 确保患者获取个体化和优质的处方重配服务，更有信心的获取和使用处方药；

● 得到完整的处方和详尽的用药指导，准确地了解如何使用和管理药品；

● 有机会与医疗专业人士讨论用药情况，了解治疗过程和重要性；

● 减少发生药品不良事件和不良反应的可能性；

● 可参与自身健康护理的决策，有助于自我管理；提高与医护人员对治疗的一致性，从而提高治疗效果，减少住院次数，缩短住院时间，减少社区就诊的次数。

运行良好的系统对诊所的益处

● 尽早明确诊断，降低病情加重的风险，减少可能的投诉和起诉；确保拥有相关的处方使用和监管系统，在不良事件发生时保护处方者免受不必要的责难；

● 提高长期用药处方系统的使用效率，工作更有计划性；

● 减少患者对诊所工作人员的询问，避免了前台的拥挤，提高了医疗服务的声誉；

● 适当和有效地发挥专业医务人员和辅助工作人员的时间和技能；

● 所涉及人员更加深入地了解处方重配过程，包括各自的作用、职责和流程；

● 通过更好地完成工作，提高医务人员和辅助工作人员的士气；

- 实现诊所运行质量目标，最大限度地提高实践收入；

- 增进与其他医护人员的合作和工作关系，比如非医学方向的处方者、护士和社区药师；

- 易于实现的新举措，这将进一步降低工作负担，提高护理质量，如电子处方的转移，长期用药处方连续调配服务。

运行良好的系统对英国国民医疗保健体系（NHS）的益处

- 保证以安全、有效和适当的方式用药；

- 有效利用 NHS 的资源，以减少浪费；

- 适当发挥每个人的技能和知识，并扩大医务人员职责；

- 降低发生内部差错和不良事件的可能性，促进整个 NHS 系统的错误学习分享机制，有助于防范不良事件的发生。

持续改进

长期用药处方系统是一个复杂的系统，涉及许多人员和流程，所以使用正确性是至关重要的。有很多容易出错的环节或者潜在出错的可能性。整个系统需要定期审查，包括整个过程中的每个步骤，以保证其服务质量，并最大限度地减少低效和不安全的风险。定时的审查作为临床管理的一部分，可以帮助诊所持续改进长期用药处方系统。当需要快速改进长期用药处方系统的时候，需要平衡系统的安全性。当我们可以认识并保持这种平衡的时候，更高效的系统是可能实现的。

系统映射和对比学习

回顾和重新设计长期用药处方流程是为了给患者提供更好的服务。实际操作者可能会发现流程回顾是很有用，它可以确定长期用药处方系统在实践中的真正工作方式，并发现哪些环节效率低并有待改进。所有系统会有很多相同的地方，但根据各个地区的政策，运行模式也具有不同的地区性。对长期用药处方系统的对比是一个识别潜在的问题或瓶颈的好方法，并允许对比和改进发现的问题。对比和回顾一个系统并不困难，但它确实需要一定的时间和整个团队的参与，包括使用者和照顾者，以及其他外围人员，例如社区药师。

当更改任何系统时，做到这两点非常重要：一是清楚地了解想要达到的目的，二是考虑好将如何鉴别改进的效果。

目前，已经有很多成功的举措，可显著改善长期用药处方药品管理，这里是一些例子：

● 有些诊所已经开发了基于网络系统来方便患者申请长期用药处方。这将减少 GP 工作量，使患者多一种申请方式，患者无需考虑诊所开门时间，随时上网申请；

● 一个地区卫生管理部门允许患者使用短信服务申请长期用药处方。此服务对于具有一定生理缺陷的患者非常适宜，如听力较差的患者；

● 同步更新患者的长期用药处方信息可以节省患者和实际操作者的时间，并潜在地减少浪费。很多医药管理网站都在研发处方同步的不同方式；

● 为了更好地利用 GP 的时间，并提高患者满意度，一些社区诊所为长期用药处方系统指定并培训了专业工作人员；

● 电子处方（简称 EPS）的使用减少了患者申请和领取处方的复杂过程，并更广泛和有效的推广了长期用药处方连续调配服务；

● 通过审查电子处方，或者签订个体化或多个电子处方，使得处方开具过程更加高效，大大减少了 GP 的工作量。

● 在患者实际领取药物前，医师可以随时取消电子处方，提高患者安全；

● 对于提供长期用药处方代理领取服务的诊所，电子处方不需要工作人员整理（或者邮寄）处方，节省了时间和资源。

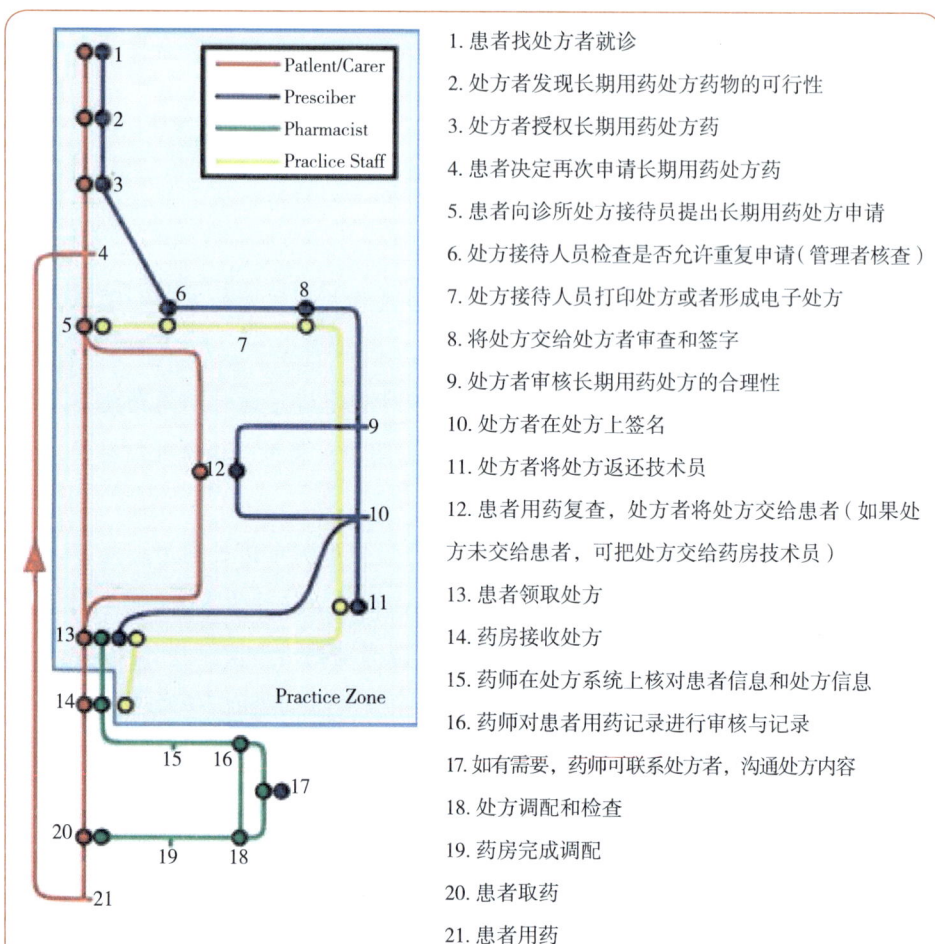

1. 患者找处方者就诊

2. 处方者发现长期用药处方药物的可行性

3. 处方者授权长期用药处方药

4. 患者决定再次申请长期用药处方药

5. 患者向诊所处方接待员提出长期用药处方申请

6. 处方接待人员检查是否允许重复申请（管理者核查）

7. 处方接待人员打印处方或者形成电子处方

8. 将处方交给处方者审查和签字

9. 处方者审核长期用药处方的合理性

10. 处方者在处方上签名

11. 处方者将处方返还技术员

12. 患者用药复查，处方者将处方交给患者（如果处方未交给患者，可把处方交给药房技术员）

13. 患者领取处方

14. 药房接收处方

15. 药师在处方系统上核对患者信息和处方信息

16. 药师对患者用药记录进行审核与记录

17. 如有需要，药师可联系处方者，沟通处方内容

18. 处方调配和检查

19. 药房完成调配

20. 患者取药

21. 患者用药

图2 英国长期用药处方的流程示意图

为了帮助理解长期用药处方的过程，并提高其管理质量，整个流程可以简化为九个关键领域：

关键领域

授权长期用药处方	申请长期用药处方
是否应该开具长期用药处方？	产生处方并由医师签字
患者用药复查	患者获取处方
社区药师的作用	患者使用药物
整个流程的质量保证	

然而，Zermansky 等提供了长期用药处方的模版[4]，在建立实践指南时，许多诊所使用了这种模板。这种模版简单描述如下。

（1）产生处方：包括接收申请和开具处方。通常委托给诊所处方接待员。

（2）管理控制：一般属于诊所管理人或者药物管理者的责任，包括四个要素：①授权检查；②符合性检查；③药物复查日期——确保每个患者知道药物复查的确切时间；④标记——确保处方者可以注意到需要药物复查的患者。

（3）临床控制：这是医师或其他处方者的责任，涉及两个任务：①授权——确保长期用药处方是合适的，药物依然有效，患者耐受性好而且需要继续使用；②定期复查——复查针对患者和药物，以确保药物治疗仍然有效、适宜，耐受性好。处方者需要决定药物是否继续，变更或停止。

更多有关开发和提高长期用药处方系统的详细信息可以参照国家处方中心（简称 NPC）网站。NPC 是现在的 NICE 的一部分，但保持原有网站上他们以前的资源库。http://www.npc.nhs.uk/repeat_medication/repeat_prescribing/index.php

长期用药处方系统模版的特点——清单

（1）通过书面形式，建立完成和清晰的政策和程序，考虑定期审核和处方运行形式的改变（比如助理处方者的使用，长期用药处方连续调配服务的使用），以及诊所的发展。

（2）监督和管理的人员须经过适当培训，建立责任制；

（3）所有工作人员，包括临时代理处方者，都要进行培训，并充分认识到工作诊所长期用药处方系统的运行模式，并注意到他们的个人责任；

（4）为每个患者提供全面、最新和准确的长期用药处方使用信息；

（5）所有的信息必须安全和保密，对全体员工进行计算机处方系统的定期培训；

（6）计算机系统通过使用个人密码对所有用户保密，包括 Caldicott 政策，数据保护法等安全政策信息法。长期用药处方信息要定期备份；

（7）未经授权的人员、患者或医药代表是看不见屏幕上的信息的，除非专门为此目的设计的，如临床知识概要"共享"屏幕；

（8）只有通过临床证明、的确对患者有益的药物，才允许增加到患者的长期用药处方药物单上，而且只有通过授权的处方者可以添加药物。

（9）只有符合资质的处方者可以授权长期用药处方；

（10）所有处方必须由了解患者或者可以直接进入患者医疗记录的处方者进行审查和签名；

（11）明确规定哪些药物不适合长期用药处方的使用，如特殊管制类药品、催眠药，牢记特殊患者群体的需要，如身患绝症者；

（12）在患者的长期用药处方药品记录中，明确的记录审计线索，包括任何药品的添加和删除；

（13）建立出院患者药品校对流程，在改变长期用药处方前，要检查患者所有住院或门诊的医嘱；

（14）对于长期用药处方的后续授权，需要明确规定适当的时间间隔，建立患者复查提醒系统，确保所有使用长期用药处方的患者得到定期复查。包括临床和药物复查，以及医患治疗一致性的评估；

（15）准确地开具处方，提供全面的行政指导，也最大限度地提高药物同步和更新，避免重复治疗；

（16）在可审计的限制范围内，检查药物申请的频率，便于迅速发现、调查和消除任何形式的药物滥用；

（17）在适当情况下，处方药品计量要考虑到每个患者的需要，考虑到他们的临床状况、安全和方便，并避免浪费；

（18）定期评估患者的病情；需要规定开具药物的时间；考虑持续治疗的受益；药物不良反应和药物相互作用；进行所有必要的监测；

（19）建立医患关系，确保患者参与对治疗的选择和决定，提高治疗一致性和满意度，并尽早反馈任何潜在的问题；

（20）为患者提供长期治疗和处方管理信息，帮助患者和护理人员了解长期用药处方系统（申请，领取药方，如何请求帮助，药物复查等），并考虑到护理人员的方便，尤其是照顾多个患者的护理人员。接受并认真考虑服务建议和回馈，并酌情采取行动；

（21）进行定期质量评估。从错误事件和投诉中学习，改善和演变处方操作系统。

（22）涉及新药的任何副作用或者临床事件，通过英国药品"黄卡方案"报告药品食品监督部门。

重复风险评估（附表1）提供了一个简单的方法，来鉴别长期用药处方系统中需要回顾和改进的领域。

参考文献

［1］Prescriptions dispensed in the community statistics for 1999–2009: England, Health and Social Care Information Centre 2010

［2］Saving time, helping patients　— a good practice guide to quality repeat prescribing. National Prescribing Centre January 2004

［3］National Prescribing Centre Medicines Management Services Collaborative Service Improvement Guide: Repeat Prescribing. NPC 2006

［4］Zermansky AG. Who controls repeats? Br J Gen Pract 1996; 46: 643–7

附表 1

重复调配风险评估工具

问题	分数
是否有书面协议？	是的 =0 否 =1
产生	
1. 申请	
如何提出申请？	打电话 =2 家属电话 = 0 写信 / 发电子邮件 / 邮寄 / 传真 = 0
如果申请是手写的，使用的什么形式？	长期用药处方药品单（处方侧联）=0 其他 =1
如果处方接待人员接受了口头申请，是否同一个人产生处方？	是的 =0 否 =1
是否标记了需要的申请药物？	是的 =0 否 =1
申请药物是否可以重复申请？	是的 =0 否 =1
2. 产生	
处理长期用药处方的工作人员的是否是指定的，是否经过培训？	是的 =0 否 =1
处方是电脑生成的吗？	是的 =0 否 =1
处方领取时间需要多久？	<48 小时 = 0 ≥ 48 小时 =1
是否建立指定的时间处理长期用药处方的申请？	是的 =0 否 =1
3. 签署	
是否有设定的签署时间？	是的 =0 否 =1
签署时是否有适当的可用资源（如计算机）？	是的 =0 否 =1
医生签署前进行检查吗？	是的 =0 否 =1

问题	分数
4. 其他	
当一个处方丢失后，怎么办？	重新打印 =0 重新开具 =1
如果处方没有被领取，怎么办？	记录 =0 无记录 =1
如果处方被重新打印，会记录？	是的 =0 否 =1
	产生合计
管理	
1 授权	
谁授权长期用药处方？	接待员 =2 护士 =0 医师 =0 专科护士 = 0
重新授权的过程是什么？	通知 GP= 0 不通知 GP= 2
授权多少张可重复的长期用药处方？	0~6=0； 6~12（对于稳定的患者）= 0 6~12（适用于不稳定的患者）= 1 >12=2
2 依从性	
处方发出前是否检查依从性？	是的 =0 否 =1
对依从性的评估，是否有书面标准规范？	是的 =0 否 =1
3 家政服务（使用 20 例患者样本）	
样本之外：是否有可以使用仿制药的原创药？	是的 =1 否 =0
样本之外：是否需要剂量优化？	是的 =1 否 =0
样本之外：是否有任何复制使用的药品？	是的 =2 否 =0
样本之外：是否有 6 个月或以上没有领取的药物？	是的 =1 否 =0

续　表

问题	分数
样本之外：是否有任何剂量说明书丢失？	是的 =1 否 =0
药物监测测试（比如血检）是最新的吗？	是的 =0 否 =1
每次的剂量都一样吗？	是的 =0 否 =1
	总管理
临床	
1 紧急申请	
谁发出紧急申请？	前台接待员提出 = 2 前台接待员根据规定协议提出 = 0 医生 = 0
先前的紧急授权允许由接待员发出吗？	是的 =2　否 =0 是的，有规定协议 = 0
2 出院	
谁来决定长期用药处方中药物的增加 / 删除？	医生 = 0 其他 = 2
谁来更新长期用药处方？	医生 = 0 接待员，医生核对 = 0 接待员，医生不核对 =2
3. 用药复查	
谁执行用药复查？	医生 = 0　药师 =0　护士 =0 在适当的时间间隔没有审查 =2
是否建立用药复查提醒？	是的 = 0 否 =1
	最大风险评分 = 46

（杨会霞　译；郑帅　审校）

附件 3　患者信息表，用于申请慢性病长期用药处方[10]

LEIGHTON ROAD SURGERY

REPEAT PRESCRIPTION ORDER FORM

Full Name...

Date of Birth...

Address ....

....

Daytime phone number...

IT TAKES TWO WORKING DAYS TO PROCESS REQUESTS

Item No	Name of Medication	Strength	Dose
e.g.	Aspirin Dispersible	75mg	1 a day
1.			
2.			
3.			
4.			
5.			
6.			
7.			
8.			
9.			
10.			
11.			
12.			

附件4 处方中不宜用其仿制药替换的药品

英国健康和社保董事会（Health and Social Care Board）2016年9月更新的《不宜用其仿制药替换的处方药》[12]

Items Unsuitable for Generic Prescribing September 2016

HSC Health and Social Care Board

The following list provides examples of drugs / preparations which would NOT be recommended for generic prescribing. This list is guidance only and practices may wish to add other categories of their own depending on practice policy. For further information refer to the BNF or contact your Pharmacy Advisor. Please note: the list of brand names given as examples is *not exhaustive*. Please refer also to HSCB guidance on using specified brands that are cost effective choices for HSC

Medicine Category	Generic name / group	Examples	Comments
Drugs with a **narrow therapeutic index**	Aminophylline	Phyllocontin Continus®	There may be differences in the bioavailability of the preparations and / or the difference between therapeutic and toxic plasma concentrations. Therefore the brand name should be prescribed.
	Lithium	Priadel®, Camcolit®, Liskonum®	
	Theophylline	Nuelin SA®, Slo-Phyllin®, Uniphyllin Continus®	
Drugs with a narrow therapeutic index for **certain indications**, e.g. renal transplant	Ciclosporin	Neoral®, Sandimmun® Deximune®	
	Mycophenolate	CellCept®, Arzip®, Myfenax®	
	Tacrolimus	Prograf®, Advagraf®	
Anti-epileptic drugs Category 1	Phenytoin	Phenytoin Flynn hard capsules	**Anti-epileptic drugs Category 1** Ensure the patient is maintained on a specific manufacturer's product **Anti-epileptic drugs Category 2** *The need for continued supply of a particular manufacturer's product should be based on clinical judgement and consultation with patient / carer taking into account seizure frequency and treatment history. **Anti-epileptic drugs Category 3** (Levetiracetam, Lacosamide, Tiagabine, Gabapentin, Pregabalin, Ethosuximide, Vigabatrin) It is usually unnecessary to ensure that patients are maintained on a specific manufacturer's product unless there are specific reasons such as patient anxiety and risk of confusion or dosing errors.
	Carbamazepine	Tegretol®, Carbagen®, Epimaz®	
	Phenobarbital	Prescribe generic name and state manufacturer	
	Primidone	Prescribe generic name and state manufacturer	
Anti-epileptic drugs Category 2 for some patients*	Valproate, Lamotrigine, Perampanel, Retigabine, Rufinamide, Clobazam, Clonazepam, Oxcarbazepine, Eslicarbazepine, Zonisamide, Topiramate		
Certain **modified-release preparations**	Diltiazem	Angtil XL®, Zemtard®, Slozem®, Adizem XL®, Tildiem LA®	The BNF states that brand names should be specified in certain instances as different versions of these modified-release (m/r) preparations may not have the same clinical effect.
	Mesalazine	Asacol MR®, Pentasa®	
	Nifedipine	Adipine MR or XL®, Coracten SR or XL®, Adalat Retard®	
	Methylphenidate	Concerta XL®, Equasym XL®, Medikinet XL®	
Certain **Controlled Drugs** including patches (Schedule 2 and 3)	Buprenorphine	Butec®, Butrans®, Transtec®, Bupeaze®, Hapoctasin®	Caution due to differing dosage regimes for SR and XL preparations. The BNF states that dosage should be reviewed if brand altered.
	Fentanyl (transdermal)	Mezolar®, Durogesic DTrans®, Fentalis®, Matrifen®, Tilofyl®	
	Morphine	MST®, MXL®, Zomorph®, Morphgesic SR®, Sevredol®	
	Oxycodone	Longtec®, Shortec®, Oxycontin®, Oxynorm®	
Certain **inhaler devices**	Beclometasone (+/- Formoterol)	Qvar®, Clenil®, Fostair®	Always state the type of device, e.g. accuhaler, turbohaler. This is to ensure that the patient continues to receive the device that they have been trained to use.
	Dry powder devices	Accuhaler®, Easyhaler®, Turbohaler®, Pulvinal®, Clickhaler®, Foradil®	
Multi-ingredient products	See examples →	Stalevo®	Generic prescribing may not be practical or may cause confusion due to multiple ingredients. Some combination products are appropriate for generic prescribing using an approved 'co-' prefix e.g. co-codamol, co-amilofruse, etc.
		Hormone replacement therapy	
		Oral contraceptives	
		Multi-ingredient GI preps. e.g. Peptac®, pancreatin, rehydration salts, laxatives etc.	
		Multi-ingredient ENT preparations	
		Creams, bath oils, antiseptics, liquids or gels	
		Bowel cleansing solutions	
Specific brands for **specific indications**	Duloxetine	Yentreve® or Cymbalta®	
	Denosumab	Prolia® or Xgeva®	
	Buprenorphine	Subutex® or Temgesic®	
Miscellaneous	See examples →	Antipsychotic depot injections	These should be prescribed using the brand name to avoid confusion / aid product identification. Generic prescribing for these drugs may affect clinical response or contribute to administration incidents
		Stoma care products and appliances	
		Wound products	
		Insulin	
		Nutritional products	
		Vaccines	
		NRT	
		Calcium salts, e.g. Natecal D3®, Adcal®	
		Pre-filled injectables – e.g. Adrenaline, somatropin, apomorphine, erythropoietin	
		Vitamin D, e.g. Desunin®, Fultium-D3®, InVita-D3®, Pro-D3®, Thorens®	

附件 5　不适合慢性病长期用药处方项目的药品 [2, 8, 15]

在英国，GP 根据自己的专业判断，决定哪些药物可以用到慢性病长期用药处方上，但是通过药理研究和患病属性，以下药品不建议用于长期用药处方：

药品类别	药品或药品种类
抗生素	口服抗生素 局部用抗生素
皮质激素	口服皮质激素药 强度局部用皮质激素
容易滥用的药物	安眠药和抗焦虑药 特殊管制类药物 赛克利嗪（止吐药和抗组胺药） 假麻黄碱
戒烟药	伐尼克兰 尼古丁替代药物
减肥药物	奥利司他
治疗窗狭窄的药物（部分地区禁用）	法华林 锂剂 氯氮平 茶碱或者氨茶碱
口服抗癌药（部分地区禁用）	环磷酰胺 巯嘌呤 甲氨蝶呤
适用于短期服用的药物	止咳药 非甾体抗炎药 维生素 D

附件 6　各种慢性病的药物治疗复查周期[2]

患者病情和治疗稳定的慢性病	建议的复查周期
哮喘	12 个月
冠心病	12 个月
糖尿病	12 个月
癫痫	12 个月
绝经症状的激素代替治疗	12 个月
75 岁以上老年患者	12 个月
精神分裂症	12 个月
甲状腺疾病	12 个月
高血压	6 个月
75 岁以上老年患者并服用 4 种或者 4 种以上药物	6 个月
长期避孕药	6 个月

附件 7　英国常用的 Ⅱ 类，Ⅲ 类和 Ⅳ 类特殊管制药品表

管制类别	药名
Ⅱ 类	Diamorphine 海洛因 Morphine 吗啡 Nabilone 大麻隆 Remifenyanil 瑞芬太尼 Pethidine 哌替啶 Secobarbital 司可巴比妥 Glutethimide 格鲁米特 Amfetamines 苯丙胺类药物 Sodium Oxybate 羟丁酸钠 Cocaine 可卡因
Ⅲ 类	Barbiturates（for example: phenobarbital; except Secobarbital in Ⅱ 类） 巴比妥类药物（例如：苯巴比妥；除外司可巴比妥属于 Ⅱ 类） Buprenorphine 丁丙诺啡 Diethylpropion 二乙胺苯丙酮 Mazindol 马吲哚 Meprobamate 甲丙氨酯 Midazolam 咪达唑仑 Pentazocine 喷他佐辛 Phentermine 芬特明 Temazepam 替马西泮 Tramadol 曲马多
Ⅳ 类第一部分	Benzodiazepine（for example: diazepam; except Temazepam, Midazolam in Ⅲ 类）苯二氮䓬类药物（例如：地西泮；除外替马西泮和咪达唑仑属于 Ⅲ 类） Zaleplon 扎来普隆 Zolpidem 唑吡坦 Zopiclone 佐匹克隆
Ⅳ 类第二部分	Androgenic and anabolic steroids 雄激素和类固醇 Clenbuterol 克伦特罗 Chorionic Gonadotrophin 绒毛膜促性腺激素 Somatotropin 生长激素 Somatrem 人蛋氨生长素 Somatropin 促生长激素

第四章 加拿大慢性病长期用药处方项目的研究与借鉴

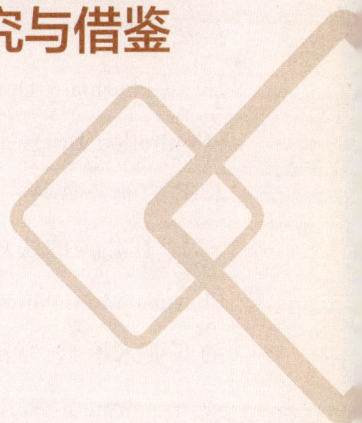

人口老龄化和慢性病高发、快速增长是全世界共同关注的社会问题。加强慢性病的有效综合防控已成为世界各国所面临的重大公共卫生问题。在加拿大医药卫生体制、机制中，设置有慢性病长期用药处方制度。长期用药处方一般是针对处于病情相对稳定的慢性病，由执业医师开具、可以连续调配一定次数的处方，药师可以根据该长期用药处方的授权和指令，以处方指定的时间间隔和次数为患者连续调配药品[1]。加拿大《卫生职业人员法实施细则》(Health Professions Act–BYLAWS),《药房开业和药品分类法》(Pharmacy Operations and Drug Scheduling Act),《管控药品和物质法》(Controlled Drugs and Substance Act) 等法律法规，以及医师、药师执业相关的业务规范，都对慢性病长期用药处方有具体规定或要求（参见附件一）。在相关的法规和规范性文件中，如《社区药房执业标准》(Community Pharmacy Standards of Practice)（参见附件二），对慢性病长期用药处方采用的专业术语是"Prescription Refills"，也有表示为"prescribing with repeats"或"renewing prescriptions"❶加拿大慢性病长期用药处方项目的制度安排、运行机制和实践，有很多成功经验，并形成一些比较科学的技术规范，可供深入研究借鉴，对正处于"深水区"的我国医改以有益的启示。

第一节　加拿大慢性病长期用药处方取药流程

加拿大各省都对医师处方出台具体的执业标准和业务规范。执业医师根

① 注：根据加拿大《药房开业和药品分类法》(Pharmacy Operations and Drug Scheduling Act)中的《社区药房执业标准》(Community Pharmacy Standards of Practice)（参见附件二），refill 与 renewal 是有所不同的。refill 是指药师根据医师开具的长期用药处方进行连续调剂药品（原文："refill" means verbal or written approval from a practitioner authorizing aregistrant to dispense additional quantities of drug（s）pursuant to a prescription）；Renewal 是指药师依法在特殊情况下根据以往调剂过的处方提供患者一定数量的药品[原文："renewal" means authorization by a full pharmacist to dispense additionalquantities of drug（s）pursuant to a previously dispensed prescription, inaccordance with section 25.92 of the Act]。但各省的执业标准和有关文献经常将两者等同起来，对应参考文献也认为两者是相同的。。

据患者评估和诊断结果开具长期用药处方时，应在处方中确定处方药品总量，每次调配量，规定可续配次数和间隔时间，以及第一次药品调配的时间（Start Date），见图 4-1。长期用药处方上注明的可续配次数是凭该处方可以直接在药房连续调配到指定量药品的次数。长期用药处方标示格式可以采取"Repeat＿＿

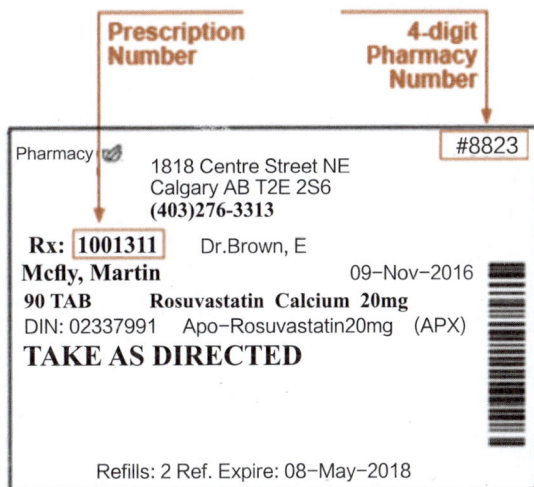

图 4-1　长期用药处方药房调剂信息样图

times at intervals of ＿＿week"、"Refill ＿＿times every ＿＿day" 或 "Dispense 100 mg at 25 day intervals" 等形式，甚至还可在处方底部采用表格形式，如

。药房在续配长期用药处方时还应注明处方号和药房编码[1]。

　　慢性病长期用药处方取药流程，在《加拿大药师执业示范标准》（Model Standards of Practice for Canadian Pharmacists）和各省医师、药师执业标准，如《萨斯喀彻温省药师执业标准》（Standards of Practice for Saskatchewan Pharmacists）都有所提及，但没有具体的长期用药处方取药流程图。从加拿大各省医师业务标准、药师业务标准来看，长期用药处方取药流程，主要包括处方开具、处方传送、处方调配和取药送药等四大环节。处方开具是执业医师对慢性病患者进行评估和诊断，根据病情开具处方。如果患者用药后，其用药反应和疗效取得预期效果，药品剂量和给药方案稳定后，在患者再次预约就诊时，医师可以开具长期用药处方。处方传送主要是指处方从医师传送到药房药师，同时也包括药师与药师之间的传送。如果长期用药处方的药品不属于特殊药品（具体品种限制见第三节内容），法律允许其从一个药房转移（Transfer of Prescriptions）到另一药房调配，但原始处方应保留在最早接收和调配的药房那里，剩余的可续配药品（remaining refills）可以根据患者要求转移❶在处方调配环节，药师在接收到长期用药处方（包括口头处方、书写处方、传真处方和电子处方）之后，需要对患者进行评估，对长期用药处方进行审核，并按规定执行长期用药处方调配。如果有不合理或者不利于患者利益最大化的相关问题，药师应该及时与处方者沟通。

患者申请长期用药处方续配和取药，可以采取本人上门、电话、传真或者网络在线申请等四种方式。本人上门是指患者或者家属亲自去药房申请续配药品，现场等待续配完成并取走药品或延后一段时间再来药房取药。患者还可以直接电话药房药师或者药房技术员，或者根据电话录音自动提示功能，或者发送传真，交代清楚处方信息和个人身份信息，完成长期用药处方续配申请。近些年，越来越多的长期用药处方可通过药房网站或者在线 APP 来申请处方续配，然后在收到续配完成通知之后亲自上药房取药或者由药房按约定方式送药（邮寄或送药上门）。值得特别说明的是，长期用药处方在线申请具有诸多优点。对患者，可以节省来去药房和等待的时间，可以随时随地检查处方续配的状态，还能很方便地选择打印需要的处方用药信息。对药房和药师，可以更直观、准确判断有效处方或失效处方，更方便检查患者用药历史，评估患者用药，监督用药依从性，提升长期用药处方调剂和续配的服务质量（见图 4-2）。

---

① 注：根据《药房开业和药品分类法（Pharmacy Operations and Drug Scheduling Act）》中的《社区药房执业标准》（Community Pharmacy Standards of Practice），处方转移的原文解释：prescription transfer means the transfer via direct communication from a registrant to another registrant of all remaining refill authorizations for a particular prescription to a requesting community pharmacy。

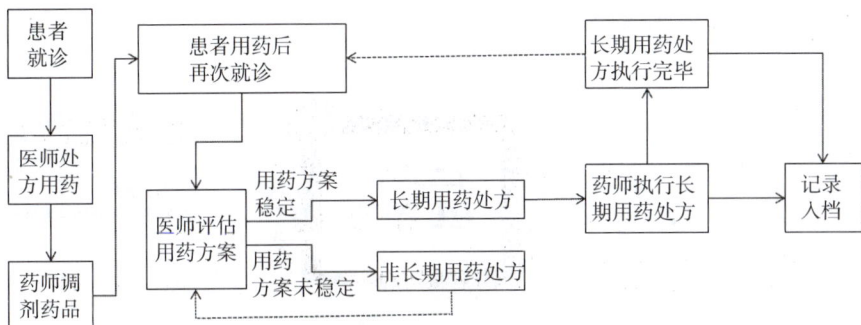

图 4-2　慢性病长期用药处方取药流程图

第二节　加拿大慢性病长期用药处方取药模式的技术支撑

从慢性病长期用药处方流程（图 4-2）来看，长期用药处方取药模式的技术支撑主要是合理用药的专业技术支持和保障，包括医师和药师以及相关技术员的专业能力和工作配合。另外还涉及医疗用药服务能力提升、处方安全、患者隐私保护等所需软硬件的技术支撑。加拿大各药师管理学会在其网站上不定期公布医院药房和社会药房管理和药品调剂所需软件供应商的名称和联系方式[3]。

慢性病长期用药处方传送，包括从医院或诊所传送到药房，以及没有续配完毕的长期用药处方从一个药房药师传递或转送（transfer）给另一药房药师。如果通过在线平台（online platform）传递处方，加拿大政府和相关法规要求只能在能保证电子病历（Electronic Medical Record, EMR）系统与药房系统（Pharmacy system）或所在省电子健康记录（Provincial Electronic Health Record, Netcare）实现信息安全传递的网络系统上开展工作，必须确保 EMR 有处方信息传送审核功能，并且能保证系统传送加密和隐私保护以及有隐私影响评估[4]。

在处方传送到药房以后，在提升药房服务能力方面所需技术支撑，主要是方便患者申请续配和取药、方便医患沟通以及能及时提醒续配药品相关的软硬件技术支持。近些年，随着通讯技术和互联网技术发展，越来越多药房装备了处方续配申请系统、提醒电子系统，患者可以登录药房主页在线申请（reorder a prescription online），或者下载智能电话客户端（smartphone apps），进一步完善处方续配服务，见图 4-3。

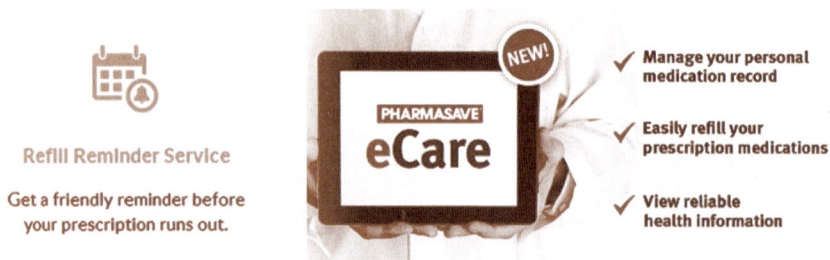

图 4-3　加拿大某药房长期用药处方提醒电子系统和 APP 界面

第三节　加拿大慢性病长期用药处方药品分类

在加拿大，药品分为特殊管理药品（麻醉药品）、处方药和非处方药。从药品管理相关法律法规分析，除麻醉药品类特殊管理药品外，几乎所有药品都允许医师根据患者治疗所需开具长期用药处方和允许药师依据长期用药处方指令进行连续调配药品。对苯二氮䓬类及其他精神药品，医师可以开具长期用药处方，但在处方开具之日起超过 12 个月药师不能继续调配。具体的长期用药处方药品分类、续配取药和处方转送（Refills & Transfers）要求见表 4-1。

表 4-1　加拿大慢性病长期用药处方的药品分类和取药要求

分类	说明	处方要求	续配和处方转移要求	购买和销售记录
麻醉药品 如：丁丙诺啡，可待因，芬太尼，氢化吗啡酮，氯胺酮，复方苯乙哌啶片，屈大麻酚，吗啡，大麻隆，氧可酮，哌替啶，氢可酮镇咳药（Tussionex）等。	列入麻醉药品目录 只含有一种麻醉药（"单一"成分）； 非肠道用药麻醉药品； 含有一种以上麻醉剂的麻醉复方制剂； 含有 2 种以下其他非麻醉成分的麻醉复方制剂；	只允许书面或传真处方 调剂记录要求包括： ◉ 患者姓名和地址 ◉ 药品名称、规格、数量、剂型 ◉ 药品生产商 ◉ 用法说明 ◉ 开药者姓名、地址	不允许长期用药处方和凭处方续配取药 在处方量内可分多次取药（part-fill）	购买记录：记录在麻醉药品和特殊管理药登记本上。至少保存两年（有些省为 3 年）备查

续　表

分类	说明	处方要求	续配和处方转移要求	购买和销售记录
麻醉药品 如：丁丙诺啡，可待因，芬太尼，氢化吗啡酮，氯胺酮，复合苯乙哌啶片，屈大麻酚，吗啡，大麻隆，氧可酮，哌替啶，氢可酮镇咳药（Tussionex）等。	含有以下 5 种麻醉剂中的任意一种成分的所有药物： ◎吗啡 ◎氢可酮 ◎美沙酮 ◎氧可酮 ◎镇痛新	◎处方 ID 号 ◎配药日期 ◎调配药师和药房技术员（如有）签名 ◎价格 ◎处方者注册号 ◎患者 ID 号和类型	不允许处方转移（包括分次取药的处方转移）	销售记录：记录在麻醉药品和特殊管理药登记本上，或保存计算机中并有打印件。记录至少保存两年（有些省为 3 年）备查
含麻醉药的复方制剂 如： Fiorina®-C1/4, Fiorina®-C1/2, Tylenol®No.2, Tylenol®No.3, Robitussin AC®, Dimetane Expectorant C®, 292® 等	在可接受的治疗剂量内，只含有 1 种麻醉药（除了上述 4 种）和 2 种或以上的非麻醉药成分的所有复方制剂	书面、传真或口头处方 口头处方可被药师或在药师监督指导下的实习生、登记在册的药学学生接收并记录 药品调剂记录应有接收口头处方的药师签名	不允许长期用药处方和凭处方续配取药 在处方量内可分多次取药（part-fill） 不允许处方转移（包括分次取药的处方转移）	购买记录：与上相同 销售记录：无要求
部分可豁免管控的可待因制剂 如：AC & C®,Mersyndol®, 扑热息痛/咖啡因/可待因 8mg,Robaxacet-8® 等	含有可待因不超过 8mg、固体口服剂型或 20mg/30ml 液体剂型，以及含 2 种及以上非麻醉药品活性成分	注意：部分可豁免管控的可待因制剂 ◎符合条件的可待因制剂可在无处方的情况下销售； ◎当根据处方调配时，应遵循与含麻醉药品制剂（口头处方）相同要求进行管理		
管控药品目录第 I 部分药品 如：安非他命，哌甲酯，右旋安非他命等	列入食品药品管理条例 G 部分中第 I 部分的药品 只含有 1 种管控药物("单一"管控药物)的药品 所有复方制剂含有 1 种以上管控药物		允许书面和传真方式开具长期用药处方和凭处方续配取药，但必须在开具处方时注明续配次数、日期和时间间隔。 口头处方不允许开具长期用药处方和续配授权 在处方量内可分多次取药（part-fill） 不允许处方转移（包括分次取药的处方转移）	购买记录：与上相同 销售记录：记录在麻醉药品和管控药登记本上，或保存计算机中并有打印件。记录至少保存两年（有些省为 3 年）备查
管控药品目录第 I 部分药物的复方制剂 （当前在加拿大已禁止流通）	复方制剂含有 1 种第 I 部分管控药物，以及 1 种或多种非管控药物成分			

分类	说明	处方要求	续配和处方转移要求	购买和销售记录
管控药品目录第Ⅱ部分药品 如：布托菲诺，大部分巴比妥类药物（如苯巴比妥米那）	列入食品药品管理条例G部分中第Ⅱ部分得药品	书面、传真或口头处方 口头处方可被药师或在药师监督指导下的实习生、登记在册的药学学生接收并记录。 药品调剂记录要求包括：	如果在开具处方时标明连续取药次数、日期或连续取药时间间隔，书面或传真处方可重复取药 在处方量内可分多次取药（part-fill） 不允许处方转移（包括分次取药的处方转移）	购买记录： 记录在麻醉药品和管控药登记本上，如按时间顺序整理的发票或相同目的的其他类似记录形式；记录至少保存两年（有些省为3年）备查。 销售记录： 无要求
管控药品目录第Ⅱ部分药物的复方制剂 如：Bellergal Spacetabs®，Tecnal®	复方制剂含有1种第Ⅱ部分管控药物，以及1种或多种非管控药物成分			
管控药品目录第Ⅲ部分药品 合成类固醇及其衍生物（如睾酮）	列入食品药品管理条例G部分中第Ⅲ部分的药品	◎ 患者姓名和地址 ◎ 药物名称、规格、数量、剂型 ◎ 药品生产商 ◎ 使用说明 ◎ 处方者姓名和地址 ◎ 处方ID号 ◎ 配药日期	如果在开具长期用药处方时标明取药次数、日期或取药时间间隔，书面或传真处方可连续取药 在处方量内可分多次取药 不允许处方转移（包括分次取药的处方转移）	购买记录： 与上相同 销售记录： 无要求
管控药品目录第Ⅲ部分药物的复方制剂 （当前在加拿大已禁止流通）	复方制剂含有1种第Ⅲ部分管控药物，以及1种或多种非管控药物成分			
苯二氮䓬类药物以及其他精神药品（Targeted Substances） 如：阿普唑仑，安定，氟胺安定，氯羟去甲安定，利眠宁，氧异安定，氯氮䓬，去甲羟基安定，羟基安定，三唑仑等	列入苯二氮䓬类及其他精神药品管理法规所示目录	◎ 调配药师和药房技术员（如有）签名 ◎ 价格 ◎ 处方者注册号 ◎ 患者ID号和类型	允许长期用药处方和凭处方续配取药 距处方开处日期一年内有效 在处方量内可分多次取药（part-fill） 在处方未转移过的情况下允许转移	购买记录： 与上相同 销售记录： 只对向其他药店销售有要求

续　表

分类	说明	处方要求	续配和处方转移要求	购买和销售记录
其他处方药	列入食品药品管理条例的处方药目录（PDL）或列入加拿大药房管理协会（NAPRA）的国家药品分类类别 I 的药品	书面、传真或口头处方 口头处方可被药师或在药师监督指导下的实习生、登记在册的药学学生接收并记录。 药品调剂记录要求见上	允许长期用药处方和凭处方续配取药 经授权的未取完药的长期用药处方可转移	购买记录：记录至少保存两年（有些省为 3 年）备查。 销售记录：不作要求

注：1. 本表主要根据加拿大安大略省管理规定进行概括总结，其他各省情况基本相近。
　　2. 来源于安大略省药师管理学会网站 2016 年 12 月发布"Prescriprion regulation summary chart"[5, 6]。
　　3. 处方调剂和药品销售记录保存期限在各省规定有所不同。如，阿尔伯塔省、安大略省要求保存 2 年，不列颠哥伦比亚省要求为 3 年。

第四节　加拿大慢性病长期用药处方运作中存在的安全隐患与风险防范措施

通过对加拿大各省发布的医师和药师的执业规范来看，相比常规处方，慢性病长期用药处方在处方开具和药品续配工作中都有一些特殊安全隐患和风险，在法规和执业规范中需要做一些特殊限制，应更多关注长期用药处方可识别性、处方传递安全、隐私保护等事项，需要更多关注长期用药处方调剂的连续性和用药依从性等问题。

一、长期用药处方用药安全风险和药学服务质量保障体系

慢性病长期用药处方的开具和药品调配，在续配过程中不需要反复预约主治医师就诊就可在药房得到连续用药。如果制度安排不当会直接影响患者用药安全和健康。为此，加拿大在长期用药处方制度设计时，通过《食品与药品管理条例》（Food and Drug Regulations）、《管控药品和物质法》

（Controlled Drugs And Substance Act）、《苯二氮䓬类及其他精神药品管理法规》（Benzodiazepines and Other Targeted Substance Regulations）等相关法律法规，在确立长期用药处方制度合法性的同时，规定长期用药处方和续配药品的分类，及具体安全风险管制措施，规定长期用药处方适用于已经过医疗机构常规治疗、病情稳定、需要继续服用相同药品的慢性病，麻醉药品和管控药品不能开具长期用药处方和续配药品，完成处方授权次数的长期用药处方不得调剂，从源头防止药物滥用，保障用药安全可控。同时，在《加拿大药师执业示范标准》及各省出台的医师、药师执业标准，如《阿尔伯塔省内外科医师管理学会医师处方实践标准》（CPSA Physician Prescribing Practices）等执业规范中，通过质量管理规范对长期用药处方的开具和调剂进行细化和标准化，保障药品质量和用药安全[7]。第一，制定处方者对长期用药处方的评估（assessment）、授权（authorization）、审核（audit）、监控（monitoring）、记录（documentation）、信息共享（sharing）等环节的质量管理规范，提升长期用药处方用药的适宜性。第二，重视社区药房和药师药学服务作用，明确药师对长期用药处方和用药的确认（verification）、用药交代、依从性帮助（compliance aids）和标签管理（label）等环节的质量管理规范，保障用药安全有效。第三，以患者为中心，强调医师、药师、诊疗部门和药房的交流沟通和合作。如果处方不正确或者不符合患者利益，应拒绝调配，并及时联系医师，如果不能及时联系到医师，应该在合理时间内写信给医师。第四，强调文件管理，要求医师治疗记录整个治疗过程和药物信息，包括可续配信息，同时应保证药师有效共享信息；长期用药处方调剂档案（Refill Documentation）中，①必须准确记录处方日期、首次调配日期，每次续配日期，药物量等信息；②说明是书写处方、口头处方还是传真处方；③长期用药处方的续配次数、间隔时间、效期应与患者资料信息相符，具有合理推断逻辑；④长期用药处方记录保存两年（有些省要求三年）备查，从最后一次续配完成之日起算，电脑系统应保存处方起始调配和续配的所有记录和历史。原则上处方开具一年以上都没有调剂的新处方，或者距首次调剂超过18个月的长期用药处方，药师不应调剂[4]。

二、长期用药处方真实性、合法性、风险与预防处方造假、欺诈

慢性病长期用药处方药品量相对较大，一般都需要从医院、诊所传递到药房，还可能在药房之间发生处方转移和多次续配。保证处方合法性、真实性和内容可识别性，预防处方信息造假（Prescription Fraud）[4]、不被篡改就显得尤为重要。在加拿大，各省法规都要求处方传送应该在保证数据信息安全和保障患者隐私的条件下进行，在各种处方指导原则中，对慢性病长期用药处方基本上都要求医师应明确填写长期用药处方指令（Refill instruction），应明确患者病历所在地址和电话。长期用药处方中有列入监管药品清单（monitored drug list, MDL）药品时，应在处方上填写药品 ID 序列号（Identifying number）。处方者如果对续配处方指令进行修改，包括说明和药品剂量，应该重新开处新处方。对同一患者开具新处方，往往意味原有药品续配指令的取消或者改变，药师应监护患者的用药情况，并及时与医师联系，确认和评估已有信息的效力和真实意思传达。另外，为尽可能预防处方欺诈问题的发生，医师应保存好空白处方，在处方打印时建议加水印及其他安全特征标记，如果条件允许应尽量选择直接传真或者电子传送到患者选定药房的方式，并尽可能加强与目标药房的沟通确认。传真处方时，应在处方中明确和确认传真接收方，处方原件在传真之后即失效（invalidated）并安全归档，不能被再次传送到其他药房（处方传真件样式见附件 3）。原则上医师不允许在非长期用药处方和已经续配完成或过期的长期用药处方上，添加（added）新的续配指令和授权。对没有续配授权和指令的处方，建议医师在处方上注明"NR"字样，避免续配指令被修改和添加。还有，处方转移（transfer）时，要求两个药房应通过传真或电话进行充分沟通。接收药房应掌握转移处方的必要信息（包括原药房的名字和地址，办理转移的药师名字，剩余可续配的次数和间隔时间，处方开具日期和最近一次的续配日期）。处方转移出去的药房，必须在电脑系统中确认已转出去的处方处于"失效（INACTIVE）"状态，避免重复调配和转移，并应当记录转移处方日期，接收药房名称、地址，接收处方的药师名字，办理转移事项的药师名字和协助办理的药学技术员的名字[8]。

三、"不能续配"政策限制和患者选择权的保障

在长期用药处方实施过程中，出现一些医师不加区分对所有患者和药品都规定"不能续配（no refill）"。为此，加拿大各省医师管理学院专门出台相关规定，禁止医师这种不负责任的行为。学会认为这与以患者为中心的价值理念不符，也没有临床支持。如果发生这种情况，医师管理学院建议医师和药师进行沟通讨论，从最大可能保障患者利益的角度来判断和决定处方续配的必要性和合理性[9,10]。同样，医师也不能在所有处方上都注明不能替换（no substitution）、不能修改（no adapt），不能延长（no extend）等标志。另外，加拿大医师执业标准还特别强调保障患者调剂药品的自主选择权。在符合医疗保障政策的条件下，患者可以自由选择符合条件的药房来调剂药品。如果是电子处方，患者也可以选择通过电子处方传递系统来传递处方，也可以要求医师打印出来，自己凭处方选择中意药房、药师进行调剂。除了法定不能续配和不能转移的处方，患者可以自主选择对没有完成续配的长期用药处方转移到其他符合条件的药师进行续配。

四、长期用药处方续配遗忘和应急药品的可获得性

慢性病长期用药处方在执行过程中，相对最容易发生的问题是续配的遗忘或延误。另外，有效长期用药处方输入电脑时，可能会因为电脑系统问题或者网络问题，显示处方医师没有得到授权（Prescriber is not authorized）或者未查询到处方医师信息（Prescriber not found）等特殊问题。这两种情况可能会涉及长期用药处方紧急续配的问题。基本上每个承接长期用药处方的药房都会提供续配提醒业务，各药师管理学会都会建议患者尽可能保持相对固定的药房和药师来办理长期用药处方业务，掌握各种申请续配药品和取药的路径和方法，避免药品短缺影响治疗效果。同时，对以上两种情况，在患者不能及时获得医师处方或授权的情况下，允许药师利用其自身专业能力对患者进行评估，判断是否提供应急药品，包括长期用药处方应急续配（Emergency prescription refills）或适当延长处方（Renew or extend prescriptions）。药师在开

展长期用药处方紧急续配业务时，应坚持以下几个原则：①药师应有优秀的专业能力和专业判断；②有足够信息确认患者实际需要，并且不会增加患者医疗风险；③应根据患者病情和以往处方给予合适量的药品；④必须保证患者或者代理人的知情同意；⑤用药师注册码登录 Pharma Care 或 PharmNet 取得学会授权并准确记录过程[11]。另外，对医师注册情况改变的长期用药处方，在大多数情况下，这种长期用药处方应该被认为无效（invalid），但是药师可以根据患者评估情况和保障患者利益最大化角度，决定是否应急续配处方[12]。

第五节　启示与借鉴

随着我国工业化、城镇化、人口老龄化进程不断加快，居民生活方式、生态环境、食品安全状况等对健康的影响逐步显现，慢性病发病、患病和死亡人数不断增多，群众慢性病疾病负担日益沉重，现有确诊患者 2.6 亿人，是严重威胁我国居民健康的一类疾病，已成为影响国家经济社会发展的重大公共卫生问题[13]。如何更好地为慢性病患者服务、方便患者治疗、提高患者生活质量是一项重要课题。加拿大慢性病长期用药处方项目的制度安排和运行机制有很多成功经验，可供我国借鉴和启示。

一、逐步建立符合我国国情的慢性病长期用药处方制度安排

加拿大的慢性病长期用药处方项目，在加拿大已经运行几十年，在平衡药品可获得性和用药安全性以及加强医药合作等方面取得了很好的社会效果。按照我国现行处方管理办法，慢性病患者每次购买药品需要开具新的处方，同时处方量和处方效期较短。心脑血管疾病、糖尿病、恶性肿瘤、慢性呼吸系统疾病等慢性病患者，欲获取连续治疗药品，需要反复多次前往医疗机构"就诊"，造成了医疗资源的浪费，加剧了"看病难"问题。另外，在实践中，因为受制于医保报销政策规定，一些地方出现慢性病患者必须到医疗机构就诊或住院治疗后，其使用的药品才能得到报销的现象，进一步加剧医疗资源和医保资金的浪费。慢性病病情相对稳定，很多疾病的用药过程，可以采取

长程的长期用药处方方式得以更好解决。建议借鉴加拿大慢性病长期用药处方制度安排，修改我国处方管理办法，对于病情稳定的慢性病患者，延长处方期限，允许医师根据专业判断，开具长期用药处方，同时完善配套管理制度和质量管理标准体系。

二、发挥医院药房和社会药房在慢性病防控网络中的重要社会功能

在加拿大的医药卫生体制中，社会药房占有重要的地位。医药卫生体制安排采取严格的医药分开制度。医院药房只对住院患者免费提供所需药品，医院药房不从事药品经营，也没有创收的任务。患者凭医生开具的处方可以到任意社区药房调配药品，非处方药更可以直接购买。社区药房调剂处方，根据法规规定收取药事服务费（政府确定定价原则，药房根据政府法规要求和市场竞争情况自主确定），药事服务费和药费由患者自付，或者由患者购买的私人商业医疗保险支付。贫困人群、丧失劳动能力的弱势群体以及65岁以上的老人在门诊购药有政府补贴。一旦患者需要入院治疗，则包括住院药费在内的一切费用均由政府医疗保障计划负担[14]。慢性病长期用药处方项目得以健康运行，主要是有医药卫生体制和相关法律法规作支持和保障。我国新医改，特别重视药品供应保障体系的建设，重视慢性病预防控制策略和工作网络建设。

对比加拿大的制度安排，我国慢性病防治只重视各级疾病预防控制机构和公立医院的功能，忽略医院药房和社会药房在慢性病防控网络中的社会服务功能，需要进一步优化工作格局。应积极发挥医院药房和社会药房资源优势，鼓励和支持社会药房开展慢性病管理、药学服务和健康教育等工作，优化资源配置，健全网络，加强慢性病防治有效协同。应赋予社会药房更多慢性病管理职责，减少患者到医疗机构复诊次数，鼓励药师开展药物治疗审核（Medication therapy reviews, MTRs）[15]、加强药物治疗管理，改善就医用药模式，充分利用医疗卫生资源，方便患者逐步获得更便捷、有效的医药卫生服务。

三、重视多学科合作，注重药师作用发挥和执业权利保障

在加拿大医药卫生服务制度安排中，尤其是慢性病防控工作中，不断聚焦多学科合作的制度设计，在发挥执业医师提供医疗卫生服务核心能力之外，不断重视医师和药师的专业合作，发挥药师的价值和作用，拓展药师社会功能和职责。从 2006 年起，加拿大各省都扩大了药师的处方权，允许药师利用其专业，依据最大化保障患者健康权益的原则，提供更多处方相关服务（Prescription related services），如长期用药处方应急续配、处方更新和延长、以及特殊情况开具新处方（Initiate new prescriptions for specified conditions）等服务[16]。鼓励药师利用自身专业开展药物治疗管理，对患者进行用药评估，参与治疗方案制定，提高患者治疗依从性和用药合理性。

在加拿大的处方标准中，明确提到医师与药师的良好关系是改善患者治疗效果的最主要因素，特别是慢性病的连续服务过程；医师和药师是专业相互补充、支持、合作的伙伴关系；医师更多关注治疗进展和治疗目标，药师更多关注药物疗效、相互作用和治疗依从性，双方需要相互信任、尊重和良好沟通，从而增强治疗效果，实现患者利益最大化[17]。

我国卫生管理中"重医轻药"问题至今没有得到很好改善。药师的社会价值并未得到充分体现。在加快建立慢性病综合防控工作机制和提供全人群生命全周期的慢性病防治管理服务的国家慢性病综合防治工作中[15]，亟需进一步发挥药师加强药品质量管理、提供合理用药指导等作用。在医药卫生管理政策中，尽快落实药师权利和责任，支持药师开展更多处方相关服务、临床用药指导、规范用药等工作。医院药师和社会药房药师应积极参与预防保健和慢性病用药疗效管理、健康教育等更有前瞻性的工作中，借以不断提升药师在公众心目中的认知度和专业形象。

（徐敢）

参考文献

［1］Alberta College of Pharmacists, College and Association of Registered Nurses of Alberta, College of Physicians and Surgeons of Alberta. Ensuring Safe & Efficient Communication of Medication Prescriptionsin Community and Ambulatory Settings［EB/OL］.https://pharmacists. ab.ca/sites/default/files/CommunicationOfMedicationPrescriptions.pdf.

［2］Alberta Pharmaceutical Association, College of Physicians and Surgeons of Alberta. Terms and Conditions for Filling Prescriptions for Ambulatory Patients［EB/OL］. http://www.cpsa. ca/physician-prescribing-practices/

［3］College of Pharmacists of BC. Pharmacy Software Vendors［EB/OL］.http://library. bcpharmacists.org/6_Resources/6-5_Pharmacy_Resources/5068-Hospital_Pharmacy_Software.pdf.

［4］CPSA.Standards of Practice［EB/OL］.http://www.cpsa.ca/standardspractice/prescribing/ March 10, 2016.

［5］Ontarion College of Pharmacist. Prescription regulation summary chart［EB/OL］. http:// www.ocpinfo.com/practice-education/practice-tools/fact-sheets/part-fills/.

［6］College of Pharmacists of BC. Prescription Regulations［EB/OL］.http://library. bcpharmacists.org/6_Resources/6-4_Drug_Distribution/5014-Prescription_Regulation_Table.pdf.

［7］CPSA. Physician Prescribing Practices［EB/OL］. http://www.cpsa.ca/standardspractice/ prescribing/.

［8］Saskatchewan college of pharmacy.pharmacy professionals(SCPP)Regulatory Bylaw［EB/ OL］. http://saskpharm.ca/site/legislationauth?nav=07.

［9］The College of Physicians and Surgeons of Ontario. Prescribing Drugs［EB/OL］. http:// www.cpso.on.ca/policies-publications/policy/prescribing-drugs.

［10］A joint letter from the OCP, CPSO, OPA, and OMA, ADVISORY NOTICE-- Pharmacists Renewing and/or Adapting Prescriptions［EB/OL］. http://www.cpso.on.ca/CPSO/ media/uploadedfiles/policies/policies/Advisory_Notice_Renewing_Adapting_Prescriptions.pdf.

［11］College of Pharmacists of BC. Policy category:profession practice-31 Policy focus:

Emergency Prescription Refills［EB/OL］. http://library.bcpharmacists.org/6_Resources/6-2_PPP/5003-PGP-PPP.pdf.

［12］Ontarion College of Pharmacist. Physician Prescribing Status［EB/OL］.http://www.ocpinfo.com/practice-education/practice-tools/fact-sheets/physician-status/.

［13］国务院办公厅. 国务院办公厅关于印发中国防治慢性病中长期规划（2017—2025年）的通知［EB/OL］. http://www.gov.cn/zhengce/content/2017-02/14/content_5167886.htm.

［14］商务部. 加拿大医药卫生体制及药品流通情况［EB/OL］. http://www.mofcom.gov.cn/article/i/dxfw/nbgz/201602/20160201262184.shtml.

［15］Canadian PharmacistsAssociation. Medication Therapy Reviews［EB/OL］. http://www.pharmacists.ca/advocacy/advocacy-government-relations-initiatives/value-for-services/medication-therapy-reviews/.

［16］College of Pharmacists of BC. Certified Pharmacist Prescriber Draft Framework［EB/OL］. http://library.bcpharmacists.org/5_Programs/5-5_CPP/5180-Certified_Pharmacist_Prescriber_Framework_Draft.pdf.

［17］Model Standards of Practice for Canadian Pharmacists［EB/OL］. http://napra.ca/Content_Files/Files/Model_Standards_of_Prac_for_Cdn_Pharm_March09_Final_b.pdf.

附件1 加拿大长期用药处方管理相关法规和执业规范、指导原则目录

主要法律法规	The Health Professions Act The Pharmacy Operations and Drug Scheduling Act Food and Drugs Act and Regulations（Federal） Controlled Drug and Substances Act（Federal） Narcotic Control Regulations Regulated Health Professions Act Drug and Pharmacies Regulation Act Drug Interchangeability and Dispensing Fee Act Personal Health Information Protection Act Benzodiazepines and Other Targeted Substances Regulations The Bylaws of the College of Pharmacists madepursuant to these Acts
主要执业规范和指导原则	NAPRA, Model Standards of Practice for Canadian Pharmacists Ontario College of Pharmacists. Standards of Practice Alberta College of Pharmacists. Standards of Practice-The Pharmacist Alberta College of Pharmacists.Health Professions Act, Standards of Pharmacist Practice College of Pharmacists of British Columbia. Code of Ethics - Detailed College of Pharmacists of British Columbia. BC Pharmacy Practice Manual College of Pharmacists of British Columbia. Framework of Professional Practice College of Pharmacists of BC. Community Pharmacy Standards of Practice, Health Professions Act – BYLAWS College of Physicians and Surgeons of Ontario.CPSO Policy—Prescribing Drugs The Royal College of Physicians and Surgeons of Canada. The CanMEDS 2005 Physician CompetencyFramework

注：为了方便查询，列英文原文，不做翻译。

附件 2　加拿大《卫生职业法实施细则》附件 F– 社区药房实践标准

卫生职业法实施细则

附件 F

第 1 部分　社区药房实践标准

目　录

1. 适用范围

本细则的规定适用于所有在社区药房提供药学服务的人员。

2.定义

社区药房：与《药房开业和药品分类法（the Pharmacy Operations and Drug Scheduling Act）》实施细则第1部分中的概念相同。

药物治疗问题：指与药物治疗目标无关的、药物潜在的或实际发生的不良反应。

诱导激励：指金钱、礼品、折扣、回扣、退款、客户忠诚度计划、优惠券、礼物或奖励等方式。

患者代理人：指受托代理患者执行某些决定或签字的人。

个人健康证号：BC省内每个人拥有的用于健康系统身份识别的终身号码。

处方复印件：调配处方的药房药师交给患者用于知晓处方内容信息的复印件。

处方转移：将长期用药处方的剩余药品续配，通过直接交流协商，从一个药房转移到患者选择的其他药房。

处方续配：经执业医生口头或书面授权，药师根据处方为患者再次调配一定数量的药品。

处方更新：依据法律25.92部分，由全职药师根据以前已配的处方进行额外的药物调配。

内科护理机构和家庭执业标准：指本细则第3部分确定的标准、限制和条件。

3.患者自由选择权

除本细则特别规定外，药师、雇主及主管不能和患者、患者代理人、执业医师、公司、合作机构、或其他任何个人、团体订立协议，用以限制患者对药房的选择。

4.社区药房技术员

（1）社区药房的药学技术员可以执行处方准备、调配和药品配制，包括

（a）接收并记录执业医师的口头处方；

（b）确认处方完整性和真实性；

（c）执行与其他药房的处方转移或接收；

（d）确认处方配制的准确性；

（e）对处方配制做最后核对；

（f）确认药品和患者在 PharmaNet 中的健康信息的准确。

（2）根据条款（1），社区药房技术员可以调配药品，但不可以进行

（a）药物使用适宜性确认；

（b）下列行为

（i）本细则 6（5），6（10），10（2），11（3），11（4），12，13（2），13（3）or 13（4）规定的行为；

（ii）本附则第 4 部分规定的行为；

（c）配制 HPA 实施细则附件 F 第 5 部分规定的药物。

（3）药房技术员必须认识和明确自己和患者或执业医生交流的级别。

5. 药房助手

如果注册者直接监督指导药房助手的操作过程，进行核查和控制，注册者可以将社区药房运行相关的技术职能委托药房助手执行，以确保社区药学服务的精确性和安全性。

6. 处方

（1）药师必须确认处方的真实性。

（2）从执业医生处接收的处方必须包含以下信息

（a）处方开具日期；

（b）患者姓名；

（c）药品名称、成分和规格（如有）；

（d）药物数量；

（e）剂量说明，包括频次、间隔时间或最大日用量；

（f）续配授权（如有），包括续配次数及间隔；

（g）书面处方须有执业医生的姓名及签名；

（3）下面（4）中"处方"，包括新处方、续配处方、更新或延期处方或药品预付（balance owning）。

（4）药品调剂时，处方必须包含以下附加信息

（a）患者的地址；

（b）执业医生在医师管理学院确定的ID号；

（c）处方号；

（d）处方调剂日期；

（e）生产厂商确定的药品识别号或药品的商品名；

（f）药品数量；

（g）药师的书面确认，包括：

（i）患者ID号确认；

（ii）患者过敏信息确认；

（iii）根据11（4）回顾和评估患者在PharmaNet数据库中存储的健康信息；

（iv）药物咨询执行情况；

（v）最终确认，包括药品预付时间；

（vi）识别和解释药物治疗问题（如有）。

（5）全职药师必须

（a）回顾和评估处方完整性，以及药品、剂量、给药途径和频次的适宜性；

（b）核查患者关于药物治疗问题、治疗成本和其他潜在问题等个人健康信息；

（c）询问患者的用药史和其他个人健康信息；

（d）适用s.25.92（2）规定时，咨询执业医生关于患者的药物治疗问题；

（e）对药物治疗问题采取适当措施。

（6）药师可以接受执业医生本人或其语音消息直接授权的口头处方。

（7）注册者必须对口头授权处方进行记录，并签名。

（8）药师不能调剂一张处方上含有多个患者用药信息的处方。

（9）对长期用药处方的续配授权

　　（a）药师可以

　　　　（i）在确信医师代理人经咨询医师并准确传达医生指示的情况下，接受医师代理人发送的 I 类管制药物的续配授权；

　　　　（ii）如果软件系统可以保留先前每次配药量的记录，在改变配药量的情况下，可以保留当前处方号；

　　　　（iii）对授权的长期用药处方原件归档，如果

　　　　　　（A）电子化交易日志有保留；

　　　　　　（B）分配了新的处方号。

　　（b）药师必须

　　　　（i）如果患者出具一张新处方申请调配，必须取消原长期用药处方中未使用药品的续配授权；

　　　　（ii）如果该未使用的续配授权在另一个药房，则必须告知其他药房；

　　　　（iii）如果药品续配授权包含有，经医师指示使用的与原处方有不同的药物 ID 号的情形，必须创建新的处方号。

（10）如果全职药师授权处方更新

　　（a）必须创建一份手写记录；

　　（b）必须分配一个新的处方号；

　　（c）必须在 PharmaNet 的处方者栏中填写在学院认证的 ID 号。

7. 处方传真传送

（1）在以下情况下，处方授权可以通过传真传送给药房

　　（a）处方只发送给患者选定的药房；

　　（b）传真设备放置在可以保护处方信息和隐私的安全区域；

　　（c）除 6（2）的要求外，处方还应包括

（ⅰ）医生的电话号码、传真号和唯一识别码（如有）；

（ⅱ）传真发送时间和日期；

（ⅲ）欲接受传真的药房名称和传真号码。

（2）药房可以通过传真向执业医师发送长期用药处方授权申请，如果药房通过传真发送续配授权申请，请求表应包含以下信息

（a）6（2）规定的信息；

（b）药房的名称、地址和10位数电话号码；

（c）执业医师姓名、医师给药房发出传真的日期和时间。

（3）药师不得调配有列入管控处方药品目录中药品的处方。

（4）处方可以通过传真传送

（a）发送传真者姓名和药房地址等符合8（4）要求；

（b）传输接收人已知，并记录在传真文档中。

8. 处方复印和传送

（1）在规定情况下，药师必须为患者、患者代理人或其他注册人员提供处方的复印件。

（2）处方复印件必须包含以下内容

（a）患者的姓名和地址；

（b）医师姓名；

（c）药品名称、规格、数量和使用方法；

（d）处方的初次和最近一次配药日期；

（e）社区药房的名称和地址；

（f）长期用药处方续配的剩余次数；

（g）提供复印件的签名；

（h）注明为复印件。

（3）经要求，药师必须将药品处方传送到在加拿大注册的药房

（a）如果该药物不含有管控药物成分；

（b）如果传输发生在已注册的药师与药师之间。

（4）在（3）的情况下，药房给其他药房传送处方时必须

　　（a）记录入患者信息

　　　　（i）传输日期

　　　　（ii）药师 ID 号

　　　　（iii）处方接收药房的 ID 号

　　　　（iv）处方接收者的 ID 号

　　（b）传送信息应含有所有列入（2）（a）到（f）的处方信息。

（5）药师必须确保处方可以用于回顾评估以及有复印件用于加拿大卫生当局授权的监察员督查。

9. 处方标签

（1）所有根据处方的调配或全职药师所做的药物调整（adaptation）必须有标签。

（2）所有处方药的标签必须包括

　　（a）药房的名称、地址和电话号码；

　　（b）处方号码和配药日期；

　　（c）患者的全名；

　　（d）医师的姓名；

　　（e）药品的数量和规格；

　　（f）医师的使用指示和说明；

　　（g）根据 GPP 要求的其他信息。

（3）对于单一品种药物，标签必须包含

　　（a）药品通用名；

　　（b）商品名、厂商名或药品识别 ID 号中的一个以上信息。

（4）对于多品种药物，标签必须包含

　　（a）商标名；

　　（b）所有有效成分和生产商或药品识别 ID 号中的一个以上信息。

（5）对于现场调配的制剂，标签必须标明所有有效成分。

（6）根据（2）要求，如果药品容器太小不能完整记录标签内容

　　（a）可在小容器上粘贴标签；

　　（b）粘贴标签必须包括：

　　　　（i）处方号；

　　　　（ii）配药日期；

　　　　（iii）患者全名；

　　　　（iv）药品名称。

　　（c）较大的包装容器上应该粘贴完整的处方标签，提示和要求患者将小包装容器放在大容器内。

（7）所有标签上的信息都应用英语记录，但指导用药的信息应该用患者习用语言。

10. 药品调配

（1）药房在配药时可以调整药品数量

　　（a）如果患者要求较小量；

　　（b）如果生厂商的单一药品规格与处方量不匹配；

　　（c）如果处方量超出了患者的用药计划量；

　　（d）如果推荐的使用剂量得到患者授权。

（2）全职药师可以调整药物数量

　　（a）如果咨询医师确认并记录咨询结果；

　　（b）如果患者记录显示依从性较差；

　　（c）如果怀疑药物误用；

　　（d）如果由于存在用药过量的风险，患者的安全无法保障。

（3）如果药师怀疑处方的真实性，可以拒绝配药。

（4）所有药物均必须配置在一个确保防止儿童误用（child-resistant）的包装容器中

　　（a）除非医师、患者或患者代理人明示不需要；

　　（b）除非根据药师判断，使用防止儿童误用容器不合理；

（c）除非药物的物理性状，或生产商的包装是为了增加患者的依从性而设计，因此不适宜防儿童误用包装；

（d）除非没有儿童保护包装；

（e）除非药品是为濒死的人开具的医学救助用的。

（5）除了口服避孕药可调配至2年之外，药师不能调剂自开具之日起超过一年的处方。

11. 患者记录

（1）应为每个使用Ⅰ类管制药品的患者建立患者记录。

（2）患者记录必须包括

（a）姓名（全名）；

（b）个人健康档案号；

（c）住所地址；

（d）电话号码（如有）；

（e）出生日期；

（f）性别；

（g）临床状况、过敏、药物不良反应和药品耐受情况（如有），包括信息来源和收集信息的日期；

（h）药物调配日期；

（i）处方编号；

（j）药物通用名、剂量及剂型；

（k）药物编码（ID号）；

（l）药物调剂数量；

（m）药物治疗持续时间（指定天数）；

（n）停药日期及原因；

（o）用药说明与指示；

（p）处方医生的ID号；

（q）处方者特殊指令（如有）；

（r）过去及现在的药物治疗情况，包括药名、剂量、剂型、频次、疗程及疗效；

（s）药物治疗问题的识别及所采取措施的描述；

（t）药物治疗依从性情况的描述；

（u）Ⅱ 和 Ⅲ类管制药物使用情况（如有）。

（3）如果药师知晓患者用药历史情况，必须采用适当方式在药历中记录下列信息

（a）医疗和健康状况及身体受限情况；

（b）过去及现在的药物治疗情况，包括药名、剂量、剂型、频次、疗程及疗效；

（c）药物治疗依从性；

（d）Ⅱ 和 Ⅲ类管制药物使用情况。

（4）药师在药品调剂之前首先应回顾和评估储存在 PharmaNet 数据库上的患者个人健康信息，并对药品和药物治疗问题采取必要和适当的措施和行动。

12. 药师 / 患者咨询服务

（1）除第（2）款另有规定外，药师在调配新处方或者续配长期用药处方时，应对患者或其代理人进行询问和提供咨询服务，包括患者亲自上门或者通过电话申请等情形。

（2）如果患者拒绝咨询，药师必须将提供咨询和被拒绝情况记录入档。

（3）药师必须以尊重患者隐私权的方式进行咨询。

（4）新处方调剂的药师 / 患者咨询服务应包括

（a）确认患者身份；

（b）药名及剂量；

（c）药物用途；

（d）药物使用说明，包括用药频次、给药途径和持续时间；

（e）潜在的药物治疗问题，包括避免措施，发生问题后的对策

建议；

（f）贮存要求；

（g）长期用药处方续配信息；

（h）其他相关信息；

（i）如何监测药物治疗反应；

（ii）预期治疗结果；

（iii）药物漏服时应采取的行动；

（iv）什么时候再次就医的提示说明；

（v）提示药师需要关注的特定药物或特殊患者。

（5）长期用药处方调剂时药师/患者咨询服务应包括

（a）确认患者身份；

（b）药名及剂量；

（c）药物用途；

（d）药物使用说明，包括用药频次、持续时间；

（e）患者是否发生或经历过药物治疗问题。

（6）药师在调剂新处方或者长期用药处方、提供患者咨询服务时，如果发现药物治疗问题，必须采取适当的措施和行动。

（7）如果发现和识别到药物不良反应（加拿大卫生部界定），药师必须通知患者主管医师的同时，登录 PharmaNet 做正确记录，并向加拿大卫生部门报告药物不良反应。

13. Ⅱ和Ⅲ类管制的药物

（1）在没有得到处方者授权的情况下，注册者不能把开具 Schedule Ⅱ和Ⅲ药物的新处方或长期用药处方归在处方医生名下。

（2）药师必须为正在购买Ⅱ类管制药物的患者或其代理人提供药物选择和使用相关的咨询服务。

（3）药师/患者对Ⅱ类管制药物的用药咨询服务必须包括潜在的药物治疗问题，包括预防措施和发生问题的应对措施。

（4）药师必须为选择和使用Ⅲ类管制药品的患者或其代理人提供用药咨询机会。

14. 独立药房服务提供者

具体以下条件，药房经理可以与在其药房内工作的他人订立合同并成为独立药房服务提供者

（a）药房服务提供符合内科护理机构和家庭执业标准；

（b）监测患者治疗结果，增强患者用药安全；

（c）有为安全有效调配、监测和管制药品制定具体制度。

15. 禁止提供诱导激励

（1）药师不能为诱导患者或代理人以下列目的开展提供或调配

（a）传送处方到指定药师或者药房执行指定药品或者器械的调配；

（b）获得其他特定注册者或药房的药学服务。

（2）第（1）规定不适用于以下项目

（a）向患者或代理人提供免费或折扣泊车；

（b）为患者或代理人提供免费或折扣的递送服务；

（c）接受带有奖励性质的信用卡或借记卡用于支付药物或器械的款项。

（3）第（1）项不适用于Ⅲ类管制药品或其他未分类药品，除非已由医生开具处方。

（徐敢　译）

附件 3 加拿大阿尔伯塔省药学会 阿尔伯塔省内外科医师学会长期用药处方传真件标准式样

处方笺头

处方者姓名 / 诊所名　　　　　　　处所地址

处方者电话号码　　　　　　　　　处方者传真号

保密传真传送到：

药房名：_____

传真号：_____ 日期：_____ 时间：_____

发送传真（打印）者姓名_____

发送传真者签名：_____

患者姓名：_____

患者地址：_____

RX #1

续配 _____ 次　每隔 _____ 天

RX #2

续配 _____ 次　每隔 _____ 天

医师认证与授权

◎本处方为处方原件。

◎本处方所示药房为本处方唯一接收方。

◎本处方原件在传真之后即失效（invalidated）并被安全归档，不能被再次传送到其他药房。

执业医师 / 处方者姓名（打印）：_____ 注册号：_____

执业医师 / 处方者签名：_____ Date：_____

（徐敢　译）

第五章 日本慢性病长期用药处方项目的研究与借鉴

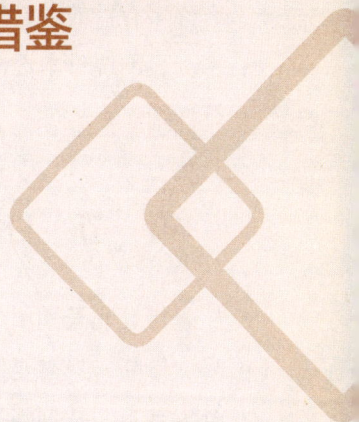

慢性病患者是广泛存在的一个群体，该类患者需要经常就医、长期治疗，复查病情变化，随访观察治疗效果，但其需要的治疗药物种类与剂量相对固定。部分慢性病患者常常会因为多种原因无法频繁到医院就诊、取药，从而影响其药物治疗效果。长期用药处方在一定程度上可以解决这类问题。日本长期用药处方仍处于早期研究和实践阶段[1-3]，并没正式全面实施，仅是在部分社区药局进行试点施行，但日本在围绕有效解决慢性病患者长期用药过程进行的探索，有许多有益的经验借鉴。本章将根据所了解到的日本长期用药处方项目的试行情况，围绕日本慢性病长期用药处方项目在日本的起源、发展与试行等内容展开详细介绍。

第一节　日本慢性病长期用药处方项目的起源与发展

慢性病长期用药处方，一般是指患者不再需要反复去医院寻找医师进行挂号、诊断，只需要使用可重复取药的处方单在药剂师指导下在药房重复取药的处方项目，药剂师需定期观察患者病情症状的变化进而判断处方是否需要进行更改[4]。该处方适合病情稳定的慢性非传染病患者便捷地获取药物、维持长期药物治疗，使医师门诊效率提高，主要接待病情变化、真正需要就诊的患者。

日本从 1974 年实施医药分家改革的同时，也在探索慢性病长期用药处方项目。从最初为解决部分药品处方期限上限问题而提出的早期分次调配处方项目（日文为"分割调剂"），发展到现在处于试行阶段的长期用药处方项目（日文为"リフィル処方せん"），均是为有效解决慢性病患者长期用药过程中的就诊、取药等繁琐手续而探索实施的，并在此过程中不断改进项目的可行性与便利性。

分次调配处方项目[2]于 2002 年开始实施，主要涉及部分药品给药日期上限的废除。相较于常规处方而言，医师开具的药物中包含较多患者自身长期保存比较困难的药品（如低温冷藏）。该处方项目的施行对患者而言，可以将药品的数量分成几次去药房领取。这样把药品总数量分成几次发给患者，可以有效避免患者一次承担过高的医疗费用，也保证了药品可以在药店规定条件下进行有效保存。因此，分次调配处方项目的引入使长期服用同一种药物的慢性病高龄患者，可以根据处方记载时间而实现长期给药的可能。从 2008 年开始，为了应对患者的需求，日本将分次取药的对象进一步扩大，具有医疗保险结算资格的药店将"通常试点药品"开始实行数日分次调配的方式（例如，90 天的处方，分成 3 次，每次取药分为 30 天的处方疗程分发到患者手中）。分次调配处方项目在服务项目中，仅限于分次调配处方的药品保管、用药指导、药品可能的副作用发现后恐惧心理的安慰以及用药合理性解释等方面，并没有药剂师介入的定期病情与用药情况的诊断与评估；同时，分次调配处方的操作和计算药品数量等过程均比较繁琐，大部分药店实施该项目的激励有限。因此，该处方项目在试行不久后就停止了。

　　随着日本慢性病老年患者急剧增多，借鉴国际引入并建立长期用药处方项目日益迫切。2010 年，日本厚生劳动省在"关于协同医疗推进研讨会"上[3]，对长期用药处方项目今后的发展展开了深入的课题讨论，对该项目的利弊与施行过程中可能遇到的问题等进行探讨。2010 年 12 月日本医学协会针对"慢性病处方有效期延长"问题展开了问卷调查[5]，统计结果显示超过 80% 的医师认为高血压、高血脂、骨质疏松、糖尿病等疾病的处方用药时间可以延长，大部分药物可以将使用期限设定在 5 周以上（52.9%）。2014 年 4 月 25 日，在日本政府举办的"经济财政咨询会议"上[6]，扩大药剂师业务的议题再次被提上议程，会议针对长期用药处方的导入与推广内容展开了深入讨论。此次会议给出了长期用药处方项目的定义，即医师开完处方后，患者被允许去药房反复取药的一种处方记录。允许的情况下，取药次数和日期都会记载。长期用药处方项目在实施的过程中，患者无明显病情变化，可以在同一个药房进行多次取药而无需反复去医院进行挂号开具处方。

　　目前，处方有效时间的延长通过了日本法律的认可，但由于日本医师协会考虑患者复诊费用减少会引起医疗机构经济受损，对长期用药处方项目并不完全支持，另外，医疗卫生人士对长期用药处方争议还较大[7, 8]，因此长期用药处方项目在日本目前并没正式全面实施，仅是在部分社区药局进行试点施行，患者开具的长期用药处方也限于定向医院的指定病种（如糖尿病、高血压），关于长期用药处方项目的开具时间、病种、医师资格、定向社区药房等相关实行细则目前也是在不断地摸索过程中[9, 10]。

第二节 日本慢性病长期用药处方项目的取药流程

一、慢性病长期用药处方的开具

慢性病长期用药处方项目的特点在于重复调配，即药剂师根据长期用药处方进行多次调配，使得患者在既定时间段内获得持续治疗的药品而无需再找医师就诊。长期用药处方约定了处方者的医疗责任及患者的知晓、依从责任，约定了医师与患者的合作关系，改变了传统医疗模式，需要医药人员、管理人员、患者及药房接待的协作配合。

长期用药处方包括患者的所有基本信息，即患者姓名、年龄、出生日期、住址，以及处方者信息、签名和日期，处方者必须注明长期用药处方的可重配次数、限制。原始长期用药处方上有医师的签字，它既是法定处方，也是社区药店履行处方重配的基础和必要条件。

二、慢性病长期用药处方的调配与取药

药房药剂师在收到长期用药处方后，应核对患者个人信息、疾病情况和用药情况，按照该处方约定的药品品种、用量和疗程及间隔，给患者调配和发放药品，收取当次的处方调配费，建立长期用药处方登记卡，登记本次重配的药品种类、剂量、疗程、日期、已重配次数，经药剂师签字。药剂师的服务是为了保证患者可安全有效地持续使用药品且不发生用药方面的问题，如果患者病情有任何变化，药剂师会建议患者咨询处方者[6, 11]。患者在指定药房取药，重配期间不得变更药房。当所有重配次数用尽或尚未全部取药但处方已过期，药房会把原始长期用药处方交还给患者。

长期用药处方项目对药剂师要求：药剂师需定期对患者的药物治疗过程进行观察与评估、监测药物的不良反应等，以对患者用药进行评估与药品调剂；如需更换药品或更改剂量时，应停止现有的长期用药处方并到医院就诊

进行病情重新诊断与处方开具。

长期用药处方项目取药流程如下图 5-1 所示：

长期用药处方的前提就是通过药剂师的持续观察，委托药剂师对药物治疗的监测，即长期用药处方为授权药剂师定期对药物治疗过程进行观察和副作用监测

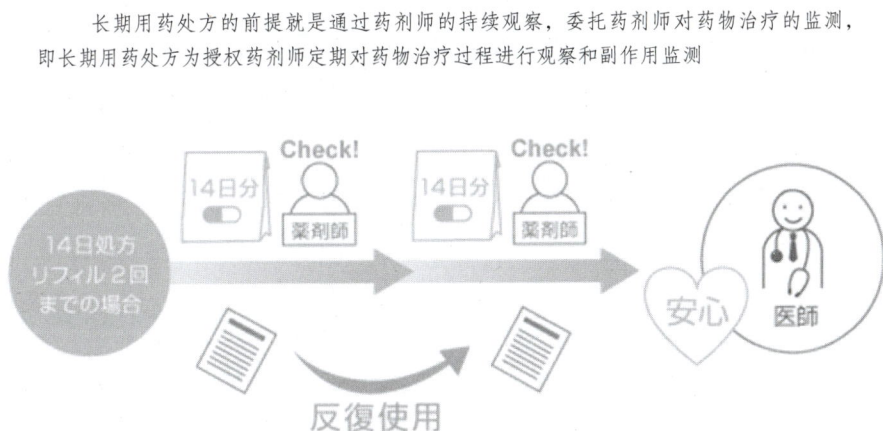

图 5-1　长期用药处方项目的取药流程[12]

1. 长期用药处方项目的取药前提

长期用药处方项目的取药前提为需通过药剂师的持续观察、并对药物治疗进行监测。在接到长期用药处方，将药品调配给患者前，药剂师需对患者的身体状态进行评估。通过对患者身体状态诊断与评估，把握患者症状与病情的发展情况，了解药物治疗与可能副作用的情况，进行继续使用该处方的评估，如果发现异常情况，则患者可能需要重新到医院就诊与处方开具。在 2010 年 3 月日本厚生劳动省展开的"协同医疗推进研讨会"上，包含药剂师在内的医疗业务扩大化议案被提上议程，该会议的报告书中关于药剂师的业务范围为"包含家庭护理，以患者为中心的药学管理（副作用状态评估、用药指导等）；针对门诊患者的知情权，参与接入式药学管理都做出了明确记载"。根据日本厚生劳动省展开的"协同医疗推进研讨会"内容，药剂师进行身体状态的诊断与评估并不属于医疗行为，但这属于"为了对患者提供必要的信息而进行比较的药物治疗管理"中重要的一个环节。

2. 根据长期用药处方的使用时间间隔进行用药情况评估，给予调配药品

药剂师根据医师给予的长期用药处方使用时长，在长期用药处方使用期

间内对患者药物治疗情况进行监测与评估，并给与药品调配。

在进行用药情况评估时，药剂师需要依据患者很多主观及客观指标。比如，药剂师需要对患者进行血压测量以确定降压类药物的疗效或是防止其他药物引起血压的变动。药剂师直接对患者进行测量的行为，是药剂师针对患者进行必要的信息采集和提供药事管理中的重要一个环节，不属于医疗行为，属于药事管理行为。

针对长期用药处方项目中药剂师接触患者进行评估的药剂师管理行为介绍如图 5-2 所示：

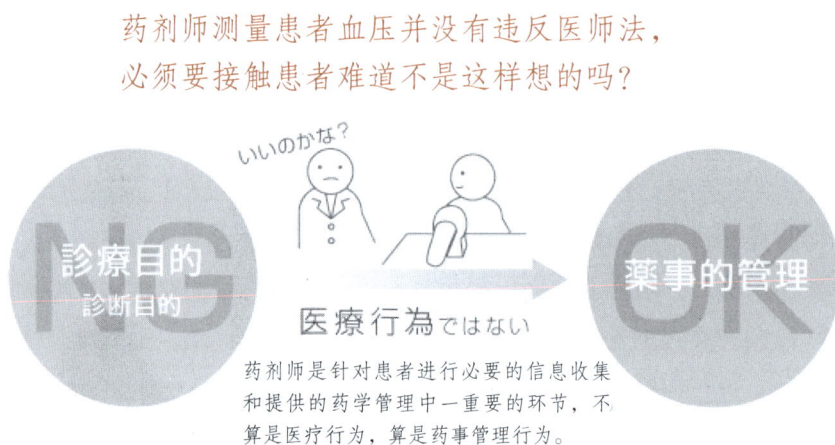

图 5-2　药剂师接触患者的药事管理行为图示[13]

3. 长期用药处方有效期满或病情出现变化，及时找医师进行病情诊断与处方确认

在长期用药处方到达有效期或者患者病情出现较大变化时，需停止使用目前的长期用药处方，及时要求患者到医院就医，进行病情重新诊断与评估，并开具新的处方。

长期用药处方项目立足于药店位置便利、取药流程快捷，加上药剂师的评估与专业指导，可以使患者能够安心、信赖该处方形式，也增加了患者对于药剂师的依赖，是药剂师逐步得到重视。因而，药剂师应不断增强自身专业技能，真正成为药学知识的专业，为长期用药处方项目的长足发展贡献一份力量。

第三节　日本慢性病长期用药处方项目的评价

一、日本慢性病长期用药处方项目的优点与缺点

（一）日本长期用药处方项目的优点[14, 15]

1.提高效率

长期用药处方项目可以有效省去患者往返重复挂号的中间环节，节约就诊时间的同时也提高了患者看病与取药的效率。

2.节约成本

长期用药处方项目可以有效节约医疗费用，包括诊疗费、处方费等，为患者节约了医疗成本。

3.减轻负担

长期用药处方项目提高了医师工作效率，减轻工作负担。医师只需要对很有必要就诊的患者进行诊断咨询即可，提高了工作效率，也减轻了医师与医院的负担。

4.分工明确

长期用药处方项目突出了药剂师作为药物专家的角色，实现了药剂师职业价值。使医疗工作者分工明确，为患者合理诊疗做出各自的贡献。

5.药剂师地位提升

长期用药处方项目使患者对药剂师的依赖与重视度得到显著提升，提高了药剂师的社会地位。

（二）长期用药处方项目的缺点

1.易引起处方管理混乱

长期用药处方项目的推行可能会出现处方管理混乱。长期用药处方在药

房重复取药的方式增加了处方管理的难度，可能会因此导致处方管理混乱。因此，长期用药处方项目需进行严格及特殊途径的管理方式。

2. 药品转售

长期用药处方项目的推行使患者可以在无医师再次判别情况下，在药剂师指导下进行重复取药，因而可能会出现药剂师转售药品的情况。长期用药处方的重复取药，药剂师是主要负责人群，因而要避免药剂师利用职能之便进行药品转售的情况，相关政策与规定需要进行细化。

3. 药剂师目前水平有待提升

长期用药处方项目的制定，将赋予药剂师较大重担与责任。目前药剂师水平与能力参差不齐，容易导致处方审核错误或病情判断不准等情况，因此，药剂师需提升自身专业水平，以适应处方的改革。

二、日本慢性病长期用药处方项目对利益相关方的影响

长期用药处方项目的试行，对于需要经常就诊、长期治疗的患者提供便利之外，对于医疗机构、患者监护人、药剂师及社区药房都有一定的影响。

（一）长期用药处方项目对于医务人员的影响

日本长期用药处方项目虽未全面开展，但其对于医务人员的影响是可以预见的，主要有以下几点[14-16]：

1. 提高工作效率

长期用药处方项目提高了医师的工作效率，使其工作更有计划性，节约了时间成本。医师根据患者的病情诊断、用药种类及时间进行长期用药处方的确认与开具，并将患者的基本信息与相关的诊疗信息提交到电子病历系统中，患者在到社区药房进行药品的重配时，药剂师会再次核对患者的个人信息、疾病诊断及用药情况及疗程，按照该处方制定的药品品种、用药剂量及疗程给患者进行调配和发放药品，并建立该患者的长期用药处方登记卡，登记每次药品重配的种类、剂量、疗程和已经重配的次数。药剂师会在每次处方重配后将上述所记录的所有问题都提交到电子病历系统中，这样医师在患者复诊的时候也会看到相应的信息，这些信息对于患者的进一步诊疗有一定

的借鉴意义，也方便了医师更加了解每一位患者的病情及用药情况。

2. 减少医疗纠纷

长期用药处方项目使医务人员可以尽早明确诊断，降低患者病情加重的风险，减少可能的投诉和起诉，在不良事件发生时免受责难。

3. 提升医院服务

长期用药处方项目使患者对辅助工作人员的质疑更少，避免了挂号的拥挤，提高了医疗服务的声誉。

4. 减少医疗成本

长期用药处方项目可以适当和有效地发挥医务人员和辅助工作人员的时间和技能，提高了医务人员和辅助工作人员的工作效率，并减少了医疗成本。

5. 明确各自职责

长期用药处方项目使所涉及人员更加深入地了解长期用药处重配过程，包括各自的作用、职责和流程，在流程管理上责任明确化，每一位医务人员及药剂师都明确自身的责任与义务，更好地配合彼此，保证了整个长期用药处方项目的顺利开展。

6. 增进医疗合作

长期用药处方项目增进了医师与其他医护人员的合作和工作关系，如非医学方向的处方者、护士和社区药剂师。

（二）长期用药处方项目对于社区药房的影响

长期用药处方项目的开展使患有慢病的患者可以定期到社区药房进行药品调剂，避免了多次到医院就诊，充分将患者分流到社区药房，既减轻了医院医师、护士、药剂师的压力，也使社区药房多了较多患者，突出了社区药房的作用，促进了医院与社区药房的合作与交流，从而促进了整个社会医疗体系的进步。

慢性病患者在疾病恢复阶段，病情在短时间内并没有较大变化，只需要治疗药物的维持治疗，因此，对于该类患者而言，长期用药处方项目是一个便利取药的过程。因为在长期用药处方项目开展前，慢性病患者需要频繁到医院进行挂号、就诊、取药等一系列过程方能拿到治疗药物，而慢性病患者大多是中老年人，甚至有些不方便行走的患者，因此，频繁到医院就诊不仅有一定难度，而且程序复杂且医疗费用昂贵。所以，长期用药处方项目不仅解决了患者不便利取药的问题，还突出了社区药房及药剂师的地位和作用，实现了医疗资源的有效分流与重新分配。

（三）长期用药处方项目对于药剂师的影响

长期用药处方项目为药剂师发挥其专业知识和专业技能提供了重要机会，使他们帮助患者恰当地使用药物、减少浪费。研究表明，由药剂师进行用药审核既有利于发现用药相关问题，也分担了全科医师的工作负荷及时间。长期用药处方项目对于药剂师的影响主要如下几点[14-16]：

1. 长期用药处方项目关系到药剂师技能提升

长期用药处方项目是建立在药剂师持续的用药效果观察与评估的前提上，也就是说药剂师要负责治疗效果的监控。具体来说，药剂师需要定期询问患者"用药后效果如何？""有没有在用药过程中出现不适或者副作用？"等类似问题来观察治疗效果以逐步介入治疗。患者一次的取药量需要提前决定好，然后定期到药房接受回访，通过药剂师判断发现问题，之后再由医师介入治疗。

2013 年日本卫生部科学研究发布的"药房应该发挥的职能和应有的形象"报告中指出，药剂师的业务范围提升迫在眉睫，不仅仅是药剂师的调配技能，药物治疗的个体化差异、疗效和不良反应确认等方面的最新信息都包含在内。因此，通过长期用药处方项目的引入与推广，药剂师需要不断提升自己专业知识与技能。

2. 药剂师职能变化，通过分级医疗的道路逐渐稳步推进

长期用药处方项目使药剂师可以与开具处方的医师协作，来精准实施药物治疗。药物治疗个体差异化，从既往病史和合并用药，体重或者肝肾功能开始，基于代谢酶和蛋白转运等特性，到个体优化形式下的诊断和治疗很有必要，这也成为药剂师工作职能变化的一大方向。

长期用药处方项目实施后，药品分发给患者不再意味着药学服务的结束，药物治疗效果的观察与评估的过程和治疗结果的确认也变的非常重要。即药物疗效的确认，不良反应的检查，患者向医师或者药剂师反馈之后，药剂师

作为医疗团队中一员，共同为患者有效治疗做出贡献，也是真正意义上的药剂师价值体现。

（四）日本长期用药处方项目对于患者及监护人的影响

长期用药处方项目需要患者的了解、理解和配合，以便提高就诊效率，节省就诊时间，并且使患者得到有针对性的治疗。随访审核取药时，药剂师会了解和整理患者的用药情况，包括处方药与非处方药，书面记录随访结果和干预措施，便于医师快速阅读。因此，患者有义务告知自己的饮食习惯与生活方式、用药史与过敏史，按照药剂师的指导服药。使用长期用药处方的患者，取药时应咨询药剂师能否继续使用。长期用药处方项目对于患者及其监护人的影响主要如下[14-16]：

1. 长期用药处方项目的实施，减少了患者到医院就诊的频率，进而减少了相应的医疗开支和时间成本，使患者及其监护人获得所需药品更加便捷。

2. 长期用药处方项目使患者及其监护人易于理解和掌握处方重配流程，知道何时、如何提出处方重配申请，知道如何获得重配处方的药品等。

3. 长期用药处方项目使患者及其监护人对正在获取的最适宜、个体化、更优质的处方重配系统所提供的医疗服务，更有信心。

4. 长期用药处方项目使患者及其监护人得到了完整的处方和详尽的用药指导，可以准确地了解如何使用和管理药品。

5. 长期用药处方项目使患者及其监护人有机会与医疗专业人士讨论用药情况，了解治疗过程和重要性，更加注重自身身体健康管理。如有些患者对于药品的服用剂量、用药时间、联合用药以及进餐对于药品使用的影响等问题都可以在处方重配时详细咨询药剂师，并在药剂师指导下进行生活方式的调节与改变，以达到更好的自我健康管理。

6. 长期用药处方项目促使药剂师更关注患者用药后的个体反应，如疗效及不良反应的发生，降低患者及其监护人发生药品不良反应和不良事件的可能性，使药物治疗过程更加安全、有效。

7. 长期用药处方项目使患者及其监护人可参与自身健康护理的决策，有助于患者自我管理，还能提高其与医护人员的行动和意识一致性，从而提高治疗效果，减少患者住院次数，缩短其住院时间，减少就诊的次数。

8.在药剂师的指导与督促下，患者的用药依从性也会增加，因为药剂师在每次重配该类药物时，都会询问患者前一阶段的用药情况并进行用法用量等问题的确认，使患者牢记用药相关的问题，保证了用药依从性。

第四节　启示与借鉴

截至目前，日本虽未全面推行长期用药处方项目，但已经进行了初步摸索与具备了基本框架。考虑到患者利益与方便，长期用药处方项目作为一种以患者为中心且能广泛推广的项目得到了社会多方的肯定。日本作为亚洲国家，与中国有较多共同之处，而且其长期用药处方项目也属于刚起步阶段，其长期用药处方项目的流程及推行方式等，有许多值得我们学习与借鉴。

一、健全相关法律法规，加强处方管理，加快长期用药处方项目的推进

长期用药处方项目的推行必须要有相关的法律法规的颁布与执行。长期用药处方的开具与实施涉及多部门、多人员、多环节、长时间，因此难免会有疏漏，为了应对安全隐患需要采取有效防范措施，完善处方重配流程与各环节人员、技术配备，制定完善的法律法规明确各方的职责，保证处方重配安全可靠。比如，需要加强对于处方的管理。长期用药处方项目的实施，有别于以往的短程处方，因此有其自身长疗程可重复取药的特点，需要加强处方分类管理，尤其是长期用药处方的单独管理，避免与正常处方之间的混乱，加强识别度，也应制定防伪方案，避免不法人员仿造长期用药处方，进而造成药物滥用等社会问题。

法律法规也应明确医师、护士、药剂师、患者各自在长期用药处方项目中的义务与责任，既让每个参与该项目中的角色明白自身应该完成的内容与责任，也让各部门人员相互间进行监督，共同促进该项目的顺利进行。如，加强患者用药教育与监督，避免患者进行药品转售情况。

二、形成长期用药处方的药品目录，规范长期用药处方项目的实施

长期用药处方项目的实施需要明确的可以进行重配的药品目录，并非所有药物都可以被列入长期用药处方药品目录中。为了保证药物治疗的连续性和安全性，避免因生物利用度不同而影响疗效，长期用药处方需要严格制定长期用药处方的药品目录。如对于病情短、病情变化的疾病用药，属于不适合重配项目的药品，包括治疗急性感染的抗生素、食欲抑制药、减肥药（奥司他韦、利莫那班和西布曲明等）、尼古丁、安非他酮、治疗急性疼痛的镇痛药、利尿药、安眠药和镇静药、口服避孕药等。因此，在制定该项目的药品目录时要综合考虑多方面的因素，从患者合理安全用药角度出发，根据药物自身治疗特点及疗效和毒性进行遴选，目录的制定可以规范长期处方项目的实施。

三、电子化处方体系的建立，患者信息的及时、同步更新

成熟的格式化长期用药处方的在线申请、在线记录和在线审核，以及在不同社区药房和医院之间信息的及时同步，既提高了医务工作人员的工作效率，又保证了资料的准确性、患者的用药安全性。目前中国的医院电子病历系统也为联网，因此，在这方面也需加强电子处方的推进。电子处方不仅可以将医师开具的长期用药处方信息及时自动传输到患者指定的社区药店，方便了社区药剂师进行基本信息和疾病诊断、用药种类剂量和疗程的确认，还可以在患者每一次进行处方重配后，将药剂师记录的患者病情变化、用药疗效、可重配药品种类、剂量和疗程等信息自动在网上进行提交更新，以便系统自对核对患者的相关信息，达到双重确认，确保了患者的用药安全，也规范了长期用药处方项目的实施流程。

四、统一长期用药处方的取药流程与定点社区药房的选定

中国医院及药房均比较多，因此，长期用药处方项目实施时需要制定统一的取药流程与定点社区药房的选定。统一的取药流程可以保证长期用药处方项目在实施过程中保持其一致性，避免了不同医院、社区药房间的差异导

致患者取药遇到问题，或不法分子利用不同地区取药流程的差异而投机取巧谋取利益。同样，并非所有的社区药房都可以进行药品处方的重配，国家应制定相应的考核与评估体系，只有满足一定的资质与要求后方能成为医院定点的长期用药处方项目的社区药房。取药流程的统一和定点社区药房的评估与选定对于医院、药房均众多的中国国情而言是十分必要的，是保证长期用药处方顺利进行的先决条件。

五、对药剂师进行定期定向培训与考核

长期用药处方项目充分体现了对药剂师专业知识、技能和经验的信任与重托，给予了药剂师处方权、审核权和患者教育权，同时还要求药剂师要对患者病情变化、用药治疗情况做出准确的判断和评估，因此，药剂师在该项目中发挥重要作用。所以，对于药剂师要进行资格审查，只有满足一定专业知识储备、技能和经验的药剂师才能胜任长期用药处方的工作。对于这类药剂师也要进行定期的相关知识内容的培训和考核，不断鞭策药剂师们增强自身专业知识与技能，以满足患者复杂变化的病情与用药情况的评估与判定，实现患者用药的安全、有效、合理。药剂师工作的成败也决定了长期用药处方项目的长远发展。

长期用药处方项目充分体现了以患者为中心的理念，能够为患者提供快捷、方便、安全的药学服务。从日本试行的长期用药处方项目的发展历程、拟实施模式及操作流程可见，该项目充分进行了医疗资源的重新分配，改善了患者的就医模式，也满足了现代人快节奏简便的生活方式；这一项目也促进了药剂师与医师的交流，大大提高了药剂师的社会地位，也促进了药剂师自我专业技能的提高，充分利用了社区药房的资源，有效提高了医疗资源的利用率。目前中国人口众多、老龄化也越来越严重，长期用药处方项目的推行对于即将面临的医疗资源配置不均、药剂师作用尚未显现有重大意义，可以有效解决慢性长期用药患者定期取药问题，因此，日本的长期用药处方项目拟实行方案也值得我们学习与借鉴。

（张劭）

参考文献

［1］Walker K. Repeat prescription recording in general practice［J］. J R Coll Gen Pract，1971，21（113）：748-751.

［2］リフィル処方箋は、日本の薬剤処方のかたちを変えます.［EB/OL］. http://www.qlifepro.com/ishin/2015/07/29/prescription-refills-japan/，2015-5/ 2016-2.

［3］チーム医療の推進について（チーム医療の推進に関する検討会報告書）［EB/OL］. http://www.mhlw. go.jp/shingi/2010/03/dl/s0319-9a.pdf 厚生労働省，2010-3/2010-9.

［4］リフィル処方箋［EB/OL］. https://ja.wikipedia.org/wiki/ リフィル処方箋，2014-9/2017-1.

［5］慢性疾患で処方期間が長期［EB/OL］. http://www.self-medication.ne.jp/pro/2010/12/000694.php

［6］"［経済財政諮問会議］「リフィル処方箋」検討を - 薬剤師の業務範囲拡大も". 薬事日報 .［EB/OL］. http://www.yakuji.co.jp/entry35741.html，2014-4-25/ 2014-12-18.

［7］専門家 5 人に聞く – リフィル処方箋導入の是非［EB/OL］. https://pcareer. m3.com/plus/article/experts opinions on the introduction of prescription-refills/，2015-6/ 2016-10.

［8］リフィル処方箋の導入 – 中医協で検討へ医師委員からは「かかりつけ医の処方変更で対応すべき」との意見も［EB/OL］.http://medical.nikkeibp.co.jp/leaf/mem/pub/di/trend/201507/543150.html，2015-7/ 2016.12.

［9］^ "日医、リフィル処方せん反対明言薬剤師による体調確認想定に「議論する状態にない」". m3.com 医療維新［EB/OL］. https://www.m3.com/open/iryoIshin/article/342298/，2015-7-23/ 2015-7-24.

［10］"リフィル処方箋、否定的意見相次ぐ - 分割調剤を含め総会で議論". 薬＋読（やくよみ）（マイナビ）［EB/OL］. https://pharma.mynavi.jp/contents/yakuyomi/industry_news/ リフィル処方箋、否定的意見相次ぐ - 分割調剤 /，2015-7-24/ 2016-3-3.

［11］"「診療報酬の算定方法の一部改正に伴う実施上の留意事項について」別添 3「調剤報酬点数表に関する事項」（平成 24 年 3 月）（PDF）厚生労働省［EB/OL］. http://www.

mhlw.go.jp/topics/2008/03/dl/ tp 0305-1g.pdf，2008-3/ 2008-10.

［12］リフィル処方せん｜薬剤師さんのためのここがポイント医療政策.

［13］薬剤師のフィジカルアセスメント｜薬剤師さんのためのここがポイント医療政策.

［14］おさらいしよう、リフィル処方箋のメリット・デメリット［EB/OL］. https://pcareer.m3.com/plus/ /article /review for the advantages and disadvantages of refilling prescriptions/，2014-8/ 2016-12.

［15］リフィル処方箋のメリット［EB/OL］. http://for-guests.com/refill-prescription/，2015-5/ 2016-12.

［16］日本でも導入されるかもしれないリフィル処方せんとは？［EB/OL］. https://www.38-8931.com/message/2016/09/post-528.html，2016-7/ 2016-9-10.

附件 1 案例介绍

一、医院就诊

（一）案例基本信息

患者男，62 岁，于半年前诊断为"T2DM"（type 2 diabetes mellitus，T2DM，2 型糖尿病），予以生活方式干预和口服格列吡嗪（商品名：瑞易宁）5mg，2 次 / 日，二甲双胍 500mg，2 次 / 日治疗，但患者饮食控制不佳，FPG（fasting plasma glucose，FPG，空腹血糖）波动于 7~8mmol/L，2 小时 PG（plasma glucose，PG，血糖）波动于 10~13mmol/L。2016 年 11 月就诊于医院门诊，查随机血糖 12.6mmol/L。有高血压病史 3 年，血压最高达 160/100mmHg，未接受药物治疗。患者否认家族甲状腺 C 细胞恶性肿瘤及胰腺炎病史，否认高血压、糖尿病家族史。

（二）体格检查结果

体温 36.9℃，身高 170cm，体重 98 kg，血压 160/91mmHg，全身无色素沉着，双肺呼吸音清，心率 75 次 / 分钟，律齐，四肢浅感觉、振动觉和位置觉无减退，双膝反射正常；双侧足背动脉搏动正常。

（三）辅助检查结果

1. 门诊查随机血糖 12.6mmol/L；

2. 血清 ICA（islet cell antibody，ICA，胰岛素细胞抗体）、GAD-Ab（glutamic acid decarboxylase antibody，GAD-Ab，谷氨酸脱羧酶抗体）、IA-2A（protein tyrosine phosphatase antibody，IA-2A，蛋白酪氨酸磷酸酶抗体）及 IAA（insulin autoantibody，IAA，胰岛素自身抗体）均为阴性；

3. 肝肾功能正常，眼底检查正常。

（四）病情诊断结果

T2DM，肥胖症，高血压，混合型高脂血症

（五）治疗药物详单

1. 二甲双胍 500mg，2 次 / 日；

2. 格列吡嗪减量为 5mg，1 次 / 晚；

3.利拉鲁肽 0.6mg，每日晨起皮下注射；

医师叮嘱开始用药 1 周后利拉鲁肽剂量增至 1.2mg/d，2 周后增至 1.8mg/d，二甲双胍增至 500mg，每天 3 次，停用格列吡嗪。

患者要求对于需要长期治疗用药的种类开具长期用药处方，以免重复就诊开药。医师根据病情判断是否可以进行重复配置，并审核可以进行可重配的药物种类。最后开具长期用药处方单，并进行签字确认，并将长期用药处方录入电脑系统备档。

二、长期用药处方单确认

经医师确认，以下药物可进行重复调配，并开具了长期用药处方单：

1.二甲双胍 500mg，每天 3 次；

2.利拉鲁肽 0.6mg，每日晨起皮下注射；

该长期用药处方单用药处方时长为 3 个月，可分 2 次患者自行持长期用药处方单到社区药店取药。

三、长期用药处方单取药流程

（一）长期用药处方单的确认并取药

在医师开具的长期用药处方单后，患者与药剂师进行长期用药处方单的确认，并进行取药。本次取药既包含非长期用药处方的药物，也包括长期用药处方的药物。药剂师应对患者用药记录进行审核与记录，方便之后的用药随访与治疗情况跟踪。药剂师将已配置好的药品发给患者后并进行适当的用药交代。具体如下：

1.生活方式干预

该患者血糖控制不佳合并肥胖，首先应给予生活方式干预措施。

患者须调整不良生活习惯，包括饮食、锻炼（如步行，每天 30 分钟，每周 5 日）及减轻体重（减轻总体重的 5%~10%）。若无法达到理想体重也不用担心，减重 4.5~6.8kg 也可带来巨大改变。并叮嘱患者自行监控血糖、尿糖和体重情况。

2. 用法用量指导

（1）二甲双胍片：餐中或餐后即刻服用，一次 500mg，一日 2 次。

（2）格列吡嗪片：餐前服用，一次 5mg，每晚 1 次。

（3）利拉鲁肽：0.6mg，每日晨起皮下注射。1 周后利拉鲁肽剂量增至 1.2mg/日，2 周后增至 1.8mg/ 日。

3. 注意事项叮嘱

（1）加用利拉鲁肽用药 3 日后患者上腹部有饱胀感，伴轻度恶心、呕吐。但随着用药时间推移，患者胃肠道的不良反应开始减轻至消失，因此告知患者不必过于担心。

（2）利拉鲁肽需经皮下注射给药，注射部位可选择腹部、大腿或者上臂。在改变注射部位和时间时无需进行剂量调整。建议每次注射的点之间应相距1.0 cm，且尽量避免在一个月内重复使用一个注射点。该药品严禁肌肉注射或静脉注射。

（3）利拉鲁肽贮藏：冷藏于 2~8℃冰箱中（勿接近冰箱的冷冻室），不可冷冻。首次使用后，应在 30℃以下贮藏或冷藏在 2~8℃冰箱中，盖上笔帽避光保存。且告知患者每次注射后应丢弃注射针头，以避免污染、感染和渗漏，同时能确保给药准确。利拉鲁肽首次使用后的效期为 1 个月，贮藏笔芯时切勿带有针头。

（4）利拉鲁肽注射方式：利拉鲁肽为可调节剂量、一次性预填充注射笔由笔型注射器和装有 3ml 液体的笔芯组成。笔芯由 1 型玻璃制成，内有一个活塞（嗅丁基橡胶），并由一个橡胶塞（嗅丁基橡胶 / 聚异戊二烯橡胶）密封。每支笔含有 3ml 溶液，可以进行 30 次 0.6mg，15 次 1.2mg 或 10 次 1.8mg 注射。

（二）长期用药处方单第一次取药

患者凭医师签字的长期用药处方到药店进行取药，药剂师接受处方者和患者的授权，接受长期用药处方后，复核患者信息，治疗情况等，该患者复查相关糖尿病指标以确定患者病情变化。复查 FPG 6.0mmol/L，2 小时 PG 8.3mmol/L，体重 96.5kg。根据上述糖尿病相关指标情况判断患者病情稳定，血糖控制尚可，体重也有所下降，可继续目前治疗方案，可继续按照原有处方取药。在电脑上核对患者基本信息与处方信息，确认无误后进行处方重配的操作。长期用药处方配置完成后，药剂师应对患者用药记录进行审核与记录，方便之后的用药随访与治疗情况跟踪，如有需要可以联系处方者沟通处方内容。最后，药剂师将已配置好的药品发给患者，并进行适当的用药交代与用药沟通。

患者咨询用药过程中加用利拉鲁肽的原因：

药剂师回复：利拉鲁肽治疗肥胖糖尿病优点

利拉鲁肽是人类胰高糖素样肽 -1（glucagon like peptide-1，GLP-1）的受体激动剂：

1. 可作用于胰岛 B 细胞，增加胰岛素合成与分泌，提高 B 细胞对葡萄糖的敏感性，并以葡萄糖浓度依赖性抑制胰高糖素分泌等方面；

2. 能产生饱腹感、减轻体重及更好地控制血糖；

3. 皮下注射吸收慢同时半衰期短，低血糖发生率低。

（三）长期用药处方单第二次取药

患者凭医师签字的长期用药处方到药店进行取药，药剂师接受处方者和患者的授权，接受长期用药处方后，复核患者信息，治疗情况等，该患者复查相关糖尿病指标以确定患者病情变化。复查 FPG 5.8 mmol/L，2 小时 PG 7.8 mmol/L，体重 94.2 kg。根据上述糖尿病相关指标情况判断患者病情稳定，血糖控制尚可，体重也有所下降，可继续目前治疗方案，可继续按照原有处方取药。在电脑上核对患者基本信息与处方信息，确认无误后进行处方重配的操作。长期用药处方配置完成后，药剂师应对患者用药记录进行审核与记录。同时告知患者本次为最后一次长期用药处方取药，叮嘱患者应该在本次用药结束后到医院重新就诊，进行身体状况与用药评估。

（以上案例来自某试行长期用药处方药店）

（张弨　译）

第六章 瑞典慢性病长期用药处方项目的研究与借鉴

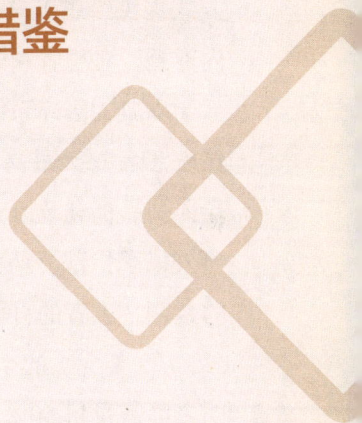

第一节　瑞典慢性病长期用药处方取药流程

瑞典的普通处方有效次数为一次，医生可以根据疾病类型和严重程度，决定患者的药物是短期或长期服用。对于大部分需要长期药物治疗的疾病，例如高血压、高脂血症类心血管疾病等，可采用"慢性病长期用药处方"的方式提供给患者。在不需要每次就诊的情况下使用长期用药处方在半年时间内取药，对患者和处方医生都是一种方便[1]。

瑞典的医疗系统对所有公民提供保障，保障的金额基于医疗费用，例如，住院患者每天最高自付费用为 100 瑞典克朗，超过部分由政府承担。相应，瑞典药品福利政策（Swedish Pharmaceutical Benefits Scheme-PBS）帮助所有瑞典公民承担部分药费。基于所购买药品价格的不同和患者当年累计购买药品的金额，患者的自付比例也不同。例如 2007 年，患者需要自付 900 瑞典克朗（约 125 美金）的全部药费，当累计自付部分在 900 瑞典克朗至 1300 瑞典克朗之间需自付 50% 药费，当累计自付部分在 1300 瑞典克朗至 1700 瑞典克朗之间需自付 25% 药费，当累计自付部分在 1700 瑞典克朗至 1800 瑞典克朗之间需自付 10% 药费，当累计自付部分达到了 1800 瑞典克朗，患者则不需要在这 12 个月报销范围内自付任何药品费用[1]。

根据瑞典对慢性病长期用药处方的相关研究，应用慢性病长期用药处方较多的药品包括：心血管类药物（例如抗血小板、β 受体拮抗剂等）、雌激素、抗抑郁药、甲状腺素、降糖药、哮喘药等[1-7]。

对于患者长期服用的药物（并未查询到资料说明如何定义长期服用，及相应的类型），处方量最多可为一年，并以三个月为一阶段。

患者从医生处获得处方后，将处方带到药店，可以获得第一次的处方药量，药房会将调配日期及数量打印在处方上。之后，患者可以根据处方限制，获取之后的药品，不需要再次联系医生。

第二节　瑞典慢性病长期用药处方取药模式的技术支撑

所有的瑞典社区药店都隶属于一个集团，叫做瑞典国家药店集团（Apoteket AB）[1]。每张处方上应标明药品名称、剂量、数量、单次剂量，以及处方医生，在处方日期一年内有效。处方医生必须在处方上标注处方可调配的次数。因此，这一张处方可以作为"长期用药处方"，不需要就诊就可以多次调配。在药店，每经过一次调配，电脑根据储存的信息，将调配日期、数量打印在处方上。当一长期用药处方的限制最多调配次数被调配完，药店会留存处方。

瑞典国家药店集团（Apoteket AB）对长期用药处方的公告[2]：

长期用药处方的使用规则

对于享受药品福利的处方，有如下规则：

1. 处方只能在上一次调配后的 2/3 用量消耗后才能再次调配。也就是说，对于一个每次调配量为 3 个月的长期用药处方，最早也要 2 个月之后才能得到下一次调配。

2. 处方开具者（医生或其他开具处方的医疗人员）的执业地址必须以条码形式印在处方上。处方开具者同时必须在处方上标示"药店应当依据药品福利政策调配"。

3. 如果您不想注册加入药品福利政策，但想得到药品福利，您需要每一次购买处方药品时，出示药品福利证明卡。

例外情况

您可以购买超过每次长期用药处方量的药品，或者是超过了药品福利限制的数量。但是您必须自付超过了每次长期用药处方量部分的全部费用。

在特殊情况下，例如长期在国外度假，您可以拿到超过 3 个月的药量并且使用福利，但是您必须出示相应特殊情况的证明。

避孕类药物（例如口服避孕药／避孕注射剂）一般作为例外，可以不在 3 个月的限定范围内。

解读

首先，这些规则仅适用于瑞典药品福利政策下的处方药物购买。也就是说，如果患者全部自费购买药物，则可以随时取长期用药处方中的药物。

第一条规则为了减少患者药物的浪费，所以要求患者的药量的确消耗了 2/3 后才允许患者再次取药。由于瑞典常规每次取药量为 3 个月，如果患者能够 2 个月内按时服用药物，则很有可能养成按时服用的习惯，在第三个月内安排再次调配很方便。这样的限制，不仅可以很好利用福利资源，也同时避免了某些患者在家"囤积"药物造成过期，或给别人使用药物等类似事件。同时，因为长期用药处方的特殊性，不使用于病情不稳定、有服药过量自杀倾向、依从性差的患者，此类情况不仅对用药安全产生影响，也因为患者不需要看医生而得到用药，失去了医生评估患者病情的机会。

第二条规则一方面确认处方的真实性（来自有处方权的医生），另一方面，有助于政府监管药品福利的使用，以预防对药品的大量囤积／骗取药品等行为。

第三节　瑞典慢性病长期用药处方运作中存在的安全隐患与风险防范措施

基于文献搜索，瑞典慢性病长期用药处方运作中研究最多的风险为患者的依从性（Refill Adherence），有多篇文献分别研究了患者的依从性的相关因素、患有多种慢性病的患者的依从性、患者的不依从性对治疗及医疗费用的影响等方面。

一、慢性病长期用药处方患者依从性相关研究

（一）评估患者依从性的方法

依从性（adherence）的定义为"一个人服用药物的行为与医疗人员建议的一致程度"[1]。衡量患者的顺应程度是很复杂的，现有的方法都有其不足。通过长期用药处方的调配来估算依从性是一个相对方便的方法，这样的数据不仅可以显示患者何时取自己的长期用药处方，也可以表示整体治疗依从性。长期用药处方调配数据比其他依从性评估的数据相比较更加有意义[1]。

根据 Kripsman 等[3]的研究结果，从处方上提取和药房记录数据上的数据在一年中并无显著差异，而四年的数据比一年的数据可以更好地了解患者的慢性病长期用药处方依从性。

LeseuEG[4]比较了两种评估长期用药处方依从性的方式。第一种为广泛使用的连续取药比率（continuous measure of medication acquisition，CMA）方式，CMA 可以由"患者取得用药量（天数）"除以"研究时间段（天数）"得出，CMA 百分比作为对依从性的衡量，常规认为 80%~120% 为依从性达标，大于 120% 为取药过多，<80% 为取药不足。第二种方式为"最长缺口期"（maximum gap method）方法，只要患者在研究时间段，按照患者服药量，没有连续超过 45 日的缺口期（45 日是基于瑞典的药品福利政策可以允许的每次最大量为 3 个月），则认为是依从性达标。两种方式有各自的利弊，应当基于具体药品类型而定，同时应当考虑是否有证据证明依从性衡量方法与最终患者疗效之间的相关性。

（二）长期用药处方的使用对依从性的影响

长期用药处方的使用与患者用药不足（包括不顺应）可能有相关性[1]。在一篇对于长期用药处方患者用药的依从性研究[1]中，取药不足定义为取药量小于 80% 所需时间段的药量，取药过多定义为取药量大于 120% 所需时间段的药量，发现 57% 的患者依从性达标，21% 的患者取药不足，22% 的患者取药过多。

（三）患者的依从性的相关因素

患者的依从性被多种相关因素所影响，可能的因素包括患者个体情况，医生情况，药品福利支付比例，以及药物的不同类型[1]。基于 16 个大型药房3636 张长期用药处方的数据统计，患者性别差异与依从性无关，不需自付药费的患者比他人更有可能有取药过多的情况。研究中还发现，社区全科医生（general practitioner）的患者比医院医生的患者长期用药处方依从性更高。对于不同类型的药物，避孕药依从性最高（81%），最低的是抗哮喘类型药物，质子泵抑制剂，非甾体类抗炎药（30%~40%）[1]。

（四）患有多种慢性病的患者的依从性

Krigsmank 等[5]调查了同时患有糖尿病及慢性呼吸系统疾病（哮喘/慢性阻塞性肺疾病）的患者，并分析了长期用药处方依从性在三年内的取药间隔。在 56 名患者中，68% 的患者的糖尿病用药依从性达标，42% 的患者的呼吸疾病用药依从性达标。糖尿病和呼吸疾病的取药间隔并没有相关性和一致性，并且患者对糖尿病用药的依从性大于呼吸疾病的依从性。这篇研究的讨论部分提出，糖尿病药物的不依从性可能导致血糖的不稳定，而呼吸疾病长期用药多为预防，可能导致急性发作频率增加。基于此原因，患者可能认为糖尿病是一个更加严重的疾病，从而更加严格顺应糖尿病用药[5]。

（五）患者的不依从性对治疗及医疗费用的影响

Krigsmank 等[6]评估了在不顺应的患者中，取药不足的情况和严重程度、取药过多的经济影响。研究结果显示，对于长期用药处方依从性不足 80% 的患者，每 90~100 天治疗期的治疗空缺期（treatment gap）中位数为 53 天，相应的调配（取药）中位数为 40 天。相对于有自费部分的患者，每个免付自费（每年已超过 1800 瑞典克朗自费门槛）的患者每年过多调配的药品金额多出32000 瑞典克朗（约 243 美金）。将此数据估计全瑞典患者的用药，每年调配过多约 1.42 亿瑞典克朗（约 1900 万美金）价值的药品。因此，取药过多、囤积药品的现象在免付自费的患者中比有自费部分的患者更为常见，这个现象导致了药品费用的浪费[6]。

Krigsmank 等[7]还评估了降糖药物的长期用药处方依从性与血糖控制的

相关性，结果显示顺应达标患者的平均糖化血红蛋白 HbA1c 为 6.5%，而顺应不达标患者为 6.8%（P=0.025）。并且，依从性达标患者不仅有更低的 HbA1c 平均值，他们对心血管药物的依从性也高于他人。因此，依从性高与患者的良性治疗结果有相关性[7]。

二、药师在提高患者依从性中的角色

药师进行的"用药审核（Medication Review）"可以有效减少与长期用药处方用药相关问题。患者用药的依从性对患者的健康是很重要的，正如一篇 Cochrane 回顾性研究表明，患者的临床结果可能在提高依从性后有改善[1]。在瑞典，药师的作用有待进一步提高，这和瑞典药店的背景以及药师教育水平有关[8]。所有瑞典社区药店都隶属于瑞典国家药店集团，虽然瑞典国家药店集团与政府协议有包括其"促进合理用药"职责，但并未开展全国性质的提高患者依从性活动。随着瑞典药店市场的管制解除，引入其他药店的竞争，药师提高患者依从性的职责将有望进一步提高[8]。

药师可以通过以下方式提高患者依从性[9]：

1. 对患者提供依从性重要性的宣教和指导，解释药物的副作用，并评估用药方案。

2. 监测用药，并对药物反应进行随访。

3. 根据协定计划（protocol）开具药物处方、将用药方案简化。

4. 对患者进行电话随访，并提供信息、解答患者咨询。

5. 通过提供患者一段强调用药依从性的视频来教育患者。

Braithcoaites 等研究[10] 表明，药师通过药物依从性干预（medication adherence Interventions）能够提高依从性，特别是目标性强的、个体化的药师与患者的互动。例如，与药师面对面沟通的药物依从性干预应用后，糖尿病患者的用药依从性可显著提高。药师同时在提供药物治疗管理（medication therapy management–MTM）服务方面有重要作用，在服务中药师深度指导患者用药，从而优化治疗结果。当提供药物治疗管理服务时，药师回顾患者所有用药（包括处方药、非处方药、甚至营养品），从而确保患者在恰当的服用，并且预防不良反应，提高治疗效果。如果有潜在问题或建议治疗更改，药师可以借此机会与处方医生沟通，从而协调患者的用药过程[10]。

第四节　启示与借鉴

一、对长期用药处方取药时间的限制

根据我国医保现状，可以对患者长期用药处方取药时间进行限制，瑞典选择 2/3 的原因是考虑大部分处方每次取药为三个月用量，所以 2/3 则是两个月的用量。我国可根据常规每次处方量，相应设定限制。例如，如果常规每次量为一个月，则选择 1/2 作为时间限制较为合适，因为 2 周的时间可以为患者出行、其他安排等作为缓冲。如果同样选择 2/3，则患者只有 10 天时间安排再次调配，显得过于紧凑。

二、预防与长期用药处方相关的患者依从性降低

患者用药治疗的依从性基于一个人对自己的药物必要性的判断，而且有多个因素。这些因素包括对疾病的认知（症状）、个人看法（对药物的消极取向）、情境（他人的观点）。Horne 认为并没有真正的典型的'不顺应患者'，而很多患者都是在有些时候"不顺应"[5]。基于此，设计慢性病长期用药处方制度时应当考虑如何尽可能提高患者的依从性，例如，设定恰当的报销额度及比例，从而避免药物的浪费，并且提高治疗的效果。

三、药师在长期用药处方中的角色

药师不仅可以作为长期用药处方的实施者（确保患者在合适的时间得到药物），还可以在提高患者治疗效果、减少药物费用浪费中发挥作用。例如，如果患者的记录体现出患者取药不足或取药过多，则可以进行药物依从性干预，了解患者不顺应的潜在问题，并进行解决。对于部分药物（例如副作用较明显的药物），药师可以预先通过用药指导对患者进行宣教，从而预防依从

性问题。最后，对于享受政府补贴的患者，药师可以评估患者的依从性，以确保药品不被浪费。

（陆浩）

参考文献

［1］Andersson K, Melander A. Repeat prescriptions: refill adherence in relation to patient and prescriber characteristics, reimbursement level and type of medication. European Journal of Public Health, Vol. 15, No. 6, 621–626.

［2］Apoteket AB. How to buy prescription medicines and other prescription products. https://www.apoteket.se/other–languages/how–to–buy–prescription–medicines–and–other–prescription–products/.

［3］Krigsman K, Nilsson JL. Refill adherence for patients with asthma and COPD: comparison of a pharmacy record database with manually collected repeat prescriptions. Pharmacoepidemiology and drug safety 2007；16：441–448.

［4］Lesén E, Sandström TZ, Carlsten A. A comparison of two methods for estimating refill adherence to statins in Sweden: the RARE project. Pharmacoepidemiology and drug safety 2011; 20: 1073–1079.

［5］Krigsman K, Nilsson JL. Adherence to multiple drug therapies: refill adherence to concomitant use of diabetes and asthma/COPD medication. Pharmacoepidemiology and drug safety 2007；16：1120–1128.

［6］Krigsman K, Melander A, Carlsten A. Refill non–adherence to repeat prescriptions leads to treatment gaps or to high extra costs. Pharm World Sci（2007）29：19–24.

［7］Kindmalm L, Melander A, Nilsson JL. Refill adherence of antihyperglycaemic drugs related to glucose control（HbA1c）in patients with type 2 diabetes. Acta Diabetol（2007）44：209–213.

［8］Södergård B. Adherence to treatment: what is done in Sweden? Practice, education and research. Pharmacy Practice（Granada）. 2008 Oct–Dec；6（4）：171–177.

［9］Al-Jumah KA, Qureshi NA. Impact of pharmacist interventions on patients' adherence to antidepressants and patient-reported outcomes: a systematic review. Patient preference and adherence. 2012；6：87-100.

［10］Braithwaite S, Shirkhorshidian I. The role of medication adherence in the U.S. healthcare system. June 2013. Avalere Health. http: //avalere.com/research/docs/20130612_NACDS_ Medication_Adherence.pdf.

第七章 澳大利亚慢性病长期用药处方项目的研究与借鉴

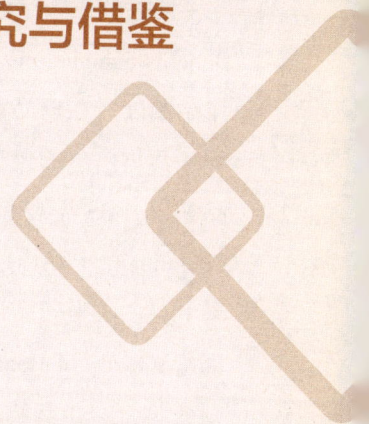

1984 年，澳大利亚通过了《全民医疗保障法》，建立了覆盖全体居民的国民医疗照顾制度（Medicare）制度，实现了全民医疗保障。所有澳大利亚公民、永久居留者以及一些与澳大利亚签订了医疗互惠协议国家的公民均可享受 Medicare 提供的福利：全免费的公立医院急诊、门诊和住院医疗服务；免费或部分补贴的私人全科和专科医疗服务；补贴的社区私人药品服务；全免费的病理检验、影像检查和治疗服务等。

澳大利亚医疗保险中最具特色的举措是实行药品津贴计划（Pharmaceutical Benefits Scheme，以下简称 PBS）。这是专门针对临床大量使用的处方药品的津贴制度。在药品津贴方案的实施过程中，药师在从药品的保管、准备、调配、药物信息的传递以及药品的高质量使用方面起到了极为关键的作用。药品进入 PBS 需要向药物报销指导委员会（Pharmaceutical Benefits Advisory Committee，PBAC）提出申请，PBAC 主要对药物的成本效益进行评估。如果 PBAC 认为药品评估结果适合进入 PBS 药品报销目录，则会向卫生和老龄部（Ministry of Health and Aging）提出建议。如果卫生和老龄部接受该建议，则药物将交由药物福利价格管理局（Pharamceutical Benefits Pricing Authority，PBPA），后者进一步与药品厂商就药物在 PBS 目录中的价格进行协商，并最终决定是否进入 PBS 目录。

药物进入 PBS 目录后，需要按事先协商的价格向药房供应。患者在得到医生开具 PBS 药品处方后，凭处方到药房购药时，只需支付部分处方药的费用，其余部分由 PBS 补贴。在购药时必须出示 Medicare 卡才能享受 PBS 药品补贴。不同药品的自付费用不同，但都是有自付限额。低收入人群可申请医疗服务卡（concession card），持卡人可以享受 PBS 报销目录中低价药品的免费试用和更低的自付上限。联邦政府通过"全民医疗保健方案"和"药品津贴方案"基本负担了澳大利亚居民的医疗费用和大部分的处方药品费用，保证居民公平地享受医疗保健服务。药房凭调配处方的记录向澳大利亚健康保险委员会（Medicare Australia）领取政府的药物津贴。澳大利亚的药品处方根据药品、可重配次数和支付类别分为三类，具体如表 7-1 所示。

表 7-1　澳大利亚处方分类、开具条件及支付方式

处方类型	开具条件	支付方式
标准 PBS 处方（Standard）	最常见的药品处方类型，无需第三方授权。处方者必须遵守相应处方开具的条件，例如使用适应证以及个人标准 PBS 药品的可重配次数	患者分摊付款额（co-payment）为 6.10~37.70 澳元，取决于其享有优惠的状态。其余的药品费用及药师费用由 PBS 支付
授权处方 *（Authority）	针对具有限制供应条件的 PBS 药品（例如，必须具有某一种适应证）或其开具的药品量较大或可重配次数比 PBS 常规情况多	
私人处方（Private）	用于开具 PBS 药品目录之外的药品，或其在 PBS 原则下不可供的药品	患者全额支付药品和药师费用。药师需要打印标准 PBS 和管制处方向 PBS 系统申请补偿

★注：授权处方目前分为 2 类，包括需授权处方（Authority required）和简化流程的需授权处方（Authority required-Streamlined）。需授权处方开具前需要获得澳大利亚民政部（DHS）或退伍军人事务部（DVA）的电话或书面批准。简化流程的需授权处方开具前无需 DHS 或 DVA 的电话或书面批准，仅需标注简化流程的授权代码。

下面将从澳大利亚的慢性病长期用药处方取药流程、技术支撑、药品分类、运作中存在的安全隐患与风险防范措施等方面进行介绍，以供参考。

第一节　澳大利亚的慢性病长期用药处方取药流程

一、药品津贴计划药品的取药流程

药师为患者调配发放药物津贴计划中的药品时，首先需要完成以下步骤：

1. 药师必须在 PBS 处方背面签字，并抄录其姓名和批准的提供方编号。

2. 在 PBS 处方及其底方上必须为 PBS 处方药品指定 PBS 处方识别码，可以使用任何数字序列。如果一张 PBS 处方上的药品数量超过一种，则应为每一种药品分配一个独立的识别码。慢性病长期用药处方授权时，则必须为相同药品分配相同的 PBS 处方识别码。同时药师必须在慢性病长期用药处方授权上分配药师的身份识别码，必须在调配药品日期和地点旁写明。

一般情况下，处方自医生开具后有效期为 12 个月，药师对 PBS 处方进行

调配发药前，需要收到以下材料：

（1）患者 / 药师副本，上面会记录处方者、患者和 PBS 药品详细信息。慢性病长期处方调配发药，需要将长期处方重配授权附在患者 / 药师副本上。该患者 / 药师副本然后由药师留存。

（2）民政部（DHS）/ 退伍军人事务部（DVA）副本，上面会记录处方者、患者和 PBS 药品详细信息。在首次发药后，该副本会转交至民政部进行处理和支付。

（3）处方者副本，书面授权副本将由 DHS 或 DVA 保存，电话或授权网站授权副本将有处方者保存 12 个月。该副本必须记录日剂量、疾病信息、临床用药指征、患者年龄以及患者之前是否获得该 PBS 药品授权。

二、慢性病长期用药处方授权

根据慢性病长期用药处方有无按照"规章第 24 条（Regulation 24）"，可分为普通处方和符合"规章第 24 条"处方。下面分别概述两种不同类型慢性病长期用药处方的授权方式。

表 7-2　慢性病长期用药处方分类、适用及不适用条件

慢性病长期用药处方类型	适用条件	不适合用条件
普通	允许药师按一定可重配次数和间隔期发放药品	不适用于牙科医生开具的 PBS 药品
规章第 24 条处方	允许药师一次性调配发放 PBS 药品	不适用于调配验光师开具的 PBS 药品

1.普通慢性病长期用药处方

当 PBS 处方申请长期用药处方调配供应时，药师将准备慢性病长期用药处方授权表格。慢性病长期用药处方可能会出现在标准的 PBS 处方、PBS 授权处方或授权处方表格或先前的慢性病长期用药处方授权上。对于先前的慢性病长期用药处方授权，必须同时具有 PBS 处方副本（底方），或新版"患者 / 药师副本"。慢性病长期用药处方授权表格必须显示：

（1）津贴类别（优惠或一般）——可在相应的复选框中标记"X"；

（2）患者的姓名和详细地址；

（3）对于慢性病长期用药处方的授权 PBS 处方，需要有授权处方编号；

（4）最初的 PBS 处方详细信息，标明药品、剂型、剂量、数量和服药说明；

（5）如果供应替代药品，则标明实际提供的药品商品名；

（6）首次调配需要标注药房名称、地址和批准编号、最初的 PBS 处方日期和分配的 PBS 处方识别号；

（7）后续供应需要标注药房批准编号、最初处方的日期以及 PBS 处方编号；

（8）长期用药处方药品的重配次数以及已提供的重配次数；

（9）药师的签名和药房批准编号；

（10）调配日期。

准备重复调配或延迟调配的慢性病长期用药处方授权时，药师必须附上一份旧版 PBS 处方副本，或者新版 PBS 处方的患者/药师复印件，并在调配供应药品时，把这两份材料提供给患者。

2. 符合"规章第 24 条"的慢性病长期用药处方

规章第 24 条允许药师一次性调配分发 PBS 慢性病长期用药处方。这类 PBS 处方必须经由执业医生、助产士或执业护士在处方背面签署"规章第 24 条"。同时执业医生、助产士或执业护士必须首先认为其符合以下条件：

（1）最大的 PBS 药品量对于患者治疗仍是不够的；

（2）患者患有慢性疾病或者居住在边远地区，其在获得 PBS 药品供应方面受限；

（3）患者在个别情况下获得药品津贴遇到很大困难。

如果该药品在 PBS 范围内，或者如果其在"军人及遗属药物津贴计划（RPBS）"范围内供应符合"存在困难条件"。规章第 24 条并不适用于调配验光师开具的药物津贴药物。

三、延迟调配的慢性病长期用药处方授权

当 PBS 处方上开具数种 PBS 药品，但是患者不需要同时服用所有的药品，则必须为每一个延迟调配药品准备单独的慢性病长期用药处方授权。在最初的 PBS 处方、副本以及慢性病长期用药处方授权上应当注明"最初调配延迟（original supply deferred）"。延迟调配药品的长期用药处方授权与普通的慢性病长期用药处方授权方式相同，但是需要在"已发药次数"处写上"0"。延迟调配的慢性病长期用药处方应按照首次调配处理。需要在后续慢性病长期用药处方授权上写明授权延迟调配的药房详细信息。

四、慢性病长期用药处方的药品接收

收到 PBS 药品的人士必须在收据上签名并标注日期。如果接收方并非患者，则其必须在 PBS 处方或慢性病长期用药处方授权背面书写其地址信息。仅当调配分发药品后方可获得收据。如果需要通过邮寄、铁路或其他方式运送 PBS 药品，且无法提供收据，则药师必须在 PBS 处方或慢性病长期用药处方授权上证明已调配该药品，且写明调配日期以及寄送的详细信息。例如，如果在 2008 年 4 月 1 日向患者邮寄了 PBS 药品，则药师应当写明："证明调配发药——已于 2008 年 4 月 1 日向患者邮寄（药师姓名）（药师签名）（证明日期）"。

如果在紧急情况下提供该药品，且接收人无法阅读或书写，则药师应在 PBS 处方或慢性病长期用药处方授权上签字并注明声明日期，说明已调配发放该药品，并注明调配的日期，并解释没有收据的原因。例如，如果在 2008 年 5 月 1 日向一名手臂骨折的患者提供 PBS 药品，则药师应当写明："证明调配发药——患者手臂骨折且无法签名（药师姓名）（药师签名）（证明日期）"。

五、特殊情况处理

情景一、如果患者的慢性病长期用药处方药品用完了，而全科医生诊所不上班怎么办？

如果患者的慢性病长期用药处方药品已用完，无法联系患者的全科医

生诊所（例如周六、周日）以获得药品，则患者应申请从药师处获得一份紧急的药品。请注意，这种服务仅适用于确实紧急的情况，且适用于大多数的处方药而非管制药品，药师将依据专业判断来决定调配该药品是否适宜。

取药时需要注意以下事项：

1. 患者必须亲自前往，不能派遣代理人至药房；

2. 患者必须能够提供其正在接受所需药物治疗的证明，例如携带药瓶等；

3. 患者应当联系药房以确保有这种服务；

4. 因为在 NHS 系统上无法显示这次药品调配服务，因此如果患者不是那所药房的长期患者的话，则药品和调配将需要收取费用；

5. 患者付费后会收到一份收据，药师需要填写患者的详细信息以及其他信息，例如患者的医生信息。

情景二、药品序列更改怎么办?

当一种药品或某个商品名的药品从序列中删除，则自删除生效日起，即使该 PBS 处方是在该日期前开具的，该药品或该商品名的药品无法作为 PBS 药品进行供应。这同样适用于慢性病长期用药处方的授权。但是，如果对于 PBS 药品处方限制改变，或者该序列药品的最大处方量或可重配次数更改时，则在此更改生效日期前开具的有效 PBS 处方可仍作为 PBS 药品供应，适用处方当日条件。

情景三、在紧急情况下，没有 PBS 处方怎么办?

在紧急情况下以及当澳大利亚下辖州法允许时，药师可为无 PBS 处方的患者提供 PBS 药品，前提是处方者通过电话或其他方式提供处方的详细信息。处方者必须在药师提供药品后 7 天内将书面 PBS 处方及副本提供给药师。当 PBS 药品需要获得民政部或 DVA 提前批准时，处方者必须获得批准，然后告知药师 PBS 处方以及批准的详细信息。这仅限于首次药品供应，而不适用于慢性病长期用药处方。

第二节　澳大利亚慢性病长期用药处方取药模式的技术支撑

澳大利亚在医疗资源信息共享方面，建立了统一高效的数据库，以实现数据的标准化、规范化，加强对各类医疗信息的总结、分析、归纳和动态管理。就诊人员的详细信息包括出生、死亡、就诊情况、药房售药记录等均可在网上直接查询，可以用来及时分析和掌握疾病谱和各个社区的健康状况。Medicare 持卡者在全国各个医疗机构就诊均可直接刷卡。

目前澳大利亚的药房配备有新版调配发药软件（Pharmacy dispensing software，PDS），使用在线报销的 PBS 处方必须使用 PDS，并满足其要求（见图 7-1）。药师在 PDS 中选择正确的患者档案并输入以下信息，并根据最初的处方进行发药，而不是根据所附的慢性病长期用药处方或延迟授权表格来发药：

- 患者姓名和地址
- Medicare 编号和有效期终止日期
- 状态编号和有效期终止日期（如适用）
- 处方开具日期
- 处方者详细信息，包括姓名、地址和处方者编号
- 药品详细信息，包括名称、剂型、剂量、数量、使用说明以及慢性病长期用药处方开具次数
- 对于授权处方药品，填写授权处方编号
- 简化流程的需授权处方药品的 4 位数授权编码

在完成上述步骤后，继续下面流程：

1. PDS 软件会向 Medicare 发出交易指令，Medicare 会将该处方的详细信息与 PBS 或 RPBS 原则进行比对，包括与 Centrelink 直接链接进行患者状态审查。

2. Medicare 会发送一条信息告知药师，这份报销申请是否可以支付。

3. 在一些情况下，药师将需要在申请报销前纠正错误或遗漏。这可以在

向患者提供药品前完成。

4. 向患者提供药品。

5. 在药房报销周期结束后，通过 PDS 系统关闭这次报销申请。药师需要保留所有处方和报销相关的纸质文件，可以是电子形式或纸质形式保存以供 2 年内备查。

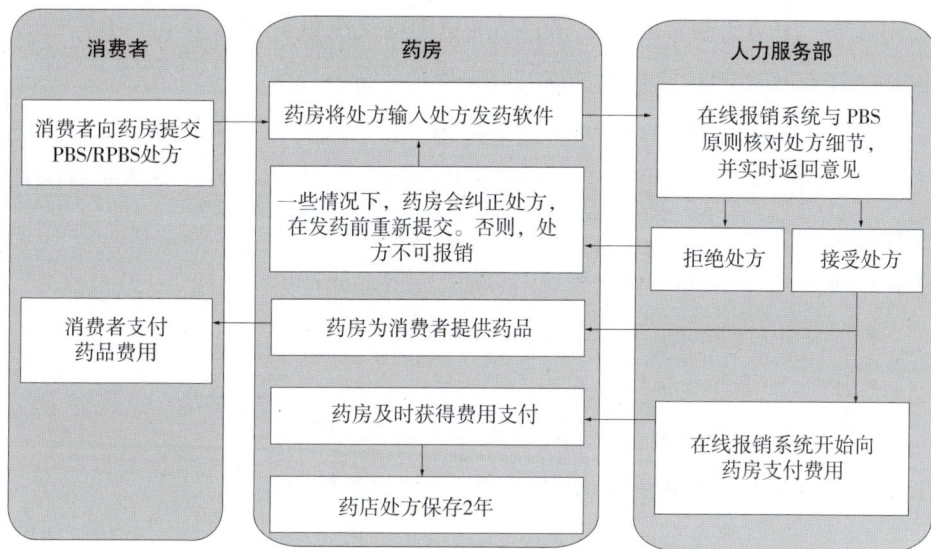

图 7-1　PDS 发药及药品报销支付流程

在线申请 PBS 报销可以提高药师的工作效率，并获得更多以下收益：

1. 获得费用支付的频率缩短，Medicare 每周支付药房费用；

2. 药师可以在为患者发药前确定 Medicare 将会支付的费用金额；

3. 在发药时看到可能的拒单，这样可以在患者离开药房前纠正任何错误；

4. 通过处方发药软件自动生成和发送电子声明单。

第三节　澳大利亚慢性病长期用药处方药品分类

一、澳大利亚药品分类

目前澳大利亚采用双分层系统对药品进行分类，包括风险分类和归序分类（Scheduling）。根据风险高低，将药品分类为注册药（Registered medicines）和上市药（Listed medicines）。注册药需要经过澳大利亚药品管理局（Therapeutic Goods Administration，TGA）评价质量的可控性、安全性和有效性，包括所有处方药、OTC 药以及部分经注册的补充药物（complementary medicines），后者包括传统药物或替代药物，包括维生素、矿物质、草药、芳香疗法和顺势疗法用品等。上市药需要由 TGA 来评估质量的可控性和安全性（不包括有效性），包括部分上市的 OTC 药和大多数上市的补充药品。

另外，归序分类（Scheduling）也是另一种澳大利亚对药品和毒药的分类系统。根据具体的方式和要求，将药品和毒药分为 10 个序列。与药品不相关的序列如下所示：

- 序列 1（Schedule 1），目前不再使用（Not currently in use）
- 序列 5（Schedule 5），危险品（Caution）
- 序列 6（Schedule 6），毒药（Poison）
- 序列 7（Schedule 7），危险毒药（Dangerous Poison）
- 序列 9（Schedule 9），违禁品（Prohibited Substance）
- 序列 10（Schedule 10），需要确保禁止销售、供应和试验的威胁健康的物质（Substances of such danger to health as to warrant prohibition of sale, supply and use）。

其中与药品相关的为第 2、3、4 和 8 四个序列。具体的分类如下表 7-3 所示：

表 7-3　澳大利亚药品序列分类及要求

序列号	药品类别	要求及说明
序列 2（Schedule 2）	只能在药房销售的药品（Pharmacy Medicine）	这类药品的安全使用可能需要药师的专业建议
序列 3（Schedule 3）	药师指导使用的药品（Pharmacist Only Medicine）	这类药品的安全使用需要药师的专业指导，不需要医师处方

续　表

序列号	药品类别	要求及说明
序列 4（Schedule 4）	处方药或处方兽药（Prescription Only Medicine or Prescription Animal Remedy）	必须凭医师处方和在药师指导下使用。这类药物包括大多数需要处方的药物，例如局部麻醉药、抗菌药物、强效止痛药，以及未被归为序列 8 的毒药，和苯二氮䓬类药物。氟硝西泮例外，其属于序列 8 的药品
序列 8（Schedule 8）	管制药品（Controlled Drug），该类药物包括阿片类镇痛药，例如哌替啶、芬太尼、吗啡（美施康定®）、羟考酮（奥施康定®）、美沙酮和丁丙诺啡等	氯胺酮是序列 8 中的管制药品，在澳大利亚执业护士可获得授权处方该药

二、澳大利亚 PBS 慢性病长期用药处方可重配次数和间隔期

PBS 药品所允许的最大数量和可重配次数是由药物报销指导委员会（Pharmaceutical Benefits Advisory Committee，PBAC）推荐的。对于军人及遗属药物津贴计划（RPBS）药品，由军人及遗属药物审评委员会（RPRC）推荐允许的最大数量和可重配次数。目前牙科医生不能开具 PBS 药品目录中药品的慢性病长期用药处方，见表 7–4。

表 7–4　PBS 慢性病长期用药处方可重配次数和间隔期

PBS 慢性病长期用药处方类型	可重配次数	间隔期
牙科处方	无法开具 PBS 药品的慢性病长期用药处方	不适用
一般处方	1~6 个月（如果临床情况适宜）	PBS 目录指定最小间隔期，如无特殊指定则为： 20 天：可允许提供 5 次或更多的可重配次数的 PBS 药品（眼用制剂除外）； 4 天：所有其他类型的药品
超长处方	6~12 个月	

PBS 处方及其慢性病长期用药处方可以根据患者需要开具适合的药品数量，但不能超过最大数量。在处方上需要注明所需的药片、胶囊数量以及所

需的慢性病长期用药处方数量，不能使用缩略语，例如"最大量（Max.Qty、M.Q. 或 M.R.)"。如果处方者认为对于某位患者应当增加调配的最大药片数量或慢性病长期用药处方数量，则处方者必须填写《PBS 授权处方表格》。在PBS 授权处方上提供增加数量和可重配次数一般是为了提供大约 1 到 6 个月的可重复性的治疗（如果临床情况适宜）。通常在所需剂量高于常规剂量的情况下会发生这种情况。批准增加授权数量和可重配次数时，PBS 授权药品和限制津贴药品仅当 PBS 处方的适应证与序列中公布的适应证相同时方可授权。批准增加授权数量和可重配次数仅可扩展至提供患者的药物津贴，而不意味着批准患者治疗的任何方面。

PBS 中列出了慢性病长期用药处方在 PBS 下获得的频率，在取药之间设定有所需最小间隔。但是在一些情况下，在间隔期未结束前，如药师认为"需要立即调配发药"，则仍可对该处方进行调配发药。如果在法律规定的时间内患者已获得相同或具有等效的药品（任意品牌），则这份处方通常不可作为PBS 处方获得补助。如果没有指定的间隔期，则：

● 在当天或过去 20 天内，如果 PBS 药品（眼用制剂除外）在 PBS 序列中可允许提供 5 次或更多的可重配次数（例如，在 6 月 4 日调配发放 PBS 药品，则患者需要到 6 月 25 日方可再次获得该 PBS 药品）。

● 或者对于所有其他药品，在当天或在过去 4 天内（例如，在周一为患者提供 PBS 药品，则在周六前不可为该患者提供 PBS 药品）

澳大利亚政府根据《2008~2009 年联邦预算》的部分内容，自 2009 年1 月 1 日起将一些药品的慢性病长期用药处方延长至 6~12 个月，旨在减少慢性病患者对慢性病长期用药处方要求。在全科医生管理计划（General Practitioner Management Plan, Medicare 项目 721 和 725）或团队监护计划（Team Care Arrangements，Medicare 项目 723 和 727）下管理的患者，根据其治疗医生的临床决定，将有资格接受这类药物长达 12 个月的定期供应。批准的慢性病长期用药超长处方药品目录见附件 1，下图示例为澳大利亚 2017 版 PBS 目录中阿托伐他汀的内容。其中"No. of Rpts"为阿托伐他汀的慢性病长期用药处方次数，如下图所示，阿托伐他汀的慢性病长期用药处方次数为 11 次。同时 PBS 目录中还列出了安全网最大可记录数值（MRVSN）。安全网指的是医疗费用支出安全网。患者可向药剂师出示处方记录表，以证明其已达到相关的 PBS 安全网启用额，这样可在任何药店申请安全网优惠卡，从而以较低价格购买或免费取得 PBS 药物。

ATORVASTATIN

Note No increase in the maximum quantity or number of units may be authorised.
Note No increase in the maximum number of repeats may be authorised.

Restricted benefit
For use in patients who meet the criteria set out in the General Statement for Lipid-Lowering Drugs
Clinical criteria:
- Patient must be receiving treatment under a GP Management Plan or Team Care Arrangements where Medicare benefits were or are payable for the preparation of the Plan or coordination of the Arrangements.

atorvastatin 10 mg tablet, 30

9230T	Max Qty Packs	No. of Rpts	Premium $	DPMQ $	MRVSN $	Brand Name and Manufacturer	Brand Name and Manufacturer
	1	11	..	12.33	13.52	ª APO-Atorvastatin [TX]	ª Atorvachol [ED]
						ª Atorvastatin Amneal [EF]	ª Atorvastatin AN [EA]
						ª Atorvastatin GH [GQ]	ª Atorvastatin Sandoz [SZ]
						ª Atorvastatin SCP 10 [RZ]	ª Atorvastatin SZ [HX]
						ª Blooms the Chemist Atorvastatin [IB]	ª Chem mart Atorvastatin [CH]
						ª Lipitor [PF]	ª Lorstat 10 [AF]
						ª Terry White Chemists Atorvastatin [TW]	ª Torvastat 10 [RW]
						ª Trovas [RA]	

Schedule of Pharmaceutical Benefits – February 2017

注：Max. Qty Packs 最大包装数量；No. of Rpts 慢性病长期用药处方次数；DPMQ：最大药品量分发价格（澳元）；MRVSN：安全网最大可记录数值（澳元）

图 7-2　示例：澳大利亚 2017 版 PBS 中对阿托伐他汀的慢性病长期用药处方次数的限制

三、澳大利亚延续调配发药（Continued dispensing）药品类别

自 2012 年 7 月起，澳大利亚发布了可在无 PBS 处方的情况下延续调配发药（Continued dispensing）的药品类别，包括：HMG–CoA 还原酶抑制剂（他汀类药物）以及口服避孕药。药师必须在提供该药品后 24 小时内，以书面方式通知患者最近一次的处方者，同时在其约房发药系统中将此次药品供应记录为"延续调配发药"供应。药师进行延续调配发药需满足以下条件：

- 需要立即提供药品以确保治疗的连续性；
- 无法获得患者处方者的处方或电话口头医嘱；
- 患者和处方者之间最近一次咨询距今不超过 12 个月；

- 之前的临床访视支持继续使用该药，且该药治疗稳定；
- 患者在过去 12 个月内未获得过该药的延续调配发药供应。

澳大利亚延续调配发药（Continued dispensing）案例 1：

一患者正在服用他汀类药物，而他的长期用药处方已到期，又即将外出度假 3 周来不及找医生开处方。其妻子来药房为他办理长期用药处方。

药师考虑：

√患者是否需要立即获得该药以维持治疗的连续性？

√该药是否属于延续调配发药的药品？

√患者最近一次在处方者处的访视距今不超过 12 个月？

√患者是否稳定地服用该药？

√患者的健康状况是否改变？

药师的选择：

这个案例适合延续调配发药。患者连续 4 年服用该药，且每 6 个月检测一次胆固醇水平（从患者妻子与药师的沟通中获悉），因此该患者治疗稳定。该患者妻子知道她丈夫需要一份处方。药师在发放该药 24 小时内以书面形式通知患者最近一次的处方者，患者取走该药，药师填写好《无 PBS 处方发药工作表单》（见图 7-3）。

澳大利亚药学会

日期：

药师：

患者信息

姓名：　　　　　　　　　　　　出生日期：

地址：

□同意提供其他来源信息（如"是"，请勾选）

　详细信息来源（例如其他药房的信息）：

	通用名	
	商品名	
	剂量	
	剂型	
申请 药品 信息	上次处方 • 　处方开具者 • 　处方开具日期 • 　上次发药日期	
	适应证	
	给药方案	
	本药在该剂量下疗程	
	规律服用，无间断？	
	在过去 12 个月内，之前的无有效处方供应	
健康 疾病 状态	上次咨询处方开具者的大概日期	
	当前用药（包括 OTC 和传统药物）	
	自上次咨询以来的健康状态是否改变？ • 　住院？ • 　药物更改 • 　疾病状态改变 • 　可能影响治疗疗效的生活方式？ • 　发生可能的不良反应？	
	影响药品供应决定的其他问题？	
	供应决定*	

*NS = 不供应；TO = 提供电话订单；ES = 紧急供应； CD = 延续调配发药； R =
转诊至处方开具者

注意：本表格作为药师用于采集患者信息的通用模板，适用于无有效处方申请药品
的情况。考虑无有效处方供应药品时，应结合药房调配发药记录（和其他信息资源）
使用本信息。在所有情况下，药师应结合专业判断使用本表格。

图 7-3　无 PBS 处方发药工作表单

第四节　澳大利亚慢性病长期用药处方运作中存在的安全隐患与风险防范措施

澳大利亚医药分开的运营模式与我国不同，医生处方行为受到行业自律组织的规范，在医师处方过程中药物最大用量和可重配次数都受到严格限制。药师行为主要包括药师处方调配行为和申请药物补贴行为两方面。药师处方行为受到药房行业协会与澳大利亚政府签订的第三、第四社区药房协议的规范。药房行业协会是澳大利亚的第三方组织，在药师行为行业自律方面发挥着重要作用。在申请药物补贴过程中，PBS 管理组织澳大利亚健康保险委员会将会对申请信息进行审核，确认药物使用人的优惠资格、处方开具是否符合药物津贴计划药物使用规范、药物治疗方法是否符合规定。

法律环境保障了药房及其监督角色的法律地位和权力。《国家卫生法》（The 1953 National Health Act）和国家卫生（药物津贴）条令（National Health–Pharmaceutical Benefits– Regulations 1960）支撑和指导了医保报销药品管理的各个方面，明确了各主体的法律地位和权力义务，有助于其分工与合作。在这样的法律环境下，使得药品报销指导委员会、医师协会、药房行业协会等第三方组织在监督各方行为方面发挥了技术监督和行为监督的作用。同时，未上升到法律层面的各种行业规范和协议，也对主体行为起到了行业自律的约束作用。例如澳大利亚联邦政府与澳大利亚药房行业协会签订的协议、规章第 24 条（Regulation 24）等。良好的信息支持使对药房行为的有效监督成为可能。在澳大利亚药品报销过程中，时刻保持了报销药品范围、政府支付药品价格、处方信息、药师、处方调配信息、患者自付信息、患者资格等相关信息在卫生部门、人力服务部门、药师等相关主体间的畅通。信息的透明加大了对主体不良行为曝光的可能，有助于主体加强自律，从而降低管理成本。

当然，不可回避的是在慢性病长期用药处方运作过程中，在一些情况下患者处方药物的可重配周期为半年至一年，这大大增加了药物治疗疗效评估问题以及副作用监测不及时的风险。澳大利亚医院药剂师学会（SHPA）在2000年发布的执业实践标准中，提到推荐用于针对接受慢性病长期用药处方治疗患者的药物咨询服务。

慢性病长期用药处方药物咨询服务

对于使用慢性病长期用药处方的患者，药师应当通过询问以下问题来检查患者对用药的理解状况：

1. 您目前是如何服用药物的？

可根据药品说明书来核对患者的回答，从而发现依从性和其他问题，并进行相应处理。

2. 您感觉服药后的效果如何？

这是为了确认在充分治疗情况下的潜在问题，给予患者机会提出任何问题。

3. 您在服用药物期间是否注意到有哪些不同之处？

这是为了发现任何副作用或相互作用。如可能，可提出相应副作用的处理办法。

第五节　启示与借鉴

一、澳大利亚不断改革的药品津贴计划

澳大利亚早在1948年就实行了药品津贴计划（PBS），最初仅免费提供数量有限的拯救生命的药品，后逐渐演变成提供广泛受补贴的药品。PBS并非一成不变的，自2007年以来，PBS也进行了一些相应的调整措施。比如，调整社会药房药品加成方法，提高多数药品加成率；建立PBS网上系统，鼓励药店网上报销，每张处方PBS支付药房0.4分澳元；在不超过患者原支付水平的情况下，鼓励药师开具PBS目录中非品牌的替代性药品，每开具一次PBS，支付药师1.5澳元；增加对社区服务基金的投入，用来补贴参加政府改

革计划的批发商，2008 年至 2011 年，增加了 6900 万澳元的投入。

除此之外，PBS 还采取了多项改革，包括简化医生处方审查流程，减少医生行政性工作量；与制造商签订供应保证条款，要求降价后必须保证 24 个月的供应；建立战略行动工作组，保证有疗效的新药能通过合适途径及时进入 PBS；加强患者教育，鼓励使用仿制药等。

二、澳大利亚独具特色的延续调配发药（Continued dispensing）

延续调配发药自 2012 年 7 月实施以来，获得了广大慢病患者的支持。澳大利亚药学会发布了《Guidelines for the Continued Dispensing of eligible prescribed medicines by pharmacists》，指导药师在实际工作中的操作。延续调配发药可避免患者治疗中断，提高患者用药依从性，同时也更好地方便患者在紧急情况下获得药品。尽管目前所涉及的药品仅限于他汀类药物和口服避孕药，但却在患者紧急需要药品的情况下，缓解燃眉之急。在一项患者对延续调配发药的态度调查中，绝大多数患者支持这种新的药品发放形式，同时也对药师表现出很高程度的信任。但是，澳大利亚的部分医生对于延续调配发药并不支持，认为这并不能给患者带来最佳利益。不可否认，延续调配发药赋予药师更大的权利和责任，如何在实际操作中给患者带来最大获益，同时控制风险、保证患者用药安全，这些都是值得我们追踪、借鉴和探讨的。

（赵　明　杨莉萍）

参考文献

［1］SHPA Standards of Practice for the Provision of consumer medicines information by pharmacists in hospitals. The Society of Hospital Pharmacists of Australia Consumer Medicines Information Working Party. The Australian Journal of Hospital Pharmacy，2000，30（5）：225-228.

［2］Australian Government Department of Health. Measure to reduce repeat prescription requirements for patients with chronic conditions.

［3］http: //www.pbs.gov.au/info/publication/factsheets/shared/2008-11-01-repeat_prescriptions.

［4］Australian Government Department of Health. Prescribing medicines-information for PBS prescribers. Available at www.pbs.gov.au/info/healthpro/explanatory-notes /section1/Section_1_2_Explanatory_Notes#Maximum-quantities.

［5］Belinda Garth，Meredith Temple-Smith，Malcolm Clark. "Your lack of organisation doesn't constitute our emergency" -repeat prescription management in general practice. Australian Family Physician，2014，43（6）：404-408.

［6］Pharmaceutical Society of Australia. Guidelines for the Continued Dispensing of eligible prescribed medicines. 2013.

［7］Abukres SH，Hoti K，Hughes JD. Avoiding Treatment Interruptions: What Role Do Australian Community Pharmacists Play? PLoS One. 2016 May 12;11（5）：e0154992.

［8］Australian Medical Association. 'Continued dispensing' not in the best interests of patients. Available at http: //ama.com.au/node/7603.

［9］Abukres SH，Hoti K，Hughes JD. Patient attitudes towards a new role for pharmacists: continued dispensing. Patient Prefer Adherence. 2014，27（8）：1143-51.

［10］Abukres SH，Hoti K，Hughes JD. Continued Dispensing: what medications do patients believe should be available? PeerJ. 2015 May 5；3；e924.

［11］杨莉萍. 浅谈澳大利亚药房与药师. 中国新药杂志［J］. 2009，18（6）：560-

563.

［12］冯修猛.澳大利亚药剂师在药学服务中的角色及对我国药学教育的启示［J］.药学教育，2007，23（1）：61-62.

［13］曹立亚.国际药师制度发展研究与借鉴［M］.北京：中国医药科技出版社，2013.

［14］刘扬.澳大利亚药品津贴计划及其对完善我国基本药物监管方式的启示［J］.卫生软科学，2013，27（12）：756-759.

［15］傅鸿鹏.澳大利亚PBS改革小有斩获［J］.中国医院院长，2013（8）：80-81

附件1　澳大利亚延长慢性病长期用药处方有效期的措施

（来源：澳大利亚 PBS 网站 http://www.pbs.gov.au/info/publication/factsheets/shared/2008-11-01-repeat_prescriptions）

自 2008 年 11 月 1 日起，以下药物可增加慢性病长期用药处方次数：

用于治疗囊性纤维化的药物：

- 胰腺提取物；

- 胰脂肪酶。

用于治疗高胆固醇血症的药物：

- 阿托伐他汀钙；

- 氟伐他汀钠；

- 普伐他汀钠；

- 辛伐他汀；

- 非诺贝特；

- 吉非贝齐；

- 消胆胺；

- 盐酸考来替泊。

用于治疗严重眼干的药物，包括干燥综合征：

- 羧甲基纤维素钠和甘油。

用于治疗严重眼干的药物，包括干燥综合征：

- 卡波姆 980；

- 羧甲基纤维素钠；

- 羟丙基甲基纤维素；

- 羟丙基甲基纤维素和卡波姆 980；

- 羟丙基甲基纤维素和右旋糖酐；

- 聚乙二醇 400 和丙二醇；

- 聚乙烯醇；

- 石蜡。

用于治疗溃疡性结肠炎的药物：

- 柳氮磺吡啶。

（赵明　译　杨莉萍　审校）

附件 2　澳大利亚延续调配发药法案

2012 年澳大利亚卫生部延续调配发药法案

2012 年 6 月 29 日

第一节　目的

本法案指定可提供的 PBS 药品以及在没有处方的情况下根据之前 PBS 处方者的处方，由一名获准供应 PBS 药品的药师（以下简称"获准药师"）提供 PBS 药品时必须满足的条件 *。

*注：在澳大利亚国家卫生法第 90 条中列出了获准成为一名提供 PBS 药品的药师所需要的条件

第二节　条件

一、一般条件

（1）对于本法案的 89A（3）（b）条，本部分列出提供申请药品供应时必须满足的条件。

（2）一名获准药师在以下情况下必须考虑 PSA 指南。

（a）满足本部分所列出的条件；

（b）决定这些条件是否符合。

（3）在本部分中：

（b）参考最近一次为该患者开具 PBS 药品的处方者

二、无法获得处方

这种情况下获准药师认为，该患者无法获得一名 PBS 处方者开具的 PBS 药品处方。

三、之前的 PBS 药品供应

这种情况指的是获准药师认为：

（a）该患者之前已基于一名 PBS 处方者开立的处方获得 PBS 药品供应；

（b）PBS 处方者为该患者至少开具一次 PBS 药品处方供应。

四、治疗稳定性

这种情况指的是获准药师认为该患者的治疗稳定。

五、PBS 处方者之前的临床审查

这种情况指的是，获准药师认为满足以下情况：

（a）该患者不间断地规律使用 PBS 药品；

（b）自该阶段开始以来，PBS 处方者已评估该患者的病情，并决定需要进行当前的 PBS 药品治疗。

六、上次供应 PBS 药品的处方

这种情况指的是获准药师认为，在此次申请供应前该患者获得的上次 PBS 供应具有一份有效处方。

七、在过去 12 个月无延续调配发药

这种情况指的是获 PBS 药品供应。

八、获得 PBS 药品供应患者的声明

这指的是，该患者或该患者的代理人（该获准药师除外）签署一份声明，成人在未提供一份有效处方的情况下获得 PBS 药品供应。

九、最大供应量

这种情况指的是获准药师认为，本法案 85A（2）（a）下 PBS 药品提供的最大量和数量。

十、准备和记录信息

（1）这种情况指的是，提供 PBS 药品时获准药师：

（a）记录药师使用支持其供应 PBS 药品的信息；

（b）准备药师将发给 PBS 处方者的信息。

（2）必须记录和准备的信息包括：

（a）声明供应的 PBS 药品符合本法案 89A（3）（a）提供 PBS 药品；

（b）声明满足 2.02 至 2.02 小节中所述条件；

（c）声明获准药师认为向该人士提供 PBS 药品以有助于治疗连续性。

第三节　药物津贴

一、药物津贴

对于本法案中 89A（3）（a）条，附表 1 中列出了可由获准药师在无处方的情况下供应法案 89A（1）条项下的药物津贴。

附表 1　药物津贴

第 1 部分　口服激素避孕药

（略）

第 2 部分　调脂药物

（略）

（赵明　译　杨莉萍　审校）

第八章 新加坡慢性病长期用药处方项目的研究与借鉴

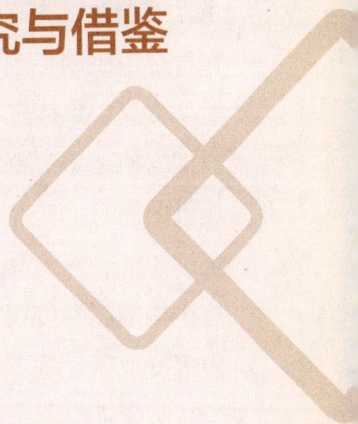

众所周知，新加坡拥有世界一流的医疗卫生体系，覆盖范围广、服务效率高、医疗品质优，据《2000 年世界卫生报告》（The World Health Report 2000）统计，其卫生系统总体绩效在 WHO 成员国中名列第 6 位，[1] 遥遥领先于众多发达国家。早在 1993 年，新加坡政府就以白皮书的形式发布了报告《可负担的医疗》（Affordable Health Care）[2]，保证全体民众都能够享受到良好的、可负担的基本医疗服务，而这本白皮书也成为指引 21 世纪新加坡医疗卫生体系发展和改善的蓝图，"以人为本"的理念贯穿始终。现今的新加坡，可以说在医疗卫生的各个领域均取得了显著的成果：公民平均寿命延长、新生儿存活率提高、癌症患者存活率与欧洲接近、心血管疾病死亡率是亚太地区大多数国家的一半。更值得一提的是，新加坡在取得与世界发达国家水平相当的成果的同时，其成本更低、满意度更高，可谓"价廉质优"。[3] 根据新加坡卫生部（Singapore Ministry of Health，MOH）于 2015 年开展的"患者对公共医疗机构的满意度调查"[4] 结果显示，85.9% 的患者对公立医院、综合诊所和国家专业医疗服务中心的服务质量感到满意，84.9% 的患者愿意向他人推荐公共医疗机构。

然而，和许多发达国家一样，目前新加坡的老年人口比例正在迅速增长。截止至 2016 年，新加坡人口总计 560.73 万人，65 岁以上人口达 48.76 万人（占比 8.70%），预期寿命 82.7 岁，[5] 预计 2030 年 65 岁以上的人口占比将达到 1/5。伴随着老龄化社会的到来，慢性病给医疗卫生体系带来了巨大的压力与挑战。药学服务作为医疗卫生服务的重要组成部分，针对病情稳定并且需要长期药物治疗的慢性病患者，新加坡的便民举措之一是采用长期用药处方的取药模式，既避免了为取药而频繁就诊给患者带来的不便，也节省了医疗资源的压力和重复浪费。

第一节　新加坡慢性病长期用药处方的取药流程

为了确保所有患者都能够在适当的时间、适当的场所，享受到适当的医疗服务，新加坡建立起公私合作的多层次医疗卫生体系，主要包括初级医疗服务和更高级别的医疗服务。病情相对简单的患者通常由私立机构中的私人全科医生（general practitioner）或公立机构，即综合诊所（polyclinics）提供初级医疗服务，而病情相对复杂的患者会由私人全科医生或综合诊所转诊至二级或三级医院接受专科医疗服务（specialist care）。[6]

根据 MOH 公布的 2015 年门诊数据统计结果[7]，专科门诊（specialist outpatient clinics）全年门诊量 465.81 万人次，综合诊所全年门诊量 487.47 万人次，而这些医院机构中的药房则是门诊患者照方取药、接受药学服务的主要场所。[8]

就长期用药处方而言，《新加坡医疗机构和药房药学实践标准》（Pharmacy Practice Standards for Healthcare Institutions and Pharmacies in Singapore）[9] 中采用的英文原文是 repeat prescription 或 prescription refills，具体是指根据医师在处方上确定的次数可以反复或重复调配的处方。原则上慢性病患者在某一医院就诊后所获得的长期用药处方是可以在新加坡的任一医院药房或社区药房进行重配的。实际上，接受政府医疗补贴（subsidy）的新加坡公民均需要在指定的医院就诊方可享受补贴；倘若在其他医院药房或社区药房重配处方，则需要完全自费。因此大部分患者选择在指定的医院就诊并重配长期用药处方。

新加坡的慢性病长期用药处方的重配（refill）由患者、药师（pharmacist）和药学技术员（pharmacy technician）共同完成，流程示意图详见图 8-1，在不同的医院中该流程大致相同，但由于各医院在优良药学实践规范（good pharmacy practice）的相关规定、自动化程度、新型拓展服务等方面的不同可能或多或少存在差异。

新加坡中央医院（Singapore General Hospital）是新加坡建立最早且规模最大的三级急性照护医院和全国转诊中心，现以该医院为例，对慢性病长期用药处方的取药流程[10] 做一介绍，见图 8-1。

• 第一步，患者手持处方来到药房的登记处（registration counter），柜台接待员对处方的有效性及合法性进行初步审核。

• 审核通过后，患者排队将处方提交给药房，获得序列号，在等候区等候取药。

● 录入处（typing station）的药学技术员根据处方识别码从医院信息系统中调取该患者的电子处方，并且在药房信息系统中创建患者的当次处方（包括当次所需的药品名称、用法、用量、数量等信息）。

● 审核处（checking counter）的药师对已创建的当次处方进行审核，复核药学技术员录入信息的准确性，并对处方用药进行临床审核（clinical review）。确认无误后，处方被传送带传送到标记处（tagging station）。

● 标记处的药学技术员将处方关联并放入到一个嵌有射频识别标签（radio frequency identification tag，RFID）的药筐中，处方及药筐随传送带进入自动化药房发药系统（automated pharmacy dispensing system，APDS）。APDS 将患者所需药品自动调配到该药筐中并传送到人工调配处（manual picking stations）。

● 在人工调配处，药学技术员会对不能通过 APDS 自动调配的药品进行人工调配，并对单个患者的所有药品进行打包，整个过程通过 RFID 技术和二维码技术确保处方、药品以及摆放位置的正确对应。

● 打包好的药品经传送带送至一名负责审核的药师处，该药师再次对照处方审核药品并再次进行患者用药临床审核。

打包好的药品被传送到发药药师，同时系统自动呼叫序列号提示患者来窗口取药。发药药师一边对患者进行用药教育一边发药，从而确保患者知晓所取的药品和用药注意事项，能够正确用药。

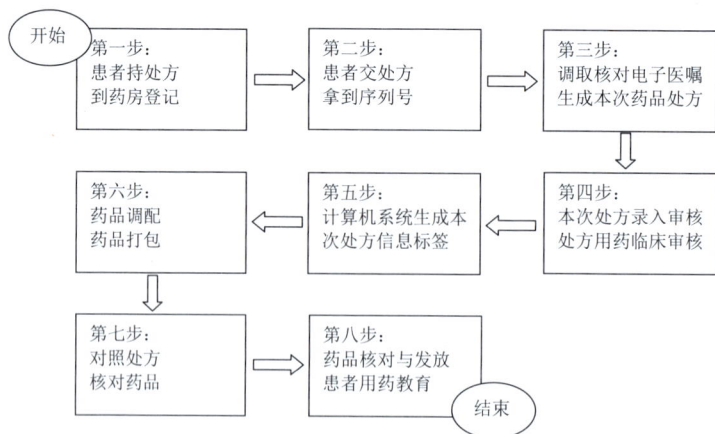

图 8-1　新加坡慢性病长期用药处方的取药流程

第二节　新加坡慢性病长期用药处方的服务模式创新

在新加坡，除了慢性病长期用药处方的常规取药模式以外，药学相关部门还运用现代化技术手段积极地拓展多种服务形式来提升服务效率、减少等候时间、促进用药安全。

一、借助自动化药房发药系统与 RFID 技术

在信息化和自动化高度发达的今天，新加坡大多数医院药房可以在患者首诊后取药时，通过药房信息系统录入医师为患者开具的药品总量，患者每次取药后，系统会自动扣除取走的药品数量，并记录可重配的剩余药量，不需人工计算，降低了计算错误的发生风险。自动化发药系统的引入也在很大程度上提高了处方调配效率、减少了差错发生率。例如新加坡中央医院门诊药房引入的 APDS 能够通过识别嵌入每个药筐的 RFID 对患者所需药品进行自动分拣与包装，APDS 中主要放置的是吸塑包装药品（blistered packaged medicines）和整盒包装药品（boxed packaged medicines），药品从机械臂收集盒到滑槽仅需要 4 秒钟，移动速度非常快。APDS 的引入使得新加坡中央医院门诊药房的未出门差错（near miss）大大减少，患者的等候时间也显著缩短。[10]

二、开展长期用药处方的快捷重配服务

为了解决药师人手相对缺乏、长期用药处方重配等候时间长以及不同患者群体对药学服务需求不同等日益凸显的问题，新加坡各级医院对改进长期用药处方取药流程进行了多种尝试与探索，其中之一即是开展长期用药处方的快捷重配服务（Express Refill Service，ERS）。快捷重配服务是针对患者常规使用并且熟知用法的药品提供的耗时更短、更为便捷的长期用药处方重配服务。该项服务的目标人群需要满足以下几方面条件：①仅限长期用药处方重配取药，换言之，处方中的每种药品都至少已经完成过一次配药。因为每一张新开具的处方都可能会有医嘱的变化，考虑到患者安全是医疗服务的重

中之重，药师必须对其进行临床审核从而确保患者取到正确的药品并且能够正确使用，所以新开具的处方不得申请 ERS。②自处方开具之日起患者没有任何用药调整；③自处方开具之日起患者没有再次住院和门诊就诊；④患者表示对自身用药方案熟悉且不需要用药教育并自愿接受 ERS。[11]

满足上述条件并且选择 ERS 的患者，在持处方前往药房登记处时告知接待员即可，药房工作人员会提供给患者专门的 ERS 序列号，等候取药。而图 8-1 长期用药处方取药流程中的第四步仅由药学技术员审核本次处方录入的正确性，如：药品名称、用法、用量、数量等，而不再进行临床审核；此外，第八步药师核对完毕后直接将药品发放给患者，而不再进行用药教育。

为了确保患者用药安全，对于选择 ERS 患者的处方用药情况，药师会在 24 小时内非高峰时段进行处方审查，以确认是否存在药品相关问题，若发现问题则及时联系患者，安排用药指导；药房还会将联系电话提供给患者，方便患者遇到疑虑随时电话咨询。研究表明[8]，ERS 提供的差异化服务，一方面提高了门诊药房的工作效率，为药师节省出更多时间关注用药较为复杂的患者；另一方面缩短了工作流程和取药等候时间，提高了患者满意度，同时安全性总体良好。

三、借助处方药自提柜为患者提供便利 [12]

新加坡保健服务集团综合诊所（SingHealth Polyclinics，SHP）为慢性病长期用药处方的重配提供了一种称为处方药自提柜（Prescription In Locker Box，PILBOX）的创新性服务，使得患者或其照护者能够在自己方便的时间取药，而不需要在药房排队耗费过多的时间。具体服务流程介绍如下：

● 首先患者需要到药房确认自身用药情况是否适合选择 PILBOX 服务，只有使用长期用药处方取药并且年龄满 18 岁的患者才适用；患者在药房登记使用该项服务，并设定未来的取药日期。

● 取药日期前一周，系统会给患者发送提醒短信，药房工作人员也会向患者再次进行电话确认。

● 取药前，患者在 SHP 收费站或网站上支付药费及服务费，获取支付收据。

- 取药日期当日选择自己方便的时间前往自提柜，扫描支付收据上的二维码并输入手机号码后，即可取到药品。
- 如果患者遇到用药品相关问题，可以随时致电药房进行咨询。
- 药房工作人员会在患者取药后第二天对患者进行电话回访，从而确保用药安全。

PILBOX 服务是针对人们生活节奏快、日常工作忙碌的一种人性化便利服务，在周末以及法定节假日均可进行。然而，需要注意的是，PILBOX 服务不支持药品退换，患者在自提柜取药时需仔细核对药品是否正确、是否完好；如果患者需要更改取药日期，可在原登记日期前至少 2 个工作日致电药房进行更改；如果取药日期当日忘记取药，则会收到短信提醒并且只能前往药房取药。

四、送药上门服务与网上药房服务 [13, 14]

在新加坡，部分医院的门诊药房还拓展了多种取药模式以方便长期用药处方的重配。例如：

- 送药上门服务（Home Delivery Service），患者通过支付一定的服务费，药房可以将重配的药品为患者快递到家。以新加坡中央医院为例，患者选择该项服务需要满足以下条件：①仅限本院开具的处方；②仅限患者常规并且重复使用的药品；③至少取 2 周量的药品在家使用；④处方没有任何变更或调整；⑤处方中不得涉及紧急治疗用药、抗生素、管制药品或对温度高度敏感的药品；体积和重量大的药品配送需要额外付费；对于不确定是否符合标准的药品，患者需事先向药房工作人员咨询确认；⑥在送药上门之前缴纳相应费用；⑦一旦申请并确认使用该项服务后，不得有任何变更；取消或变更需支付额外的费用。符合上述条件的患者填写送药上门服务申请单并将申请单和原始有效的处方一并提交给药房，处方由药房保管。
- 网上药房服务（Online Pharmacy Service），当患者已在医院或诊所中与医生进行过面对面的沟通、有初始的健康检查记录，并且原始处方的首次配药已在实体药房中进行后，长期用药处方后续的重配可以通过网络下单，药房将药品调配、打包后寄送到患者家中。这些服务能够减缓医院就诊压力、节约医疗资源，也为慢性病患者提供了诸多便利。

第三节　新加坡慢性病长期用药处方的药品分类

在新加坡的药品管理中，药品分为处方药品（Prescription Only Medicines，POM）、药房药师准售药品（Pharmacy Only Medicines，P）和普通非处方药品（General Sale List，GSL）。POM 是指仅能够从医师或牙医处获得或由医师或牙医开具处方并由药师调配后获得的药品；P 是指不需要处方但可以从零售药房的药师处获得的药品；GSL 是指从药房以外的一般零售商处也能购买到的药品。长期用药处方管理涉及的药品分类主要针对处方者开具的处方药品（POM）。根据各类药品能否开具可重配的长期用药处方以及具体管理要求的不同，可进一步分为管制药品、苯二氮䓬类等镇静催眠药和其他慢性病治疗用药等三种情形进行具体说明。

一、管制药品

在新加坡，吗啡、芬太尼等麻醉镇痛药属于管制药品，只能由具有麻醉药品处方权的医师分次开具处方，而不得以长期用药处方的形式开具，患者只能从药房拿到严格限量的药品。

二、苯二氮䓬类等镇静催眠药

MOH 非常关注苯二氮䓬类等镇静催眠药的用药安全，因此无论是对处方开具还是对药品监管都提出了具体要求。根据《新加坡卫生部关于开具苯二氮䓬类药物的临床实践指南》（MOH Clinical Practice Guidelines—Prescribing of Benzodiazepines）[15]（详见附件 1），苯二氮䓬类药物应以最低剂量间断给予（例如：每 2~3 晚服药 1 次），以期短疗程缓解失眠，疗程控制在 2~4 周，即使是短半衰期的苯二氮䓬类药品也不推荐长期服用；用药前和每次就诊时，均需告知患者服用此类药物可能产生依赖、影响情绪、记忆和认知，提醒服药期间不得饮酒；用药期间需要监测药品不良反应、滥用情况、耐受性、依赖性及停药反应等；因此要求患者尽量在同一位医师指导下诊治和处方苯二氮䓬类药品，以便临床观察其成瘾性或依赖情况；必须要经过临床审核、明确适应证和详细记录备案后，方可重配此类药品；唑吡坦和佐匹克隆的注意事项同苯二氮䓬类药物。口服咪达唑仑和硝甲西泮（nimetazepam）不得用于门诊患者。MOH 还发布了《关于开具苯二氮䓬类药物及其他镇静催眠药的管理指南》(Administrative Guidelines on The Prescribing of Benzodiazepines and Other Hypnotics)[16]（详见附件2），强调开具有苯二氮䓬类药物及其他镇静催眠药的长期用药处方若不经临床审核不得重配；此外，无论该类药品是首次还是重复开具，均应将下列信息详细记录于患者的病历中：①所开具苯二氮䓬类药物或其他镇静催眠药的品种或药品名称、使用剂量、用药疗程；②开具苯二氮䓬类药物或其他镇静催眠药的适应证和 / 或正当理由；③使用苯二氮䓬类药物或其他镇静催眠药后出现药物耐受性、生理或心理依赖性以及不正当使用或滥用等情况的相关生理指标或证据（例如：皮肤上的针迹、不正常的嗜睡等）。

三、慢性病治疗用药

对于口服降糖药、降压药、调脂药等慢性病长期治疗用药，医师会根据患者病情需要选择使用单次用药处方或长期用药处方，以及长期用药处方取药的最大时限[17, 18]。在新加坡，对于非慢性病用药，医师也可以按照临床需求开具长期用药处方并注明取药间隔，然而这毕竟只是少数情况。

第四节　新加坡慢性病长期用药处方的安全隐患与风险防范

尽管慢性病长期用药处方在新加坡已经实施了几十年，但在处方质量和运作环节上仍存在一些安全风险，主要体现在处方开具时重配信息不规范、患者上交伪造处方、重配处方流程中出现差错这几个方面。以下是新加坡防范风险的举措：

一、有立法和规章制度支持

从法律层面上，为了保证长期用药处方运作过程的安全有效，新加坡《药品法》[Medicines Act（Chapter 176）][17] 和《健康产品法》[Health Products Act（Chapter 122D）][19] 对长期用药处方的开具、调配、发药等环节均作出了明确规定：①在处方开具时，若所开处方为长期用药处方，则处方者需要在处方中注明治疗药物重配的次数以及重配的时间间隔；②在处方调配及发药时，若处方者未注明该处方为长期用药处方，则只能调配一次，药师在调配及发药时需明确注明药师姓名、调配地点和日期，处方保留至少2年；③若处方者注明该处方为长期用药处方，则在处方调配及发药时，药师重配药品次数不得超过处方规定的总次数，并且在每次调配及发药时均需明确注明药师姓名、重配地点和重配日期，最后一次重配后，收回处方并且保留至少2年；④在处方调配及发药时，若处方为长期用药处方，但未注明重配次数，则重配不得超过3次；若处方为长期用药处方，但未注明重配时间间隔，则时间间隔不得少于3天。

二、有规范的操作流程和责任分工

从实践操作上，医院药房的工作人员会通过诸多环节对处方进行审核，以避免风险，确保用药安全：①在登记处，接待员会对处方的有效性及合法性进行初步审核，并与患者确认此次要取的药品数量以及希望使用何种支付方式等信息。处方需完全符合法律规定，若发现有伪造或篡改之嫌，药师应当收集足够证据并立即向警方和新加坡卫生科学局合规部门（Compliance Branch of the Health Science Authority）报案[18]。②在录入处，药学技术员会根据处方识别码从医院信息系统中调取该患者的电子处方，进一步确保处方的真实有效，核对是否为正确的患者、正确的药品、正确的用量、正确的用法、正确的疗程、对处方药品无过敏史记录等，并且在药房信息系统中创建患者的当次处方。③在审核处，药师对录入处药学技术员创建的当次处方所有信息的准确性进行复核，并对处方用药进行临床审核，如果有问题，药师会与处方者进行电话沟通。④药学技术员打印出药品标签，同时与处方药品信息进行核对。⑤调配并打包好的药品经传送带传送至一名负责审核的药师处，该药师会再次对照处方审核药品并且对患者用药进行临床审核。⑥窗口药师在发药前，进行药品的最终核对，将药品发给患者并进行用药指导。

三、有药师的用药辅导和书面说明

药师将药品发给患者时，需要将充足的信息提供给患者来保证药品安全、正确、有效的使用，这是一种专业而且必要的药学实践。为了有效地进行患者用药教育，药师对每一位患者均需要同时使用语言和文字两种方式进行。若只用文字注释而不用语言解释，则可能导致患者的误解或困惑；反之，若只用语言交流而不进行文字注明，则患者很容易遗忘。

按照新加坡药学会发布的《优良药学实践规范》(Good Pharmacy Practice Guide)（详见附件3）[18]，药师对患者的用药教育需要包括以下要点：①药品名称及其适应证；②用药方案（剂量、频率、疗程）；③特殊准备说明（例如：抗生素混悬剂需要使用常温饮用水进行配制后使用）；④特殊用法说明（例如：正确使用吸入剂和透皮贴剂）；⑤药物与药物、药物与食物之间可能发生的相互作用或其他配伍禁忌；⑥可能发生的药物副作用，包括当出现副作用时患者应该做些什么和避免做些什么；⑦药物不良反应；⑧漏服药品该如何处理；⑨正确的药品贮存方式；⑩对于特殊患者或特殊药品需要特别关注的信息。

第五节　启示与借鉴

在新加坡，慢性病长期用药处方的模式已经融入到医院门诊药房和社区药房药学服务之中，并且药学相关部门积极采用各种现代化技术去更新、改进目前现有的模式，从而解决医疗从业人员的压力、满足患者日益增长的医疗需求。新加坡目前的诸多探索和理念对我国慢性病患者门诊取药流程的改进创新和长期用药处方制度的建立有着重要的借鉴意义。

一、树立以患者为中心的理念

新加坡已经建立起并且有效维持着一个高质量的医疗卫生体系，从其建立之初的目标"所有人都能负担的医疗"，到现今政府部门每年都进行的患者满意度调查以期促进对公共医疗的完善和改进，无处不体现着以人为本、以患者为中心的理念。药学服务作为医疗卫生体系的重要组成部分，无论是其现有的服务模式还是正在开展的创新性探索，出发点均是为患者提供更加快捷、更加简便、更加安全的药学服务。从《优良药学实践规范》对患者用药教育的指导条文中亦可以看出，为了有效地进行患者用药教育，药师对每一位患者均需要同时使用语言和文字两种方式，这样既能保证患者明确理解用药教育的内容，又不至于回家后遗忘；新加坡是一个多文化民族的国家，所以适宜的患者教育尤其重要。此外，对于患者用药教育有详细的项目要求，值得我国借鉴和学习。

二、充分体现药师的价值

新加坡有世界一流的医疗服务设施和优秀的医师，并且有注册药师在工作时间内提供专业的药学服务。从慢性病长期用药处方的工作流程中可以看出，在新加坡的药房中，同时有药师和药学技术员两种人员，分工明确，配合默契。药学技术员主要负责接收处方、打印序列号、初步审核处方、药品调配及打包、打印并粘贴药品标签等工作，而药师需要负责处方重配前临床用药适宜性的审核、复核已调配的药品、与患者进行面对面的用药教育等需要药物治疗学背景和深入的药学知识的工作。

目前在中国大多医院的药房中，药师主要负责处方审核和药品调配、发药工作，尽管在发药后对于部分药品的特殊注意事项会进行交代，但迫于门诊量和等候时间等各方面的压力，还未能做到详尽的患者用药教育。开展慢性病长期用药处方工作，能够使药师真正参与到患者的用药管理中，增加与患者的沟通，及时发现患者在用药过程中可能出现的问题及后续的注意事项，将药师的作用更加充分地发挥出来。

三、多环节审核确保用药安全

新加坡有着完善的法律法规和行业规范，明确医务人员和药师的法律意识和专业职责，从源头守住医疗安全的底线。由新加坡门诊药房对慢性病长期用药处方的调配过程可以看到，在患者提交处方等待的过程中，药房工作人员完成了六个环节的审查与核对，加之自动化发药系统的精准分拣，将差错风险降至最低。而在长期用药处方的新型服务模式的介绍中亦可发现，为患者提供便捷、节省时间的同时，药师并没有放弃确保用药安全的职责，无论是后台的调配与复核，还是药师的电话回访，以及答疑解惑等药学服务，都在为患者用药安全保驾护航。药师在促进临床合理用药、保障药物质量和合理使用方面具有非常重要的作用。而目前我国关于药师的管理，在立法层面上仍需进一步加强。新加坡与我国一样，面临着人口老龄化的社会压力，无论是快捷重配服务、处方自提柜、送药上门、送药到社区药房还是网上药房服务，均是期望能够缓解医疗压力、在满足患者实际需求的前提下为患者提供更多的便捷。我们研究[20, 21]发现，国内三甲医院亦存在慢性病患者长期药物治疗的需求，而单次处方开药量过大存在诸多安全风险，因此以慢性非传染性疾病为突破口，通过开药门诊、分级诊疗、社区药房购药、慢性病长期用药处方甚至网上支付后定期代邮寄等多种形式和服务，恰当解决慢性病患者开药的实际需求，是亟须解决的问题，新加坡的慢性病长期用药处方取药模式给予了我们良好的启示。

（范倩倩，朱珠，Helen Zhang）

参考文献

［1］World Health Organization. The World Health Report 2000: Health Systems: Improving Performance［EB/OL］.（2000-05-10）. http://www.who.int/whr/2000/en.

［2］Ministry of Health. Affordable Health Care-A White Paper［M］. Singapore: Singapore National Printers for the Ministry of Health，1993: 70.

［3］William A. Haseltine 著，王丹译. 价廉质优 - 新加坡医疗的故事［M］. 北京：化学工业出版社，2016：16.

［4］Ministry of Health. 2015 Survey of Patient Satisfaction with Public Healthcare Institutions［EB/OL］.（2016-06-13）.https://www.moh.gov.sg/content/moh_web/home/pressRoom/pressRoomItemRelease/2016/2015-survey-of-patient-satisfaction-with-public-healthcare-insti.html.

［5］Singapore Department of Statistics. Latest Data［EB/OL］.（2017-02-28）. http://www.singstat.gov.sg/statistics/latest-data#17.

［6］Singapore General Hospital. Patient Service Overview［EB/OL］.（2016-08-12）.https://www.sgh.com.sg/patient-services/specialist-outpatient-services/pages/subpage.aspx.

［7］Ministry of Health. Admissions and Outpatient Attendances［EB/OL］.（2016-06-09）.https://www.moh.gov.sg/content/moh_web/home/statistics/Health_Facts_Singapore/Admissions_and_Outpatient_Attendances.html.

［8］Ong KY,Chen LL,Wong JA,et al. Dispensing medication refills without counseling［J］. Int J Health Care Qual Assur，2016，29（8）：846-852.

［9］Ministry of Health，Singapore Pharmacy Board. Pharmacy Practice Standards for Healthcare Institutions and Pharmacies in Singapore［M］. Singapore: Ministry of Health. 2001: 14.

［10］Singapore General Hospital. Pharmacy［EB/OL］.（2017-01-16）. https://www.sgh.com.sg/patient-services/specialist-outpatient-services/pages/pharmacy.aspx.

［11］Singapore General Hospital. Express Refill Service［EB/OL］.（2017-01-09）.https://www.sgh.com.sg/patient-services/specialist-outpatient-services/outpatientpharmacy/pages/

express-refill-service.aspx.

［12］SingHealth Polyclinics. Prescription In Locker Box［EB/OL］.（2017-03-03）. https://polyclinic.singhealth.com.sg/Pages/prescription-locker-box.aspx.

［13］Singapore General Hospital. Home Delivery Service［EB/OL］.（2017-01-14）. https://www.sgh.com.sg/patient-services/specialist-outpatient-services/outpatientpharmacy/pages/ home-delivery-service.aspx.

［14］Today Online. Pharmacies poised to offer prescription refills online［EB/OL］.（2015- 12-04）. http://www.todayonline.com/business/pharmacies-poised-offer-prescription-refills-online.

［15］College of Family Physicians，Academy of Medicines，Singapore Sleep Society，et al. MOH Clinical Practice Guidelines 2/2008 Prescribing of Benzodiazepines［EB/OL］.（2008-10-24）. https://www.moh.gov.sg/content/moh_web/home/Publications/guidelines/cpg/2008/prescribing_of_ benzodiazepines.html.

［16］Ministry of Health. Administrative Guidelines on The Prescribing of Benzodiazepines and Other Hypnotics［EB/OL］.（2008-10-24）.https://www.moh.gov.sg/content/moh_web/home/ Publications/guidelines/cpg/2008/prescribing_of_benzodiazepines.html.

［17］Medicines Act（Chapter 176）Medicines（Prescription Only）Order［EB/OL］. （2008-05-01）. http://statutes.agc.gov.sg/aol/search/display/view.w3p;ident=89d4917a- 6fc4-4797-a0b0-26b2055da970;page=0;query=DocId%3Ace1dda35-2048-4872-917f- 65899143140d%20%20Status%3Ainforce%20Depth%3A0;rec=0#legis.

［18］Pharmaceutical Society of Singapore. Good Pharmacy Practice Guide（Version，2009 March）［EB/OL］.（2009-03-22）. http://www.pss.org.sg/sites/default/files/good_pharmacy_ practice_guidelines.pdf.

［19］Health Products Act（Chapter 122D）Health Products（Therapeutic Products） Regulations 2016［EB/OL］.（2016-07-15）.http://statutes.agc.gov.sg/aol/search/display/view. w3p;page=0;query=DocId%3Aee5a72da-98e9-453d-ac1a-3d9e29359335%20Depth%3A0%20 ValidTime%3A15%2F07%2F2016%20TransactionTime%3A15%2F07%2F2016%20 Status%3Apublished;rec=0;whole=yes.

［20］范倩倩，杨根治，朱珠，等. 通过门诊处方开药量谈其安全风险［J］. 中国医

院药学杂志，2016，36（15）：1233–1236.

［21］范倩倩，杨根治，朱珠，等．门诊开药6个月量的处方必要性分析与风险探讨［J］．中国医院药学杂志，2016，36（21）：1831–1834.

附件 1　新加坡卫生部关于开具苯二氮䓬类药物的临床实践指南（节译）

药理学方面的考虑

应常规告知患者服用镇静催眠药或抗焦虑药可能会引起嗜睡并影响从事需要精神集中或身体协调的危险活动的能力（例如：操作机器或驾驶机动车辆）。同样，在服药期间也应避免饮酒。

Grade B，Level 2++

告知患者，服用苯二氮䓬类药物或佐匹克隆/唑吡坦时，可能会对记忆力产生影响（例如：健忘）。在服药期间若出现任何行为或精神不适（例如：抑郁症），应向医生报告。

Grade B，Level 1+

精神病学用途——失眠、精神分裂症、抑郁和焦虑

使用唑吡坦和佐匹克隆的注意事项，与苯二氮䓬类药物相同。

Grade A，Level 1+

如患者出现失眠，并怀疑与身体、心理或苯二氮䓬类药物滥用或依赖性问题有关，应将其转至适宜的专科医师处就诊。

Grade D，Level 4

如果患者出现急性失眠（不足 4 周）且病情较重，感到痛苦并影响日常生活，并且希望能够快速好转，此时可以考虑短疗程（最多 2~4 周）使用苯二氮䓬类药物或其他类似的镇静催眠药。

Grade A，Level 1+

当使用苯二氮䓬类药物作为催眠药时，为减少药物副作用和依赖性风险，应使用最低有效剂量和最短疗程。

Grade D，Level 4

对于长期失眠（长于 4 周）的患者，应以非药物疗法为主。

Grade A，Level 1+

对于伴有焦虑和 / 或失眠的抑郁症患者的初始治疗，可以联合使用抗抑郁药和苯二氮䓬类药物（疗程不超过 4 周）。

Grade A，Level 1+

苯二氮䓬类药物滥用和依赖

由于疗效尚不明确，不推荐长期使用苯二氮䓬类药物（例如：用于治疗失眠或焦虑症状）。因此苯二氮䓬类药物的长期用药处方，必须要有临床审核、明确的适应证，且需要详细记录备案后方可重配药品。

Grade A，Level 1+

苯二氮䓬类药物应以最低有效剂量间断给予(例如：每 2 或 3 晚服药 1 次)，以期短疗程缓解失眠（2~4 周）。

Grade D，Level 4

即使以治疗剂量服用苯二氮䓬类药物，也不建议疗程超过 2~4 周（特别是半衰期短的药物）。

Grade A，Level 1+

对于所有接受苯二氮䓬类药物治疗的患者，应常规告知该类药有形成依赖性的风险。

Grade A，Level 1+

如可能，应建议患者尽量在同一医师指导下诊治和处方苯二氮䓬类药物，以便临床监测其滥用和依赖的风险。

Grade D，Level 4

苯二氮䓬类药物不适用于多药滥用的患者。因此，医师在开具苯二氮䓬类药物之前，应检查患者是否有任何静脉用药的迹象。

Grade D，Level 4

口服咪达唑仑（例如：Dormicum®）和硝甲西泮（例如：Erimin®）成瘾性高并且在新加坡常被吸毒者滥用，因此不建议常规用于门诊患者。

Grade D，Level 3

为减少戒断症状，苯二氮䓬类药物应在监测下逐渐减量。

Grade A，Level 1+

（范倩倩 译 Helen Zhang 审校）

附件 2　关于开具苯二氮䓬类药物及其他镇静催眠药的管理指南（节译）

1.每一位执业医师都应当合理使用苯二氮䓬类药物。该类药物在治疗失眠、焦虑和其他精神疾病时，有时会出现不合理使用的情况，因而造成一些不期望看到的结果，比如药物耐受性和依赖性的发生。

2.为了帮助执业医师合理使用苯二氮䓬类药物，卫生部联合相关专家和专业机构对 2002 年发布的《关于开具苯二氮䓬类药物的指南》进行更新和修订。

3.建议所有执业医师熟知并遵守 2008 年修订的关于开具苯二氮䓬类药物及其他镇静催眠药的指南。

4.此外，从该管理指南生效之日起，要求所有执业医师立即遵守（见附件 A），目的是为了协助卫生部监测并记录所有患者苯二氮䓬类药物使用的合理性。

5.提醒所有执业医师，根据《药物滥用条例》第 19 条，当执业医师在诊疗过程中认为或有合理证据怀疑患者有药物滥用之嫌时，需在就诊后的七日内，同时向医疗服务主任以及禁毒中心主任提供该患者的以下信息：

（a）姓名；

（b）身份证号码；

（c）性别；

（d）年龄；

（e）地址；

（f）该患者成瘾的药物。

通报表格样本见附件 B。

医疗服务主任：K SATKU 教授

附件 A　关于开具苯二氮草类药物及其他镇静催眠药的管理指南

患者病历的记录与维护

（a）与某位患者相关的所有信息必须合并记录到该患者的唯一病历中。这些信息必须清晰地备案。

（b）当卫生部或新加坡医疗委员会有需求时，必须能够复制每位患者的病历。

（c）对于使用苯二氮草类药物或其他镇静催眠药的患者，以下信息必须记录在其病历中：

（i）全面的病史，包括社会心理学方面的病史和以前使用苯二氮草类药物或其他镇静催眠药的用药史；

（ii）全面的查体结果，包括滥用苯二氮草类药物或其他药物的证据；

（iii）如果患者使用苯二氮草类药物或其他镇静催眠药后出现戒断症状，也需要记录在案。

（d）无论是首次还是重复开具处方，每一次为患者开具苯二氮草类药物或其他镇静催眠药时，均须将以下信息记录于患者病历中：

（i）所开具苯二氮草类药物或其他镇静催眠药的品种或药品名称、使用剂量、用药疗程；

（ii）开具苯二氮草类药物或其他镇静催眠药的适应证和/或正当理由；

（iii）使用苯二氮草类药物或其他镇静催眠药后出现药物耐受性、生理或心理依赖性以及不正当使用或滥用等情况的相关生理指标或证据（例如：皮肤上的针迹、不正常的嗜睡等）。

苯二氮草类药物的使用

（e）强烈不建议医师开具成瘾性高的苯二氮草类药物，例如：咪达唑仑和硝甲西泮（咪达唑仑用于外科手术的情况除外）。

（f）当使用苯二氮草类药物或其他镇静催眠药治疗失眠时，应间断给予（例如：每 2 或 3 晚服药一次），并且只在必要时使用。

（g）执业医师应常规告知患者使用苯二氮䓬类药物可能会出现反跳性失眠，并做好相应记录。

（h）苯二氮䓬药物或其他镇静催眠药的用量应是能够缓解症状所需的最低有效剂量。

（i）应避免同时开具两种或多种苯二氮䓬类药物。

（j）苯二氮䓬类药物或其他镇静催眠药的长期用药处方若不经临床审核不得重配。

（k）如果对苯二氮䓬类药物或其他镇静药的用量或如何减量有疑问，应咨询精神科医师或其他专科医师。

（l）应当谨慎使用苯二氮䓬类药物或其他镇静催眠药，避免过度镇静（例如：可能会给驾驶、操作重型机械等的患者带来危险）。

（m）对于有饮酒史或有酒精或其他药品滥用证据的患者，开具苯二氮䓬类药物时应小心谨慎。

转诊至专科医师

（n）对于有以下情况的患者，不应再开具苯二氮䓬类药物或其他镇静催眠药，而需转诊至相应的专科医师处接受进一步治疗：

（i）需要或已经开具苯二氮䓬类药物或其他镇静催眠药累计超过8周的患者；

（ii）已经在先前就诊的专科或综合医院接受过高剂量和/或长疗程的苯二氮䓬类药物治疗的患者。应将这些患者转回各自的专科医师处接受进一步治疗，直到可以戒断苯二氮䓬类药物或其他镇静催眠药；

（iii）不接受专科医师所提出的减少苯二氮䓬类药物或其他镇静催眠药用量的建议或警告的患者。

（o）对于拒绝接受转诊至专科医师的患者应给予适当的教育，并将这种拒绝行为记录在患者的病历中。对于拒绝转诊和转向激怒型的患者，应当报警。

（范倩倩　译　Helen Zhang　审校）

附件3　优良药学实践规范（节译）

（F）药品的调配

药师负责并直接监督一切与药品调配相关的工作，包括药品的选择、配制以及用药咨询。

1）接收医嘱或处方

药师应在调配前对每条医嘱或每张处方进行审核，如有任何问题或疑问应立即解决。药师需要审核并确认的信息如下：

ⅰ）处方或医嘱无伪造或篡改。如有伪造或篡改之嫌，药师应当收集足够的证据并立即向警方和新加坡卫生科学局合规部门报案。

ⅱ）完全符合法律要求。

ⅲ）有明确的药物使用适应证。

ⅳ）用药方案（剂量、频率和疗程）合理。

ⅴ）用药方案中无重复用药。

ⅵ）无药品使用禁忌证，如：过敏等。

如药师认为医嘱或处方存在不清晰或用药方案不合理的情况（例如：大剂量用药或超说明书适应证用药），则应在调配前与相关医师沟通并做好干预记录。

2）干预

任何形式的干预都应在医嘱或处方上做好记录。需要记录的具体信息应包括以下内容：

ⅰ）所涉及医生的姓名，若医生姓名无法获得应记录诊所助理的姓名。

ⅱ）写明用药干预的原因。

ⅲ）用药干预的结果。

ⅳ）用药干预的时间和日期。

ⅴ）进行用药干预的药师姓名并由本人签字。

3）包装和标签

ⅰ）标签信息

所有调配并发放给患者的药品，其标签必须包含以下信息：

a）药品的通用名称或专有名称、剂型、重量和质量。

b）用法用量的相关说明。

c）患者姓名，若是给动物使用的药品，则注明该动物所有者的姓名。

d）调配日期。

e）处方号或其他可识别的号码。

f）调配药品的药房名称，地址和电话号码。

g）关于药品正确贮存的方法（哪里适宜贮存）和有效期（哪里可以找到）的说明。

h）相关警示说明（例如：英国国家处方集中所列出的内容）和其他特殊注意事项。

ii）标签的可读性

所有标签应使用计算机或打字机打印，文字整洁，大小均匀，确保打印效果清晰。如果出现打印错误，则应重新打印标签。

iii）语言和表达

a）注意所使用的措辞不会出现模糊不清或存在歧义的情况。

例如：表达药品使用剂量与频率的词句要分开——"每次一片，每日三次"；

避免使用小数——应使用"服用 $1\frac{1}{2}$ml"而不是"服用 1.5ml"

b）尽可能使用通俗易懂的非专业语言，例如：使用"ear"而不是"otic"或"aural"，使用"eye"而不是"ophthalmic"。

c）使用恰当的语言，例如"每晚"与"晚上"意义不完全相同；"需要时使用"与"必要时使用"意义不完全相同。

d）酌情使用描述性语言，例如："搽"搽剂，"敷"洗液，"啜"糖浆。

iv）药房药师准售药品的用药说明

药房药师准售药品的标签必须包含用药的适应证和各个年龄段的用量信息。

v）调配时使用的药品包装

a）应尽可能使用厂家的原包装。

　　b）对于再次分装的药品，所使用的包装应与厂家的规格或官方标识一致。

vi）包装上标签的粘贴

　　a）所有标签均应牢固粘贴于药品的主包装上，但计量型喷雾剂除外，其标签可粘贴于外部容器或盒子上。

　　b）注意确保标签粘贴于包装上时不起皱或弯曲。

　　标签应包括以下信息：

　　厂家名称

　　有关药品使用、贮存和适应证的说明

　　药品的通用名称和专有名称

　　有效期（一些不适宜的情况除外，例如：重组抗生素混合物和滴眼剂）

　　批号

4）指导

药师向患者提供充足的药品信息从而确保患者能够安全、正确、有效地用药，这是一种专业而必要的药学实践。

药师应采用语言和文字两种形式来更加有效地完成这项任务，因为若只用文字注释而不用语言解释，则可能导致患者的误解或困惑；反之，若只用语言交流而不进行文字注明，则患者很容易遗忘。

药师对患者的用药教育需要包括以下要点：

i）药品名称及其适应证

ii）用药方案（剂量、频率、疗程）

iii）特殊准备说明（例如：抗生素混悬剂需要使用常温饮用水进行配制后使用）

iv）特殊用法说明（例如：正确使用吸入剂和透皮贴剂）

v）药物与药物、药物与食物之间可能发生的相互作用或其他配伍禁忌

vi）可能发生的药物副作用，包括当出现副作用时患者应该做些什么和避免做些什么

vii）药物不良反应

viii）漏服药品该如何处理

ix）正确的药品贮存方式

x）对于特殊患者或特殊药品需要特别关注的信息，应常规使用各个药品的患者信息小册子和厂家提供的患者用药指导小册子。最好在向患者调配药品前，将主要面向专业医务人员的产品说明书提前取出。

（范倩倩　译　Helen Zhang　审校）

第九章　中国台湾地区慢性病长期用药处方项目的研究与借鉴

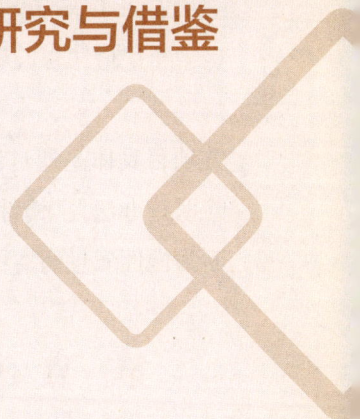

随着人口老龄化加快，我国台湾地区慢性病患者日益增多。根据台湾地区"健康保险局"（以下简称"健保局"）2007年的统计数据表明，整个台湾地区有超过700万的人罹患慢性疾病，其中有三分之一的患者病情稳定。由于慢性病患者需要定期看医生及长期服药控制，因此每次看诊均需要经历挂号、看诊、开药等流程，不仅为患者带来许多不便，而且增加了患者经济负担。因此，台湾地区自1995年开始实施"全民健康保险医疗办法"，在此社会大背景下，与全民健保制度同步推行慢性病连续处方项目（注：依台湾地区"全民健康保险医疗办法"，本书的慢性病长期用药处方即台湾地区的慢性病连续处方笺，本章沿用慢性病连续处方笺。）[1]。台湾地区的慢性病连续处方项目具体是通过慢性病长期用药处方政策实施，主要表现为"全民健康保险医疗办法""慢性病连续处方笺释出制度"的发布，规定针对那些经医生诊断为慢性病且病情稳定的患者，可以开立长期用药处方笺。

第一节　中国台湾地区慢性病连续处方取药流程

一、慢性病连续用药处方取药流程

根据台湾地区"全民健康保险医疗办法"（见附件1），当医生评估慢性病患者病情稳定且须长期使用相同处方药品治疗时，可以开立慢性病连续处方笺。此外，该类患者也可主动要求医生开立慢性病连续处方笺，特约药局❶可受理特约医院及诊所慢性病连续处方笺调剂作业。自处方开立之日算起，慢性病连续处方笺有效期为3个月；最多能调剂92天的药量[2]，但需分次调剂，每次可给予30天以内的用药量。患者持慢性病连续处方笺再次取药时，既可以在原就诊医院或诊所取药，也可以到其他"健保局"特约的药局或医院拿药，

---

① 注：药局即国内的药房或药店。在台湾地区，药局与药房是不同的两个概念，药局负责人必须具有药师或药剂生资格，而且需执业登记；药房负责人则可以不是药师或药剂生，但是必须聘请药师或药剂生当管理人，也需有执业登记；此外，药房不可出售医师处方用药，而药局则可以在有医师处方的前提下出售处方用药。

从而可以进一步节省患者时间与交通费用。

慢性病连续处方笺基本取药流程如下：

处方者开出连续三个月处方笺→初次在原就医机构进行首月药品调剂→第二、三月份交给家庭所在地周边的"健保局"授权的药局进行药品调配→由"健保局"授权的药局进行划价（划价柜台写入健保卡）、调剂→药师将调剂好的药品交付患者，患者核对领药。

慢性病连续处方笺的具体调剂流程如下：

1.处方确认：包括患者姓名、性别、年龄、保险资格，处方者姓名、住址、电话、医师证书与执业执照号码及开立处方日期等事项。

2.处方审核：包括疾病名称、药品名称、用法、用量、天数、剂型、剂量、配伍禁忌等事项。

3.药品调配：包括书写药袋、标签，并依处方内容调配。

4.核对药品及交付药品：包括核对药品、用法、用量、给药途径及使用指示等事项，并交付药品予患者（"健保保险对象"）。

5.用药指导：指导患者（"健保保险对象"）服用方法、储存方法、药品的副作用及注意事项。

6.处方调剂完成后，应于处方笺签注调剂日期及签名，并依规定保存。

二、慢性病连续处方笺作业注意事项

根据台湾地区"全民健康保险医疗办法"，慢性病连续处方笺在实施时尚需要注意以下注意事项：

1.慢性病连续处方笺至有效截止日内有效。

2.患者（保险对象）持慢性病连续处方笺调剂时，须至上次给药期届满前七日内，凭原慢性病连续处方笺进行再次调剂。

3.进行慢性病连续处方笺调剂时需持处方笺、健保 IC 卡及身份证件领药。

4.如有遗失慢性病连续处方笺或超过有效截止日，应再次就诊重新开立处方；若遇第二次领药超过时限，可持第三次领药处方进行领药，第二次领药处方作废。

5.患者就医或住院时应向医生出示慢性病连续用药处方笺，以免重复用药。

6.如患者因即将出境而预估所领药品不够使用时，可于药品划价时出具足以证明出境的相关文件（如机票复印件等），可多领取一个月的药品，但当次全部给药量以二个月为限。

7.如果患者存在以下特殊情况之一：预定出境超过2个月、返回离岛地区、远洋渔船或国际航线船舶船员，出海作业期间、或为罕见疾病患者，无法或不便领取第2个月及第3个月用药时，可与医院（诊所、药房）签订"切结书"（类似"协议书""声明文件"）（见附件2），从而可以一次性领取慢性病长期用药处方总给药量。

8.如患者因下列特殊情况之一：行动不便或远洋渔船或国际航线船舶船员，出海作业期间，导致本人无法亲自就医领药时，可与医院（诊所）签订"切结书"（见附件3），可委托他人向医师陈述病情，并由医师依专业决定是否再开给相同处方。

9.慢性病长期用药处方划价后应于三天内（不含节假日）至药房领药。

10.持慢性病长期用药处方者，服药期间如病情发生变化，应立即就医。

第二节　中国台湾地区连续处方笺取药模式的制度及资源支撑

一、中国台湾地区医药分业制度

中国台湾地区自1997年3月1日起由台北市和高雄市率先施行医药分业，除澎湖县、台东县、花莲县属台"卫生署"（现为"卫生福利部"）公告的偏远地区外，其他地区在1999年年底前均已实施医药分业[3]。"医药分业"是指在疾病治疗过程中，医生负责诊断、治疗及开立处方笺，而药师则依医师的处方调剂并交付药品，同时为患者提供药物咨询，医药共同负起照顾患者的责任[4]。

中国台湾地区对医药分业制度大力推行，尤其是实施慢性病连续处方笺释出政策，充分彰显了医药分业制度的优点。慢性病连续处方笺政策在实施过程中离不开两个关键的环节，即医生评估患者病情并开立连续处方笺和药师对后续的连续处方笺的调剂工作。由于"医药分业"制度的实施，病患在医院或诊所看完病、拿到慢性病连续处方笺后，即使在自己看不懂的情况下，也可以拿着这张处方笺到任何一处自己信任的"健保特约药局"进行药品调剂及领取，从而保障了患者"知"与"选择"的两项权利[5]。此外，药师在调剂过程中除了认真核对药单、调配药品外，还会告诉患者药物合理使用的相关信息并提供相应的用药咨询，并将患者使用过的药品做成记录，形成个人或家庭的用药档案[6]。由此可见，医药分业制度的实施，不仅提高了药师的专业形象，使其得到社会认知及肯定，而且能为患者提供更详细的用药指导，从而使其在慢性病连续处方笺调剂过程中发挥重要的作用。

二、中国台湾地区"药事服务费"制度

中国台湾地区的药事服务费起源于 20 世纪 80 年代末，包括药品调剂费、药品耗损及管理等费用。1995 年台湾地区实施"全民健康保险医疗办法"，并于 1997 年开始推行"医药分业"政策，规定由药师负责调剂药品及提供用药指导咨询。早期的药事服务费即为药品调剂费[7]，但随着药师职业的不断发展及其专业素养的不断提高，中国台湾地区药师越来越多的参与到其他药事服务当中，药师照护服务也逐步得到社会认可，并进入健保的支付项目。"台湾健保署"颁发的"全民健康保险医疗服务给付项目及支付标准"对"药事服务费"的收取做出了明确规定[8]。

中国台湾地区药师调剂费用主要包括处方确认、处方审核、药品调配、核对及交付药品、用药指导、药历管理及药品耗损、包装、仓储及管理等费用，以浮动点数计算，费用水平根据处方的种类和提供药事服务机构的级别来确定。台湾地区的医疗机构级别包括特约药局、基层院所、地区医院、区域医院和医学中心；处方种类主要分为普通处方给药 7 日内、慢性病处方（7~13 日、14~27 日内以及 28 日以上）、放射性药品处方、全静脉营养注射剂处方（TPN）和化学肿瘤药品处方。所在的医疗机构级别越高，单张处方调剂

的费用越高；处方调配难度越大，处方调剂费用越高，处方种类不同对应的费用也不同[9]，详细可参见表9-1（2015年"健保"门急诊处方调剂费用规定）。

表9-1　2015年"健保"门急诊处方调剂费用规定[8]

诊疗项目	特约药局	基层院所		地区医院	区域医院	医学中心	支付点数
		医生调配	药师调配				
门诊药事服务费（医院部分）							
一般处方给药（7天内）					√	√	50
				√			45
慢性病处方给药（13天内）					√	√	50
				√			45
慢性病处方给药（14~27天）					√	√	59
				√			52
慢性病处方给药（28天以上）					√	√	69
				√			64
门诊药事服务费（诊所及药局部分）每人每天80张内（山地离岛地区100张内）							
一般处方给药（7天内）	√						48
			√				33
		√					14
慢性病处方给药（13天内）	√						48
			√				33
		√					14
慢性病处方给药（14~27天）	√						59
			√				35
		√					24

续　表

诊疗项目	特约药局	基层院所		地区医院	区域医院	医学中心	支付点数
		医生调配	药师调配				
慢性病处方给药（28 天以上）	√						69
			√				45
		√					35
门诊药事服务费（诊所及药局部分）每人每天 81~100 张内（山地离岛地区 101~120 张内）	√		√				18

注：支付点数是台湾健保局核算药品支付标准时使用的一种计算方法，依据不同的服务成本和技术而规定不同的点数值，根据每年的保险基金规模换算出每个点数对应的金额。每个点数对应的金额随着台湾健保总支出预算水平变化而变化。

由此可见，随着慢性病处方给药时间的延长，健保支付比例也逐渐增加，另外，在诊所及药局门诊药事服务费中，医生调配药品支付的点数均明显低于药师调配支付点数，从侧面也反映了健保政策对医药分业制度的推行和对药师价值的肯定。药事服务费制度的实施，一方面体现了药师在药事服务中的重要性，激发了药师工作的积极性，另外一方面对慢性病连续处方笺制度的执行也提供了相应的政策保障。

三、中国台湾地区社区药局众多，药事人员充裕

中国台湾地区于 1997 年实施医药分业制度，将药品调剂和药物咨询工作定位于主要由社区药局的药事人员负责，并将社区药局的功能与定位定义为以下几个方面：一是药品调剂服务和处方判断性服务，接受各层级医院、诊所释出的健保处方笺，按照医生处方为病患调剂药品；二是在调配完处方后提供专业的药物咨询和用药指导服务；三是为民众提供轻微症状和非处方药物的咨询服务；四是对慢性病患者的疾病风险评估和疾病管理服务；五是对外的居家药事照护[3]。要充分发挥药师的作用，特别是保证慢性病连续处方

笺的调剂和相关用药服务能够得到确切实施，离不开数量众多的社区药局和充裕的药事服务人员。

根据中国台湾地区《2012 年版公共卫生年报》显示，中国台湾地区 2011 年底共计有 7699 家药局[5]。这些药局除了负责传统的药品供应服务还积极发展其他药事照护服务如健康促进、慢性病用药咨询、居家药学服务等。另根据文献报道，中国台湾地区 2011 年底药师执业人数 31300 人，平均每万人药事人员数 13.87 人，约为全球平均值 3.4 倍，约为经济合作与发展组织（Organization for Economic Co-operation and Development，OECD）平均值 1.8 倍，充分体现了中国台湾地区药事服务人员的充裕[10]。根据"台湾卫生署"规定，社区药局提供的服务包括：药品、营养品、医疗器械、妇儿用品等商品销售；提供慢性病连续处方笺领药与咨询服务；小区关系经营；提供简易健康体检；小区卫教讲座；建立 POS/CRM 系统，记录顾客用药习惯与过敏病史。正是有如此数量众多、功能全面的社区药局及充裕的药事人员的存在，才使慢性病连续处方笺制度的推行和实施有力充分的保障。

此外，由社区药局调剂慢性病连续处方笺还有许多优点，如方便病患，省时、省钱、节省整体社会医疗资源；在后续调剂时可再次充分确认处方合理性，并且更容易了解及监测药品的后续治疗效果；方便患者就近进行用药咨询，从而使药物发挥更佳疗效；此外，还有助于医患关系更为和谐的发展。文献研究表明，社区药师作为基层医疗服务的提供者之一，有助于提升治疗质量，对促进人民健康有直接且正面的影响[11]。

第三节　中国台湾地区连续处方笺慢性病范围和药品分类

根据中国台湾地区"全民健康保险医疗办法"，保险对象罹患慢性病，经诊断须长期使用同一处方药品治疗时，除"管制药品管理条例"所规定的第一级及第二级管制药品外，医师可以开给慢性病连续处方笺，但同一慢性病只允许开立一张慢性病连续处方笺。给予支付的健康保险慢性病范围涉及内分泌及代谢疾病、精神疾病、神经系统疾病、循环系统疾病、呼吸系统疾病、消化系统疾病等十五大类，包括常见的糖尿病、高血压、痛风、癫痫、肝硬化、慢性贫血、偏头痛等共98种。具体疾病种类详见（附表）。

第四节　中国台湾地区慢性病连续处方笺运作中存在的安全隐患与风险防范措施

一、药品替代引发的用药相关风险

根据中国台湾地区"全民健康保险医疗办法"第四十四条规定，"药品之处方，医师如未注明不可替代，药师（药剂生）得以相同价格或低于原处方药品价格之同成分、同剂型、同剂量其他厂牌药品替代。"即患者在后续第二次及第三次持慢性病连续处方笺去其他特约药局或诊所领取药品时，如该药局或诊所无首次领药时处方笺上对应厂牌的药品，但有相同成分、剂型的药品，且医师并未注明该药品不可替代的情况下，药师可以将该药品替换为相同成分、剂型、剂量且价格低于或等于原处方药品价格的其他厂牌的药品。虽然这有利于患者及时取到长期服用的药品，保证治疗的连贯性；但另一方面，也可能存在潜在的风险。这是因为患者可能对药品的具体名称及成分、剂型、剂量并不清晰，对药品的认知也十分模糊，可能无法正确理解处方笺上面的药品；另外一方面，由于药师的专业水平也可能参差不齐，对药物理解存在一定差异，即便是同一类药品，所应用的适应证也可能存在差异，因此在替代过程中也可能导致用药错误或治疗效果差异。

针对于此，可以采取的防范措施包括：对治疗效果影响重大的药品，由医师在首次开立慢性病连续处方笺时便注明"不可替代"；其次对各个特约药局或诊所的药师进行统一培训，提升专业水平，尤其是对名称相似或外观相似的药品，以及药理分类相同但适应证有所差异的药品要重点培训，从而降低药品替代风险，避免用药错误的发生。

二、社区药局药师执业能力

正如前文所述，中国台湾地区社区药局是执行慢性病连续处方笺调剂的重要场所之一，社区药局的药师也是完成慢性病连续处方笺调剂及后续用药咨询及指导的主要执行者。然而相关调查表明[12]，目前中国台湾地区民众仍认为社区药局或诊所与医院的药事服务存在差异，包括专业形象、专业服务或药品质量等方面，民众对医院的药事服务认可度更高。由此可见，社区药局药师的执业能力尚有待加强，如对处方合理性的审核、对药品禁忌证的掌握、对药品相互作用的分析等，如不能及时发现，难免在执行慢性病连续处方笺调剂时出现风险。针对的防范措施一方面可以加强慢性病连续处方笺调剂药师的资格确定，确定只有具备一定执业能力的药师才能调剂慢性病连续处方笺；另外一方面则应对社区药局药师加强培训，并定期考核，进一步加强药师的专业水平和执业能力。

三、医疗纠纷责任区分不明

尽管中国台湾地区慢性病连续处方笺制度已经实施了二十余年，然而慢性病连续处方笺释出率却仍未达目标，"台湾中央健康保险局"公布的数据显示，2008 年慢性病连续处方笺释出的平均值为 20.5%，虽然较之前有所增长，但仍不如预期[13]。研究显示[5]，台湾地区基层医师不愿开立慢性病连续处方笺的主要原因前五项原因依次为"医疗纠纷责任区分不明"、"领药流程造成民众不便"、"药师可能私自更换药品"、"药品支援系统不成熟"、"降低医患关系的密切性"，其中约 60% 的医师认为"医疗纠纷责任区分不明"是影响其开立慢性病连续处方笺的主要原因。从另一角度分析，"医疗纠纷责任区分不明"也是慢性病连续处方笺政策运行中的一个潜在风险。由于慢性病连续处方笺的开立及后续调剂由医师和药师共同完成，且民众可以到各个特约药局进行调剂，因此一旦出现医疗纠纷，法律责任的区分可能会造成分歧。此外，医师和药师的配合及相互信任也很重要，如果开立处方笺的医师和药师没有充分信任和良好的沟通，在整个慢性病连续处方笺的执行过程中就可能出现问题，特别是存在争议的疑义性处方。由此可见，在慢性病连续处方笺开立及执行过程中，相应的法律责任归属及划分也需要相应的制度进行限定，而医生和药师之间也必须保证充分的信任和及时、有效的沟通，真正达到共同协作，才能保证慢性病连续处方笺制度的良好执行。

第五节　启示与借鉴

一、方便患者，以人为本

对于病情稳定但需要长期服药的慢性病患者来说，慢性病连续处方笺政策的实施无疑为这些患者们提供了极大的便利以及费用上的节约。实施慢性病连续处方笺政策不仅可以让患者减少看诊次数，而且能够就近领药，节约路程和时间，而对于那些行动不便的患者，有的药局还提供药品邮寄服务，或者在与医院或诊所签订"切结书"后由他人代领，甚至有药师送药到家等措施[14-17]。这些措施无不体现了"以人为本"的理念，同时也有利于慢性病连续处方笺政策的实施，值得我们学习和借鉴。

二、药师在药物经济学上发挥更多的作用

药师参与整个慢性病连续处方笺的调剂，无疑整体彰显了药师的价值。研究显示，在病患实际用到药品前，药师是患者较易接触到的医疗人员，是可执行再次确认或追踪药品治疗的最佳专业[18]。我们需要借鉴的是中国台湾地区对药师参与慢性病连续处方笺调剂的相关规定和制度，如中国台湾地区"全民健康保险医疗办法"、中国台湾地区的"药事服务费制度"等，都从法律层面给予药师参与慢性病连续处方笺调剂及应获报酬做了详细而具体的规定，在制度层面对药师的地位给予相应的肯定。此外，不可否认，中国台湾地区药师的专业水平和参与药事服务的能力也值得我们学习，这从中国台湾地区药师照护取得的成效上可以得到充分体现。根据"台湾药师公会全联会"统计药事照护计划执行成果的数据表明，受照护人数在2010年、2011年、

2012 年分别为 808 人、4032 人和 4966 人，门诊就医次数降低了 29%、17%、17%。门诊医疗费用也下降了 20%、10% 和 11%，而截止 2012 年底"健保"的总医疗点数下降 15%，总药费点数也下降 11%，所节省的医疗支出总计超过新台币 5000 万元，成效显著[20]。

三、完善的配套制度及慢性病连续处方笺服务团队

自"台湾行政院卫生署"所辖"健康保险局"在"全民健康保险医疗办法"中规定慢性病长期用药处方相关调剂内容后，又先后公告"慢性病连续处方笺释出制度"、"全民健康保险慢性病连续处方笺调剂作业要点"等制度，此外，还推行了"医药分业"制度及"药事服务费"制度，从多个层面保证慢性病连续处方笺政策的顺利执行。2003 年中国台湾地区重建健保体系改造计划将推动医学中心及区域医院开立慢性病连续处方笺比率达到 15% 作为 2004 年度目标[21]，也显示了主管机关对慢性病连续处方笺政策的长期重视与导引。

此外，"台北市卫生局"、联合医院、药师公会的共同合作，于 2004 年间邀集 167 家社区药局成立慢性病连续处方笺服务团队，并于该年 8 月在当时台北市各市立医院门诊药局领药窗口旁设置慢性病连续处方笺咨询服务站，由社区药局药师志愿者们为持慢性病连续处方笺民众提供第二、三次调剂选择社区药局服务的相关倡导[22-24]。

由此可见，慢性病连续处方笺的实施和执行不仅需要相关政府机关的高度重视，制定并完善相应的配套制度，而且需要全社会包括大型医院、社区医院、政府机构及各专业学会的团队合作才能使政策更好的推行、实施。

四、充分发挥社区药局作用

如前文所述，中国台湾地区社区药局资源十分丰富，据统计，截止 2005 年 4 月底与中国台湾地区全民健康保险局完成签约的特约社区药局已有 3990 家，分布密度不亚于一般医疗先进国家[25]。中国台湾地区社区药局的发展及其在慢性病连续处方笺政策实施中的重要地位离不开行政支持。中国台湾地区"全民健康保险医疗办法"（第 4 章第 31 条）与"全民健康保险医疗办法"（第

19 条）分别载明"医师并得交付处方笺予保险对象至药局调剂"及"保险对象持特约医院、诊所医师交付之处方笺，应在该特约医院、诊所调剂或至特约药局调剂"，赋予社区执业药师处方调剂、药品发放的权利及其发挥专业技能的机会[26]。

此外，中国台湾地区社区药局功能齐全、服务全面，不仅负责基本的药品供应、药物咨询和用药指导等，还负责慢性病连续处方笺政策的宣传和推进。"台北市卫生局"、市立联合医院与药师公会间在积极合作模式下，通过设置慢性病连续处方笺咨询服务站、成立社区药局慢性病连续处方笺服务团队、建立药品物流机制等措施，极大的提升了民众对慢性病连续处方笺政策的认知、以及对慢性病连续处方笺的使用知识掌握[12]。这使中国台湾地区社区药局不仅成为慢性病连续处方笺政策的执行者，还是慢性病连续处方笺政策的推行者和倡导者，使基层民众对政策更为了解，从而大大提升了医疗服务的效率和质量。

五、慢性病连续处方笺质控及管理

为了加强慢性病连续处方笺的管理，避免重复用药及医疗资源的浪费，中国台湾地区实施了严格的质控方案和精细的管理模式。首先，为了鼓励各医院实施慢性病连续处方笺政策，"卫生署健康保险局"将"各区同院所慢性病开立连续处方笺百分比"列为每年的《医院总额专业医疗服务质量报告》（附件 4，指标 17）中的监测指标，要求各区同级院、所慢性病开立长期用药处方笺百分比应高于近 3 年全局值平均值 x（1–20%），如 2012 年该监测值为 28.81%。其次，为避免重复用药，"台湾卫生福利部"针对高血压、高血脂、糖尿病慢性病连续处方笺用药日数重复率进行监控，规定"院、所门诊高血压慢性病连续处方笺用药日数重复率如超过阈值，不予支付超过部分之高血压、高血脂、糖尿病药品费用"（见附件 4、附件 5）。其中高血压药品费用不予支付点数 =（用药日数重复率 –5.50%）× 总用药日数 ×（总药费点数 / 总用药日数）；高血脂药品费用不予支付点数 =（用药日数重复率 –5.19%）× 总用药日数 ×（总药费点数 / 总用药日数）；糖尿病药品费用不予支付点数 =

（用药日数重复率 –6.80%）× 总用药日数 ×（总药费点数 / 总用药日数）。我们可以借鉴的是中国台湾地区在慢性病连续处方笺的管理方面，一方面通过监测各医院开立慢性病连续处方笺率，规定该值的下限，以鼓励医院开立连续处方笺；另一方面，又通过监测常见慢性病如高血压、糖尿病、高血脂重复用药率，从而降低重复用药，进而减少医疗资源浪费。由此，不仅可以顺利推行慢性病连续处方笺政策，而且又避免了因该政策可能引起的重复用药的问题。

总之，历经 20 余年，台湾地区慢性病连续处方笺项目的实施极大的方便了慢性病患者，同时也在一定程度上节约了医疗资源，取得的成效显著，这与台湾地区配套制度和措施的完善、全社会团队协作、以及社区药局的发展和药师执业能力的提升密不可分。尽管慢性病连续处方笺政策实施过程中还存在一定不足，但其发展模式和宝贵经验仍值得我们借鉴，对我国慢性病连续处方笺政策的实施具有一定的参考价值和指导意义。

（胡永芳　张微微）

参考文献

［1］健康保险局：全民健康保险医疗办法．健保医字第 84004210 号．1995. Retrieved from http://dohlaw.doh.gov.tw/Chi/FLAW/FLAWDAT0201.asp?lsid=FL014028.

［2］健康保险局：全民健康保险慢性病长期用药处方笺调剂作业要点．健保医字第 88007070 号．1999. Retrieved from http://www.nhi.gov.tw/resource/Webdata/Attach_15894_1_99 法规要辑 .pdf.

［3］陈肖虹，鄢英慧，潘艳琳，等 . 台湾药事照护发展历程及现况探析［J］. 海峡药学，2013, 25（12）：184–186.

［4］张瑞芳 . 医院慢性病患者对医药分业、慢性病长期用药处方笺之认知、态度与取药行为及其相关因素［D］. 指导教授：杨铭钦教授（台湾大学），2001.

［5］白璐 . 医师、药师、民众对实施医药分业之认知、态度与经验及其对民众用药认

知，行为之影响［J］."行政院卫生署"委托研究计划，2000.

［6］黄文鸿.医药分业制度下诊所及药局良性互动之研究［J］."行政院卫生署"委托研究计划，2002.

［7］王雅静.台湾药事服务费收费情况［J］.药学评价，2010，7（6）：8-11.

［8］全民健康保险医疗服务给付项目及支付标准［EB/OL］. Retrieved from www.nhi.gov.tw/webdata/webdata.aspx?menu=20&menu_id=710&webdata_id=3633.

［9］喻鹏久，肖翔林.我国台湾地区药事服务费实践分析［J］.药品评价，2015（12）：11-14.

［10］郭奕廷.台湾药事人力资源分析［J］.药学杂志，2012，28（4）：27-31.

［11］Anderson C. Health promotion in community pharmacy: The UK situation［J］. Patient Educ Couns, 2000, 39: 285-291.

［12］董千仪，林慧玲，林昌诚等.民众对医院与社区药局慢性病长期用药处方调剂服务的观感［J］.台湾医学，2008，12: 635-643.

［13］健康保险局：九十七年医院总额专业医疗服务质量报告［J/OL］. 2008. Retrieved from http://www.nhi.gov.tw/Resource/.../19639_1_99年报医院专业版-0908.doc

［14］林昌诚.台北市慢性病长期用药处方笺释出与医药分业［R］.卫署药字第0940314639号.2005年4月28日.

［15］许炳昌.台北县慢笺e化团队.药师周刊2004年8月2日，1386期：第五版.

［16］陈本源.台中市推动慢性病长期用药处方笺释出之经验分享.台中荣总药讯，2004，11: 1.

［17］陈锦宝.桃园县药师公会国军桃园总医院-慢性病长期用药处方笺释出咨询站启动典礼.药师周刊，92年10月13日，1346期，第六版.

［18］Cranor CW, Bunting BA, Christensen DB. The Asheville Project: long-term clinical and economic outcomes of a community pharmacy diabetes care program［J］. J Am Pharm Assoc（Wash），2003, 43: 173-84.

［19］Buurma H, De Smet PAGM, Leufkens HGM, et al. Evaluation of the clinical value of pharmacists' modifications of prescription errors［J］. Br J Clin Pharmacol, 2004, 58: 503-511.

［20］药事居家照护少重复用药［N］.台湾时报，2013-06-30（11）.

［21］曲同光，医院及基层总额支付制度之实施与展望．台湾药品营销暨管理协会主办：掌握健保总额支付制度现况研讨会，台北市，台湾．2003 年 9 月 25 日．

［22］张光是，"台北市慢性病长期用药处方笺服务团队"正式启动．药师周刊 93 年 7 月 12 日，1383 期：第六版．

［23］张光是，仁爱医院咨询服务站 – 推动慢性病长期用药处方笺的前哨．药师周刊 93 年 11 月 1 日，1399 期：第四版．

［24］林昌诚，台北市慢性病长期用药处方笺释出与医药分业［R］．卫署药字第 0940314639 号．2005 年 4 月 28 日．

［25］"卫生署"，卫生统计信息网 –94 年全民健康保险统计（特约医事服务机构家数）。Available at: http://www.doh.gov.tw/statistic/data/ 全民健康保险统计 /94/3/94–T26.XLS（accessed 2007 December 9）．

［26］健康保险局：全民健保法相关法规．Available at: http://www.nhi.gov.tw/webdata/ webdata.asp?menu=1&menu_id=9&webdata_id=2091（accessed 2007 December 9）．

附件 1　中国台湾地区《全民健康保险医疗办法》及附表"全民健康保险慢性疾病范围"

全民健康保险医疗办法

"行政院卫生署" 2013 年 11 月 6 日卫署健保字第 1012660268 号令修正

第一条　本办法依"全民健康保险法"（以下称本法）第四十条第二项规定订定之。

第二条　全民健康保险（以下称本保险）保险对象之就医程序、就医辅导、保险医疗服务提供方式及其他医疗服务必要事项，依本办法之规定。

第三条　保险对象至特约医院、诊所或助产机构就医或分娩，应缴验下列文件：

一、全民健康保险凭证（以下称健保卡）。

二、身份证或其他足以证明身分之文件。但健保卡已足以辨识身分时，得免缴验。

前项第二款文件，于未满十四岁之保险对象，得以户口簿、户籍誊本等复印件或其他足以证明身分之相关文件代之。

保险对象至第一项以外之保险医事服务机构接受医疗服务，除应缴验第一项之文件外，并应缴交特约医院、诊所交付之处方。

保险对象有接受居家照护服务必要时，应由特约医事服务机构诊治医师先行评估，开立居家照护医嘱单，并由各该医院、诊所径向设有居家护理服务务部门之保险医疗机构或护理机构提出申请。

第四条　保险对象就医，因故未能及时缴验健保卡或身份证件者，保险医事服务机构应先行提供医疗服务，收取保险医疗费用，并开给符合医疗法施行细则规定之收据；保险对象于就医之日起十日内（不含例假日）或出院前补送应缴验之文件时，保险医事服务机构应将所收保险医疗费用扣除保险对象应自行负担之费用后退还。

保险对象因无力缴纳保险费，于保险人暂行停止保险给付期间，具有下列情形之一者，得检附户籍所在地村（里）长出具之清寒证明书，以保险对象之身份先行就医；因情况特殊取得清寒证明书显有困难者，得由就医之保险医事服务机构先行治疗：

一、因伤病须急诊就医或住院医疗。

二、因罹患非立即就医将危及生命之急症，或本保险重大伤病等急重症，须门诊治疗。

第五条 因不可归责于保险对象之事由，致保险对象未能依前条规定期限内，补送应缴验之证明文件时，得检附保险医事服务机构开具之保险医疗费用项目明细表及收据，依本法第五十六条规定，向保险人申请核退自垫医疗费用。

第六条 特约医院、诊所应将门诊处方交由保险对象，自行选择于该次就医之特约医院、诊所或其他符合规定之保险医事服务机构调剂、检验、检查或处置。

特约医院、诊所限于专长或设施不足，对于需转由其他保险医事服务机构提供调剂、检验、检查、处置等服务之保险对象，应开立处方，交其前往其他保险医事服务机构，接受医疗服务。

前项检验、检查之提供，得改开给保险对象转检单，提供转检服务；或开立代检单，以采取检体之委托代检方式办理。

第七条 保险医事服务机构接受保险对象就医时，应查核其本人依第三条第一项应缴验之文件；如有不符时，应拒绝其以保险对象身分就医。但须长期服药之慢性患者，有下列特殊情况之一而无法亲自就医者，以继续领取相同方剂为限，得委请他人向医师陈述病情，医师依其专业知识之判断，确信可以掌握病情，再开给相同方剂：

一、行动不便，经医师认定或经受托人提供保证文件。

二、已出海，为远洋渔业作业或在国际航线航行之船舶上服务，经受托人提供保证文件。

三、其他经保险人认定之特殊情形。

第八条 保险医事服务机构于提供门诊、急诊或住院之诊疗服务或补验健保卡时，应于健保卡登录就医纪录及可累计就医序号之就医类别一次后发还。

前项诊疗服务属同一疗程者，应仅登录可累计就医序号之就医类别一次，如为同一医师并行其他诊治，亦不得再重复登录。

前项同一疗程，指下列诊疗项目，于一定期间施行之连续治疗疗程：

一、以三十日内治疗为疗程者：洗肾、精神疾病小区复健治疗、精神科心理治疗、精神科活动治疗、精神科职能治疗、高压氧治疗、减敏治疗、居家照护及其他经保险人指定之诊疗项目。

二、自首次治疗日起至三十日内，六次以内治疗为疗程者：西医复健治疗、皮症照光治疗、简单伤口换药、非化学治疗药物同一针剂之注射、同牙位治疗性牙结石清除、同牙位牙体复形（补牙）、同牙位拔牙治疗、术后拆线、尿失禁电刺激治疗、骨盆肌肉生理回馈训练、肺复原治疗、中医针灸、伤科及脱臼整复同一诊断需连续治疗者及其他经保险人指定之诊疗项目。

三、自首次治疗日起六十日内治疗为疗程者：牙医同部位之根管治疗。

同一疗程最后治疗日为例假日者，顺延之。

第九条　保险医事服务机构于保险对象有下列情形之一者，应于其健保卡登录就医纪录，但不得登录为可累计就医序号之就医类别：

一、出院。

二、接受同一疗程内第二次以后之诊疗。

三、接受排程检查、排程检验、排程治疗、排程手术或转检服务。

四、接受第三条第四项之医疗服务。

前项排程检查、排程检验、排程治疗、排程手术或转检之检查过程中，因病情需要并行相关处置，得视同另次诊疗，登录可累计就医序号之就医类别一次。

第十条　特约医院于保险对象办理住院手续时，除精神科日间住院外，应留置其健保卡，于其出院时发还。保险对象入住慢性医院或精神科医院，如因不同诊疗科别疾病，经诊治之医师分析确须立即接受诊疗，而该医院并无设置适当诊疗科别以提供服务时，得将健保卡交还给保险对象，供其外出门诊；透析患者住院期间，经诊治之医师认定确须立即接受透析，而该医院无法提供透析之服务时，亦同。

保险对象住院期间，入住之特约医院不得以门诊方式提供其医疗服务。但入住之特约医院限于设备或专长不足，无法提供完整之检验（查）时，得以转（代）检方式，委托其他特约医事服务机构提供检验（查）服务。

第十一条　保险对象有下列情形之一者，特约医院不得允其住院或继续住院：

一、可门诊诊疗之伤病。

二、保险对象所患伤病，经适当治疗后已无住院必要。

第十二条　特约医院对于住院治疗之保险对象经诊断认为可出院疗养时，应即通知保险对象。保险对象拒不出院者，有关费用应由保险对象自行负担。

第十三条　保险对象住院后，不得擅自离院。因特殊事故必须离院者，经征得诊治医师同意，并于病历上载明原因及离院时间后，始得请假外出。晚间不得外宿。

未经请假即离院者，视同自动出院。

第十四条　保险对象罹患慢性病，经诊断须长期使用同一处方药品治疗时，除管制药品管理条例所规定之第一级及第二级管制药品外，医师得开给慢性病长期用药处方笺。

前项慢性病范围，如附表。

同一慢性病，以开一张慢性病长期用药处方笺为限。

第十五条　保险对象持特约医院、诊所医师交付之处方笺，应在该特约医院、诊所调剂或选择至特约药局调剂。但持慢性病长期用药处方笺者，因故无法至原处方医院、诊所调剂，且所在地无特约药局时，得至其他特约医院或卫生所调剂。

前项处方笺以交付一般药品处方笺及管制药品专用处方笺并用时，保险对象应同时持二种处方笺调剂。

第十六条　保险医事服务机构诊疗保险对象，有本法第四十七条应自行负担之住院费用，第五十一条或第五十二条规定不给付项目或情形者，应事先告知保险对象。

第十七条　保险对象完成诊疗程序后，保险医事服务机构应依本法规定，向保险对象收取其应自行负担之费用，并开给符合医疗法施行细则规定之收据及依药事法规定为药袋标示，其无法标示者，应开给药品明细表。

特约医院、诊所当次诊疗，未开立药品处方或处方为交付调剂者，得免开给药品明细表。

第十八条　保险对象至保险医事服务机构就医时，应遵行下列事项：

一、遵守本保险一切规定。

二、遵从医事人员有关医疗上之嘱咐。

三、不得任意要求检查（验）、处方用药或住院。

四、住院者，经特约医院通知无住院必要时，应即出院。

五、依规定缴交应自行负担之费用。

第十九条　保险对象需要输血及使用血液制剂时，应优先使用其家属、亲友捐赠或捐血机构供应之血液及其制剂。

因紧急伤病经医师诊断认为必要之输血及使用血液制剂，而捐血机构无库存血液及其制剂供应时，特约医院、诊所得向评鉴合格医院之血库调用捐血机构之血液及其制剂。

第二十条　保险对象住院，以保险病房为准；其暂住之病房等级低于保险病房时，不得要求补偿差额；暂住之病房等级高于保险病房时，亦不得要求补助差额。

特约医院应优先提供保险病房，若限于保险病房使用情形，无法提供保险病房时，应经保险对象同意，始得安排入住非保险病房，并应事先告知其应自付之病房费用差额；其后保险病房有空床时，特约医院并应依保险对象之请求，将其转入保险病房，不得拒绝。

保险对象不同意自付病房费用差额者，特约医院应为其办理转院或另行排定及通知其入住保险病房。

第二十一条　本保险病房费用，自保险对象住院之日起算，出院之日不算。

第二十二条　本保险处方用药，每次以不超过七日份用量为原则；对于符合第十四条第二项慢性病范围之患者，得按病情需要，一次给予三十日以内之用药量。

第二十三条　本保险处方笺有效期间，自处方笺开立之日起算，一般处方笺为三日（遇例假日顺延），慢性病长期用药处方笺依各该处方笺给药日数计，至多九十日；处方笺逾期者，保险医事服务机构不得调剂。

同一慢性病长期用药处方笺，应分次调剂；每次调剂之用药量，依前条规定。

第二十四条　保险对象持慢性病长期用药处方笺调剂者，须俟上次给药期间届满前十日内，始得凭原处方笺再次调剂。

前项保险对象如预定出境、返回离岛地区、为远洋渔船船员出海作业、国际航线船舶船员出海服务或罕见疾病患者，得于领药时出具保证文件，一次领取该慢性病长期用药处方笺之总给药量。

第二十五条　医师处方之药物如未注明不可替代，药师（药剂生）得以相同价格或低于原处方药物价格之同成分、同剂型、同含量其他厂牌药品或同功能类别其他厂牌特殊材料替代，并应告知保险对象。

第二十六条　为保障保险对象用药安全，药剂之容器或包装上应载明保险对象姓名、性别、药品名称、数量、天数、剂量、服用方法、调剂地点、名称、调剂者姓名及调剂年、月、日等资料。

第二十七条　保险对象如有重复就医或不当利用医疗资源之情形，保险人应予以辅导，进行就医行为了解、提供适当医疗卫教、就医安排及必要之协助，并得依其病情指定其至特定之保险医事服务机构接受诊疗服务。

前项保险对象未依保险人辅导，于指定之保险医事服务机构就医者，除情况紧急外，不予给付。

第一项辅导，得以邮寄关怀函、电访、访视或运用相关社会资源等方式进行。

第二十八条　本办法自二零一三年一月一日施行。但第六条、第七条、第十条、第二十四条自发布日施行。

附表　全民健康保险慢性疾病范围

	疾病名称（特定诊疗项目代号）
一	癌症（12）
二	内分泌及代谢疾病 甲状腺机能障碍（05） 糖尿病（01） 高血脂症（19） 威尔逊氏症（48） 痛风（07） 天疱疮（30） 皮肌炎（31） 泌乳素过高症（43） 先天性代谢异常疾病（52） 肾上腺病变引发内分泌障碍（70） 脑下垂体病变引发内分泌障碍（71） 性早熟（72） 副甲状腺机能低下症（80） 性腺低能症（Hypogonadism）（93）
三	精神疾病 精神病（47）
四	神经系统疾病 脑瘤并发神经功能障碍（73） 巴金森氏症（16） 肌僵直萎缩症（49） 其他中枢神经系统变质及遗传性疾病（54） 多发性硬化症（55） 婴儿脑性麻痹及其他麻痹性症候群（56） 癫痫（15） 重症肌无力（51） 多发性周边神经病变（74） 神经丛病变（75） 三叉神经病（76） 偏头痛（77） 脊髓损伤（81）
五	心脏病（11） 高血压（02） 脑血管病变（14） 动脉粥样硬化（57） 动脉拴塞及血拴症（58） 雷诺氏病（26） 川崎病并发心脏血管异常者（78）

续 表

	疾病名称（特定诊疗项目代号）
六	呼吸系统疾病 慢性鼻窦炎（45） 慢性支气管炎（10） 肺气肿（20） 哮喘（06） 支气管扩张症（22） 慢性阻塞性肺炎（21） 肺沉着症（59） 外因所致之肺疾病（60） 过敏性鼻炎（82）
七	消化系统疾病 消化性溃疡（08） 肝硬化（25） 慢性肝炎（03） 胃肠机能性障碍（含慢性胰脏炎、 各种胃肠息肉症、急躁大肠症候群、 胃肠糜烂性炎症、慢性大肠炎症）（23） 慢性胆道炎（18）
八	泌尿系统疾病 慢性肾脏炎（04） 肾脏感染（61）
九	骨骼肌肉系统及结缔组织之疾病 关节炎（09） 多发性肌炎（50） 骨质疏松症（27） 红斑性狼疮（24） 慢性骨髓炎（95）（须依 X 光片予以判定，如需服用抗生素，需有 CRP、ESR 检查作为判定依据）
十	眼及其附属器官之疾病 青光眼（33） 干眼症（34） 视网膜变性（35） 黄斑部变性（36） 葡萄膜炎（37） 玻璃体出血（38） 角膜变性（39）

续　表

疾病名称（特定诊疗项目代号）	
十一	传染病 结核病（17） 甲癣（29）
十二	先天畸形 先天性畸形疾病（62）
十三	皮肤及皮下组织疾病 干癣（28） 全身性湿疹（32） 乌脚病（79） 白斑（83） 脂漏性皮肤炎（84） 类淀粉沉积症（限病灶超过体表面积百分之三十以上者）（85） 类天疱疮（86） 疱疹性皮肤炎（87） 家族性良性慢性天疱疮（88） 表皮分解性水疱症（89） 严重性鱼鳞癣（含层状鱼鳞癣及鱼鳞癣状红皮症）（90） 毛囊角化症（91） 进行性全身硬皮症（92） 慢性荨麻疹（98） 异位性皮肤炎（99）
十四	血液及造血器官疾病 慢性贫血（40） 紫斑症（41） 持续性血液凝固障碍（血友病）（63） 骨髓分化不良症候群（96） Refractory Anemia RARS CMMOL RAEB RAEB-t 原发性血小板增生症（97）
十五	耳及乳突之疾病 慢性中耳炎（46） 内耳前庭病变（44） 神经性耳鸣（100）

疾病名称（特定诊疗项目代号）
其他
器官移植后药物追踪治疗（13）
汉生病（64）
痔疮（65）
摄护腺（前列腺）肥大（66）
子宫内膜异位症（42）
停经症候群（67）
尿失禁（68）
油症（多氯联苯中毒）（69）
先天性免疫不全症（53）
慢性摄护腺炎（需经摄护腺按摩取摄护腺分泌液证实者）（94）

注：表格左侧栏为"十六"

附件2　中国台湾地区《一次领全部用药保证书参考格式》

> ## 一次领取慢性病连续处方笺总给药量者　　适用

切 结 书（参考格式）

本人持慢性病连续处方笺领药，因有下列特殊情况：

□预定出境（预定出境超过2个月）

（出境目的地：　　　　　预定出境：　　　　　预定返回日期：　　　　）

□返回离岛地区

（返回离岛之地区别：　　　　　地址：　　　　　　　　）

□远洋渔船或国际航线船舶船员，出海作业期间

（服务船公司：　　　　　出海日期：　　　　　预订返回日期：　　　　）

□罕见疾病病人

（罕见疾病名称：　）

（医院、诊所如得径依病人健保卡重大伤病身分注记辨识，则可免为保证）

无法或不便领取第2个月及第3个月用药，拟一次领取本慢性病连续

处方笺之总给药量，特立书为凭，此致

医院（诊所、药局）

立书人：＿＿＿＿＿＿＿＿　　（身分证号：　　　　　　　）

　　（签名或盖章）　　　　（出生日期：　　　　　　　）

　　　　　　　　　　　　（联络电话：　　　　　　　）

年　　　月　　　日

领药日期：（医院、诊所、药局填载）

附件3 中国台湾地区《无法亲自就医保证书参考格式》

> ### 长期服药之慢性病人无法亲自就医者 适用
>
> ### 切 结 书（参考格式）
>
> 本人因属须长期服药之慢性病人，因下列特殊情况
>
> □行动不便
>
> （原因或伤病情形简述：）
>
> □远洋渔船或国际航线船舶船员，出海作业期间
>
> （服务船公司：出海日期：预订返国日期：）
>
> 无法亲自就医，同意委托_____（与本人之关系：　　），向医师
>
> 陈述病情，由医师依专业决定，是否再开给相同处方，特立书为凭，
>
> 　此致
>
> ### 医院（诊所）
>
> 　立书人：_____　（身份证号：　　　　　　　　　）
>
> 　　　　（签名或盖章）　（出生日期：　　　　　　　　　）
>
> 　　　　　　　　　　　（联络电话：　　　　　　　　　　）
>
> 受托人：_____　（身份证号：　）
>
> 　　　　（签名或盖章）　（联络电话：　　　　　　　　　　）
>
> 　　　　　　　　　　　　　　　年　　　　月　　　　日
>
> **就医日期：**　　　　　（医院、诊所填载）

附件4　中国台湾地区《2012年医院总额专业医疗服务质量报告(专业版)》

2012年

医院总额专业医疗服务质量报告

专业版

台湾"行政院卫生署"

"健康保险局"

2013 年 6 月

一、前言

制定原因：

本报告所载专业医疗服务质量指标，系依"行政院卫生署"2012年7月2日卫署健保字第1012600114号公告修正的"全民健康保险医院总额支付制度质量确保方案"附表之专业医疗服务质量指标项目呈现，并利用健保特约医疗机构申报之医疗费用申报资料，进行各指标之趋势统计。本报告区分「民众版」与「专业版」。「民众版」系供一般民众使用，介绍各指标名称主要意涵、为什么要建立这项指标及整体趋势统计；「专业版」则提供医疗与健康服务领域人员使用，呈现各指标之操作型定义、整体与6个健保分区1及各医院层级之监测统计。

意义：

本报告指标项目依其特性区分为正向指标、负向指标、及非绝对正向或负向指标。对正向指标之监测目的，在于期待指标数值呈上升或平稳但维持高于某一数值之趋势，若呈现明显下降趋势，则需进一步了解原因；反之，对负向指标，则期待指标数值呈下降或平稳但维持低于某一数值之趋势，若呈现明显上升趋势，则需进一步了解原因；对于非绝对正向或负向指标之监测目的，在于期待指标数值呈平稳趋势，若呈现巨幅变动，则需进一步了解原因。

特别声明：

本报告指标系以健保医疗费用申报资料作计算。考虑健保申报数据字段有限，无法反应完整医疗过程与结果，因此，指标数字的表现可能为多重原因造成，医疗适当性仍需就患者情形由医疗专业认定，不应直接认定反应质量，请用户解读时审慎。

注1："健保局"6个分区业务组，系指台北、北区、中区、南区、高屏及东区等六个服务范围。

二、专业医疗服务质量指标项目及定义（节选）

指标4：各区同院所门诊同一处方使用2种以上制酸剂比率（1148.01）

一、定义：

（一）数据范围：每季所有属医院总额之门诊给药案件（药费不为 0，或给药天数不为 0，或处方调剂方式为 1、0、6 其中一种）。

（二）公式说明：

分子：制酸剂药理重复案件数。

分母：制酸剂药理案件数。

1. 制酸剂：系指 ATC 码前四码为 A02A（ANATACIDS），惟下列药品参考"卫生署"药品许可证之适应症，不列入制酸剂重复使用之计算：a. ATC 码前五码为 A02AH（ANTACIDS WITH SODIUM BICARBONATE）之单方药品（程序逻辑不需处理单复方）：适应症为「酸中毒之碱化剂」

b. 医令代码为 A001046100 及 A023521100：适应症为「软便」。

2. 制酸剂重复案件：同一处方，含有两笔不同制酸剂医令，方计为重复案件。

二、监测值：以最近 3 年全局值平均值 ×（1+20%）作为上限值，2012 年监测值为 1.07%。

用药日数重复率：

指标包括「降血压药物（口服）」、「降血脂药物（口服）」、「降血糖药物（包含口服及注射剂）」及「精神疾病用药（包括精神分裂、忧郁症及安眠镇静剂三类）」等费用占率高之药品，进行同一医院同一病患不同处方开立同类药物之用药日数重复率统计。

用药日数重复率指标，自 2011 年起定义调整「允许慢性病长期用药处方笺提早拿药」，即同 ID、同院所给药日数 >=28 天，且该笔给药产生重复的原因是与另一笔给药日数 >=28 天的用药比对所产生，则在此原因下，该笔用药允许 7 天的空间不计入重复日数，另，2012 年 11 月 06 日「全民健康保险医疗办法」修正第 24 条「保险对象持慢性病长期用药处方笺调剂者，须等上次给药期间届满前 10 日内，始得凭原处方笺再次调剂，配合前述办法，修正慢笺不纳入重复日数计算之案件，2012 年 11 月起由 7 天修订为 10 天。

「给药日数」撷取该药品医令 之「医令档给药日份字段」，若同案件同药理下有多笔相关药品医令，则以给药日份最大的那一笔来代表该案件的给药日数。

指标5：各区同院所再次就医处方之同药理（降血压药物（口服））用药日数重迭率（1157.01）

一、定义：

（一）数据范围：限定为西医医院之降血压药物（口服）给药案件。

（二）公式说明：

分子：同ID不同处方之血压药物（口服）开始用药日期与结束用药日期间有重复之给药日数（允许慢性病长期用药处方笺提早拿药）。

分母：降血压药物（口服）之给药日数总和。

降血压药物（口服）：ATC前三码为C07或ATC前五码为C02AC、C02CA、C02DB、C02DC、C02DD、C02KX、C03AA、C03BA、C03CA、C03DA、C08CA、C08DA、C08DB、C09AA、C09CA，且医令代码第8码为1。

二、监测值：以可撷取数据计算最近3年全局平均值×（1+20%）作为上限值，2012年监测值为0.76%。

指标6：各区同院所再次就医处方之同药理（降血脂药物（口服））用药日数重复率（1158.01）

一、定义：

（一）数据范围：限定为西医医院之降血脂药物（口服）给药案件。

（二）公式说明：

分子：同ID不同处方之降血脂药物（口服）开始用药日期与结束用药日期间有重复之给药日数（允许慢性病长期用药处方笺提早拿药）。

分母：降血脂药物（口服）之给药日数总和。

降血脂药物（口服）：ATC前五码=C10AA、C10AB、C10AC、C10AD、C10AX，且医令代码第8码为1。

二、监测值：以可撷取数据计算最近3年全局平均值x（1+20%）作为上限值，2012年监测值为0.40%。

指标7：各区同院所再次就医处方之同药理（降血糖（不分口服及注射））

用药日数重复率（1159.01）

一、定义：

（一）数据范围：限定为西医医院之降血糖药物（不分口服及注射）给药案件。

（二）公式说明：

分子：同 ID 不同处方之降血糖药物（不分口服及注射）开始用药日期与结束用药日期间有重复之给药日数（允许慢性病长期用药处方笺提早拿药）。

分母：降血糖药物（不分口服及注射）之给药日数总和。

降血糖药物（不分口服及注射）：ATC 前五码 =A10AB、A10AC、A10AD、A10AE、A10BA、A10BB、A10BF、A10BG、A10BX。

二、监测值：以可撷取数据计算最近 3 年全局平均值 ×（1+20%）作为上限值，2012 年监测值为 0.49%。

指标 8：各区同院所再次就医处方之同药理（抗精神分裂症）用药日数重复率（1160.01）

一、定义：

（一）数据范围：限定为西医医院之抗精神分裂药物给药案件。

（二）公式说明：

分子：同 ID 不同处方之开始用药日期与结束用药日期间有重复之给药日数（允许慢性病长期用药处方笺提早拿药）。

分母：抗精神分裂药物之给药日数总和。

精神分裂药物：ATC 前五码 =N05AA、N05AB、N05AD、N05AE、N05AF、N05AH、N05AL、N05AN、A05AX。

三、监测值：以可撷取数据计算最近 3 年全局平均值 ×（1+20%）作为上限值，2012 年监测值为 0.85%。

指标 9：各区同院所再次就医处方之同药理（抗忧郁症）用药日数重复率（1161.01）

一、定义：

（一）数据范围：限定为西医医院之抗忧郁症药物给药案件。

（二）公式说明：

分子：同 ID 不同处方忧郁症药物之开始用药日期与结束用药日期间有重复之给药日数（允许慢性病长期用药处方笺提早拿药）。

分母：抗忧郁症药物之给药日数总和。

抗忧郁症药物：ATC 前五码 =N06AA、N06AB、N06AG、N06AX。

二、监测值：以可撷取数据计算最近 3 年全局平均值 ×（1+20%）作为上限值，2012 年监测值为 0.73%。

指标 10：各区同院所再次就医处方之同药理（安眠镇静）用药日数重复率（1162.01）

一、定义：

（一）数据范围：限定为西医医院之安眠镇静药物给药案件。

（二）公式说明：

分子：同 ID 不同处方之开始用药日期与结束用药日期间有重复之给药日数（允许慢性病长期用药处方笺提早拿药）。

分母：安眠镇静药物之给药日数总和。

安眠镇静药物：（不含抗焦虑药物）：前五码为 N05BA、N05BE、N05CC、N05CD、N05CF、N05CM。

二、监测值：以可撷取数据计算最近 3 年全局平均值 ×（1+20%）作为上限值，2012 年监测值为 1.42%。

指标 11：各区跨院所再次就医处方之同药理（降血压药物（口服））用药日数重复率（1163.01）

一、定义：

（一）数据范围：限定为西医医院之降血压药物（口服）给药案件。

（二）公式说明：

分子：降血压药物（口服）重复用药日数，同分区、跨院所、同 ID 不同处方之就医日期与结束用药日期间有重复之给药日数。

分母：降血压药物（口服）之给药日数

降血压药物（口服）：ATC 前三码为 C07 或 ATC 前五码为 C02AC、

C02CA、C02DB、C02DC、C02DD、C02KX、C03AA、C03BA、C03CA、C03DA、C08CA、C08DA、C08DB、C09AA、C09CA，且医令代码第 8 码为 1。

二、监测值：未订监测值，待实施 1 年后再订。

指标 12：各区跨院所再次就医处方之同药理（降血脂药物（口服））用药日数重复率（1164.01）

一、定义：

（一）数据范围：限定为西医医院之降血脂药物（口服）给药案件。

（二）公式说明：

分子：降血脂药物（口服）重复用药日数，同分区、跨院所、同 ID 不同处方之就医日期与结束用药日期间有重复之给药日数。

分母：降血脂药物（口服）之给药日数

降血脂药物（口服）：ATC 前五码 =C10AA、C10AB、C10AC、C10AD、C10AX，且医令代码第 8 码为 1。

二、监测值：未订监测值，待实施 1 年后再订。

指标 13：各区跨院所再次就医处方之同药理（降血糖（不分口服及注射））用药日数重复率（1165.01）

一、定义：

（一）数据范围：限定为西医医院之降血糖药物（不分口服及注射）给药案件。

（二）公式说明：

分子：降血糖药物（不分口服及注射）重复用药日数，同分区、跨院所、同 ID 不同处方之就医日期与结束用药日期间有重复之给药日数。

分母：降血糖药物（不分口服及注射）之给药日数

降血糖药物（不分口服及注射）：ATC 前五码 =A10AB、A10AC、A10AD、A10AE、A10BA、A10BB、A10BF、A10BG、A10BX

二、监测值：未订监测值，待实施 1 年后再订。

指标 14：各区跨院所再次就医处方之同药理（抗精神分裂症）用药日数重复率（1166.01）

一、定义：

（一）数据范围：限定为西医医院之抗精神分裂药物给药案件。

（二）公式说明：

分子：抗精神分裂药物重复用药日数，同分区、跨院所、同 ID 不同处方之就医日期与结束用药日期间有重复之给药日数。

分母：抗精神分裂药物之给药日数

精神分裂药物：ATC 前五码 =N05AA、N05AB、N05AD、N05AE、N05AF、N05AH、N05AL、N05AN、A05AX

二、监测值：未订监测值，待实施 1 年后再订。

指标 15：各区跨院所再次就医处方之同药理（抗忧郁症）用药日数重复率（1167.01）

一、定义：

（一）数据范围：限定为西医医院之忧郁症药物给药案件。

（二）公式说明：

分子：抗忧郁症药物重复用药日数，同分区、跨院所、同 ID 不同处方之就医日期与结束用药日期间有重复之给药日数。 分母：抗忧郁症药物之给药日数。

抗忧郁症药物：ATC 前五码 =N06AA、N06AB、N06AG、N06AX。

二、监测值：未订监测值，待实施 1 年后再订。

指标 16：各区跨院所再次就医处方之同药理（安眠镇静）用药日数重复率（1168.01）

一、定义：

（一）数据范围：限定为西医医院之安眠镇静药物给药案件。

（二）公式说明：

分子：安眠镇静药物重复用药日数，同分区、跨院所、同 ID 不同处方之就医日期与结束用药日期间有重复之给药日数。

分母：安眠镇静药物之给药日数。

安眠镇静药物（不含抗焦虑药物）：ATC 前五码为 N05BA、N05BE、

N05CC、N05CD、N05CF、N05CM。

二、监测值：未订监测值，待实施 1 年后再订。

指标 17：各区同院所慢性病开立慢性病长期用药处方笺百分比（1318）

一、定义：

（一）数据范围：每季所有属医院总额之门诊案件。

（二）公式说明：

分子：开立慢性病长期用药处方笺案件数。

分母：慢性病给药案件数。

开立慢性病长期用药处方笺的案件：（诊察费项目代码为慢笺）或（案件分类 =E1 且慢性病长期用药处方笺有效期间处方日份 > 给药天数且慢性病长期用药处方笺有效日份为给药天数的倍数）。

诊察费项目代码为慢笺：00155A、00157A、00170A、00171A、00131B、00132B、00172B、00173B、00135B、00136B、00174B、00175B、00137B、00138B、00176B、00177B、00139C、00140C、00158C、00159C、00141C、00142C、00160C、00161C、00143C、00144C、00162C、00163C、00145C、00146C、00164C、00165C、00147C、00148C、00166C、00167C、00149C、00150C、00168C、00169C、00178B、00179B、00180B、00181B、00182C、00183C、00184C、00185C、00187C、00189C、00190C、00191C。

慢性病给药案件：案件分类 =04、E1。

排除条件：

妇产科专科医院：医院型态别为专科医院（03），且门诊就医科别妇产科（05）之申请点数占率为各就医科别中最高者。

小儿专科医院：医院型态别为专科医院（03），且门诊就医科别小儿科（04）之申请点数占率为各就医科别中最高者。

呼吸照护病房（有申报医令 P1011C 或 P1012C 之案件）申请点数占全院申请点数 80%（含）以上之医院。

二、监测值：本项指标为正向指标，以最近 3 年全局值平均值 x（1–20%）作为下限值，2012 年监测值为 28.81%。

附件 5　中国台湾地区《增订全民健康保险档案分析审查异常不予支付指标及处理方式》

增订全民健康保险档案分析审查异常
不予支付指标及处理方式

西医基层总额部门

指标名称	038- 西医院所门诊高血压慢性病长期用药处方笺用药日数重复率
实施目的	降低不当之用药型态，降低重复用药。
指标定义	分子 - 门诊高血压慢性病长期用药处方笺重复日数 分母 - 门诊高血压慢性病长期用药处方笺给药日数 门诊高血压慢性病长期用药处方笺重复日数：指高血压同一患者同院所同品项用药日数重复。 慢性病长期用药处方笺提前 10 日领药部分不列入重复日数计算。 高血压：系指主次诊断前 3 码为 "401"（ESSENTIAL HYPERTENSION）、"402"（HYPERTENS Ⅳ E HEART DISEASE）、"403"（HYPERTENS Ⅳ E RENAL DISEASE）、"404"（HYPERTENS Ⅳ E HEART AND RENAL DISEASE）、"405"（SECONDARY HYPERTENSION）。 高血压用药：系指 ATC7 码前三码为 "C02"（ANTIHYPERTENS Ⅳ ES）"C03"（DIURETICS）"C07"（BETA BLOCKING AGENTS）"C08"（CALCIUM CHANNEL BLOCKERS）"C09"（AGENTS ACTING ON THE RENIN-ANGIOTENSIN SYSTEM） 当季医疗院所申报门诊高血压慢性病长期用药处方笺件数小于等于 10 件者不列入计算。
指针属性	负向
分析单位	依院所按季分析
分析范围	西医基层总额部门门诊案件
处理方式	院所门诊高血压慢性病长期用药处方笺用药日数重复率如超过阈值，不予支付超过部分之高血压药品费用。 不予支付点数公式＝（用药日数重复率－ 5.50%）× 总用药日数 ×（总药费点数 / 总用药日数）
核准日期及文号	2013 年 8 月 14 日卫部保字第 1020101635 号函
公告日期及文号	2013 年 8 月 22 日健保审字第 1020028087 号
实施起日	2013 年 11 月 1 日（费用年月）

指标名称	039- 西医院所门诊高血脂慢性病长期用药处方笺用药日数重复率
实施目的	降低不当之用药型态，降低重复用药。
指标定义	分子 - 门诊高血脂慢性病长期用药处方笺重复日数 分母 - 门诊高血脂慢性病长期用药处方笺给药日数 门诊高血脂慢性病长期用药处方笺重复日数：指高血脂同一患者同院所同品项用药日数重复。 慢性病长期用药处方笺提前 10 日领药部分不列入重复日数计算。 高血脂：系指主次诊断前 3 码为 "272"（DISORDERS OF LIPOID METABOLISM）。 高血脂用药：系指 ATC7 码前三码为 "C10"（SERUM LIPID REDUCING AGENTS）。 当季医疗院所申报门诊高血脂慢性病长期用药处方笺件数小于等于 10 件者不列入计算。
指针属性	负向
分析单位	依院所按季分析
分析范围	西医基层总额部门门诊案件
处理方式	院所门诊高血脂慢性病长期用药处方笺用药日数重复率如超过阈值，不予支付超过部分之高血脂药品费用。 不予支付点数公式＝（用药日数重复率－ 5.19%）×总用药日数 ×（总药费点数 / 总用药日数）
卫生福利部核准日期及文号	2013 年 8 月 14 日卫部保字第 1020101635 号函
健保署公告日期及文号	2013 年 8 月 22 日健保审字第 1020028087 号
实施起日	2013 年 11 月 1 日（费用年月）

指标名称	040- 西医院所门诊糖尿病慢性病长期用药处方笺用药日数重复率
实施目的	降低不当之用药型态，降低重复用药。
指标定义	分子 - 门诊糖尿病慢性病长期用药处方笺重复日数 分母 - 门诊糖尿病慢性病长期用药处方笺给药日数 门诊糖尿病慢性病长期用药处方笺重复日数：指糖尿病同一患者同院所同品项用药日数重复。 慢性病长期用药处方笺提前 10 日领药部分不列入重复日数计算。 糖尿病：系指主次诊断前 3 码为 "250"（DIABETES MELLITUS）。 糖尿病用药：系指 ATC7 码前三码为 "A10"（DRUGS USED IN DIABETES）。 当季医疗院所申报门诊糖尿病慢性病长期用药处方笺件数小于等于 10 件者不列入计算。
指针属性	负向

指标名称	040- 西医院所门诊糖尿病慢性病长期用药处方笺用药日数重复率
分析单位	依院所按季分析
分析范围	西医基层总额部门门诊案件
处理方式	院所门诊糖尿病慢性病长期用药处方笺用药日数重复率如超过阈值，不予支付超过部分之糖尿病药品费用。 不予支付点数公式＝（用药日数重复率—6.80%）×总用药日数 ×（总药费点数 / 总用药日数）
卫生福利部核准日期及文号	2013 年 8 月 14 日卫部保字第 1020101635 号函
健保署公告日期及文号	2013 年 8 月 22 日健保审字第 1020028087 号
实施起日	2013 年 11 月 1 日（费用年月）

附　录

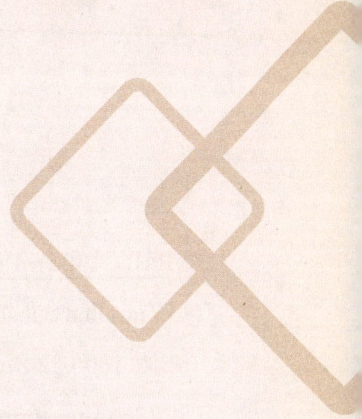

附录 1　US Code of Federal Regulations; Section 1306.22（第二章附件 1）

〔Code of Federal Regulations〕

〔Title 21，Volume 9〕

〔Revised as of April 1，2016〕

〔CITE: 21CFR1306.22〕

TITLE 21—FOOD AND

DRUGS

CHAPTER Ⅱ —DRUG ENFORCEMENT

ADMINISTRATION

DEPARTMENT OF JUSTICE

PART 1306—PRESCRIPTIONS

Controlled Substances Listed in Schedules Ⅲ，Ⅳ，and Ⅴ

Sec. 1306.22 Refilling of prescriptions.

（a）No prescription for a controlled substance listed in Schedule Ⅲ or Ⅳ shall be filled or refilled more than six months after the date on which such prescription was issued. No prescription for a controlled substance listed in Schedule Ⅲ or Ⅳ authorized to be refilled may be refilled more than five times.

（b）Each refilling of a prescription shall be entered on the back of the prescription or on another appropriate document or electronic prescription record. If entered on another document，such as a medication record，or electronic prescription record，the document or record must be uniformly maintained and readily retrievable.

（c）The following information must be retrievable by the prescription number:

（1）The name and dosage form of the controlled substance.

（2）The date filled or refilled.

（3）The quantity dispensed.

（4）The initials of the dispensing pharmacist for each refill.

（5）The total number of refills for that prescription.

(d) If the pharmacist merely initials and dates the back of the prescription or annotates the electronic prescription record, it shall be deemed that the full face amount of the prescription has been dispensed.

(e)The prescribing practitioner may authorize additional refills of Schedule III or IV controlled substances on the original prescription through an oral refill authorization transmitted to the pharmacist provided the following conditions are met:

(1) The total quantity authorized, including the amount of the original prescription, does not exceed five refills nor extend beyond six months from the date of issue of the original prescription.

(2) The pharmacist obtaining the oral authorization records on the reverse of the original paper prescription or annotates the electronic prescription record with the date, quantity of refill, number of additional refills authorized, and initials the paper prescription or annotates the electronic prescription record showing who received the authorization from the prescribing practitioner who issued the original prescription.

(3) The quantity of each additional refill authorized is equal to or less than the quantity authorized for the initial filling of the original prescription.

(4) The prescribing practitioner must execute a new and separate prescription for any additional quantities beyond the five-refill, six-month limitation.

(f) As an alternative to the procedures provided by paragraphs (a) through (e) of this section, a computer application may be used for the storage and retrieval of refill information for original paper prescription orders for controlled substances in Schedule III and IV, subject to the following conditions:

(1)Any such proposed computerized application must provide online retrieval(via computer monitor or hard-copy printout) of original prescription order information for those prescription orders that are currently authorized for refilling. This shall include, but is not limited to, data such as the original prescription number; date of issuance of the original prescription order by the practitioner; full name and address of the patient; name, address, and DEA registration number of the practitioner; and the name, strength, dosage form, quantity of the controlled substance prescribed (and quantity dispensed if different from the quantity prescribed), and the total number of refills authorized by the prescribing practitioner.

(2) Any such proposed computerized application must also provide online retrieval (via computer monitor or hard-copy printout) of the current refill history for Schedule Ⅲ or Ⅳ controlled substance prescription orders (those authorized for refill during the past six months) . This refill history shall include, but is not limited to, the name of the controlled substance, the date of refill, the quantity dispensed, the identification code, or name or initials of the dispensing pharmacist for each refill and the total number of refills dispensed to date for that prescription order.

(3) Documentation of the fact that the refill information entered into the computer each time a pharmacist refills an original paper, fax, or oral prescription order for a Schedule Ⅲ or Ⅳ controlled substance is correct must be provided by the individual pharmacist who makes use of such an application. If such an application provides a hard-copy printout of each day's controlled substance prescription order refill data, that printout shall be verified, dated, and signed by the individual pharmacist who refilled such a prescription order. The individual pharmacist must verify that the data indicated are correct and then sign this document in the same manner as he would sign a check or legal document (e.g., J.H. Smith, or John H. Smith) . This document shall be maintained in a separate file at that pharmacy for a period of two years from the dispensing date. This printout of the day's controlled substance prescription order refill data must be provided to each pharmacy using such a computerized application within 72 hours of the date on which the refill was dispensed. It must be verified and signed by each pharmacist who is involved with such dispensing. In lieu of such a printout, the pharmacy shall maintain a bound log book, or separate file, in which each individual pharmacist involved in such dispensing shall sign a statement (in the manner previously described) each day, attesting to the fact that the refill information entered into the computer that day has been reviewed by him and is correct as shown. Such a book or file must be maintained at the pharmacy employing such an application for a period of two years after the date of dispensing the appropriately authorized refill.

(4) Any such computerized application shall have the capability of producing a printout of any refill data that the user pharmacy is responsible for maintaining under the Act and its implementing regulations. For example, this would include a refill–by–refill audit trail for any specified strength and dosage form of any controlled substance (by either brand or generic name or both). Such a printout must include name of the prescribing practitioner, name and address of the patient, quantity dispensed on each refill, date of dispensing for each refill, name or identification code of the dispensing pharmacist, and the number of the original prescription order. In any computerized application employed by a user pharmacy the central recordkeeping location must be capable of sending the printout to the pharmacy within 48 hours, and if a DEA Special Agent or Diversion Investigator requests a copy of such printout from the user pharmacy, it must, if requested to do so by the Agent or Investigator, verify the printout transmittal capability of its application by documentation (e.g., postmark).

(5) In the event that a pharmacy which employs such a computerized application experiences system down–time, the pharmacy must have an auxiliary procedure which will be used for documentation of refills of Schedule Ⅲ and Ⅳ controlled substance prescription orders. This auxiliary procedure must ensure that refills are authorized by the original prescription order, that the maximum number of refills has not been exceeded, and that all of the appropriate data are retained for online data entry as soon as the computer system is available for use again.

(g) When filing refill information for original paper, fax, or oral prescription orders for Schedule Ⅲ or Ⅳ controlled substances, a pharmacy may use only one of the two applications described in paragraphs (a) through (e) or (f) of this section.

(h) When filing refill information for electronic prescriptions, a pharmacy must use an application that meets the requirements of part 1311 of this chapter.

附

录

附录 2　Multicare Health System: Pharmacist Refill Authorization（第二章附件 2）

MultiCare **⚏** BetterConnected	*Medication Guideline Ver. 1.7-1*

Title: PHARMACIST REFILL AUTHORIZATION

Scope:

This policy applies to all MultiCare Health System outpatients who are under the care of MHS providers.

Policy Statement:

To establish the MHS guideline for appropriate and safe refill authorization. The guideline also provides a collaborative practice agreement between MHS providers and pharmacists for the prescriptive authority for refill authorization and corresponding laboratory orders when appropriate.

Background/Rationale:

Refill requests present a significant disruption to MHS clinics with increased physician and nurse workload. In addition, delays in refill authorization interrupt the continuity of patient care. Pharmacists are an important resource for medication knowledge and can be used to determine the appropriateness of drug therapy. Considering the pharmacist's expertise, a variety of integrated health systems have successfully utilized pharmacists to manage medication refill authorizations. The aim of the pharmacist collaborative refill authorization is to help expedite the refill process, alleviate provider time spent on refill requests, and promote patient safety with a pharmacist drug review and enter immunizations into the patient chart received from outside sources. The use of the pharmacist refill authorization program is designed to help support the organizational goal for a Medical Home Model with improved patient health and satisfaction under a close collaboration within the healthcare team.

Special Instructions:

1. Inclusion Criteria: Patients with prescription refill requests for maintenance medications as defined in **section IV**.
2. Exclusion Criteria: Patients who are requesting prescription refills for Controlled medications, warfarin, and prescriptions for an acute treatment. Medications listed as Historical, Home health verbal order, or medications discontinued from the active drug list. Excluded criteria will be staged and forwarded to the provider.
3. Special Handling: Prescriptions listed as On-Hand, No script, Sample in EPIC. The Pharmacist will review chart notes and provide documentation. The Refill center will fill if documentation is present. If no documentation is present encounter will be forwarded to the provider.

Procedure: Determine Eligibility:
    A.　Identify if the patient's refill request meets inclusion criteria.
    B.　If refill request satisfies inclusion/exclusion criteria proceed to **section II** of policy; otherwise request is referred to primary provider.

II. Epic Chart Review:

A. Identify date of <u>last appointment</u> and review relevant progress notes from MHS health care providers.

B. <u>Check laboratory results</u> if indicated for the prescription refill.

C. The pharmacist will use their clinical judgment to determine additional information necessary to evaluate the appropriateness of the refill authorization and document into the encounter. Potential considerations may include:

    1. Indication for the medication

    2. Adherence to medication therapy

    3. Patient co-morbidities

    4. Medication profile for potential drug interactions or duplications

D. If comprehensive review is satisfactory provide refill authorization as outlined in **section III**. If insufficient information is available to safely determine the appropriateness of a refill the following actions will be taken depending on the situation:

    1. A message will be sent to the provider if the pharmacist determines that further clarification is required. Potential concerns may include length of treatment, drug interactions, medication duplication, contraindications to therapy, or other factors that may require further evaluation from the primary provider.

    2. The pharmacist will place an order for laboratory tests when indicated for the requested medication per current practice standards.

    3. Patients requiring an appointment with the provider will be directed to schedule an office visit via a forwarded encounter and if indicated a sufficient amount of medication will be approved until the next appointment.

III. Authorization Process:

A. Document request in Epic (i.e. telephone encounter). Information to include in note:

    1. Date of last appointment

    2. Date of last laboratory results if indicated

    3. Brief assessment and rationale for refill authorization and quantity approved *

B. Update medication list in Epic and send order to the patient's pharmacy using Surescript, fax, or phone.<u>* If appropriate, refills may be approved for up to a maximum of one year from the last appointment/labs based on the prescription requested.</u>

IV. Maintenance Medications

Pharmacists will have a collaborative prescriptive authority to refill prescriptions considered maintenance medications. Maintenance medications for the following indications will be evaluated for refill eligibility:

Disease State or Drug Class*	
Acne	Erectile Dysfunction
Allergies	Gastrointestinal Medications
Alzheimer's Disease	Gout, Hyperuricemia
Anemia	Hormone Therapy
Antianginals	Hyperlipidemia
Antiarrhythmics	
Anticoagulation	Hypertension
Anticonvulsants	Migraines
Antipsychotics	Nutritional Supplements
Arthritis	
Anxiety	Osteoporosis
BPH	Pain
Chronic Antibiotics/Antivirals	Parkinson's Disease
Congestive Heart Failure	Smoking cessation
Contraception	Respiratory (Asthma/COPD)
Depression	Thyroid Disorders
Dermatologic	Vascular Disease- Antiplatelet
Diabetes	

* Other indications will be considered with appropriate provider documentation available for the treatment plan.

V. Controlled Substances

Controlled substances will be staged and forwarded to the provider.

VI. Monitoring Guidelines

Appropriate laboratory results will be reviewed based on the refill medication requested using current evidence based practice standards. Guidelines for laboratory monitoring for more common medication classes are included in **Appendix A**.

VII. Quality Measures

The quality and appropriateness of pharmacy interventions will be evaluated by periodic peer review of refill encounters by a clinical pharmacist or physician.

	Related Policies: MHS P & P: Pharmacy: Electronic Prescription Transmission MHS P & P : Pharmacist Refill Authorization Guideline
	Related Forms: none **Patient Education: A description of how pharmacists can support clinical care is provided at this link.**

References:

Cassidy IB, Keith MR, Coffey EL, Noyes MA. Impact of Pharmacist-Operated General Medicine Chronic Care Refill Clinics on Practitioner Time and Quality of Care. Ann Pharmacother. 1996 Jul-Aug;30(7-8):745-51.

Cram DL, Stebbins M, Eom HS, Ratto N, Sugiyama D. Peer Review as a Quality Assurance Mechanism in Three Pharmacist-Run Medication-Refill Clinics. Am J Hosp Pharm. 1992 Nov;49(11):2727-30.

Cram DL, Maesner AT, Witmore DM. Medication Refill Clinics: The Veterans Administration Medical Center Experience. Journal of Pharmacy Practice. 1992 February; 5(1):12-21

McKinnon A, Jorgenson D. Pharmacist and Physician Collaborative Prescribing for Medication Renewals within a Primary Health Centre. Can Fam Physician 2009; 55:e86-91.

Micromedex Healthcare Series: Thomson Micromedex, Greenwood Village, CO[Accessed 8/2014].

Riege VJ, Henriksen K, Battles JB, Marks ES, Lewin DI. A Patient Safety Program & Research Evaluation of U.S. Navy Pharmacy Refill Clinics. Advances in patient safety: from research to implementation. Vol. 1, Research findings. AHRQ Publication No. 05-0021-1. Rockville, MD: Agency for Healthcare Research and Quality; Feb. 2005.

Virginia Mason Refill Protocol. Prescriptive Authority Guidelines Department of Pharmaceutical Services.

	Point of Contact:	
	Ambulatory Pharmacy Manager, 403-5542	
Approval By:		*Date of Approval:*
Pharmacy and Therapeutic Committee		*11/20/2014*
CQCC Approval		*11/05/14*
MHS Policy and Procedure		
Medical Staff Operations		
PILOT		9/16/10
QSC		12/14
Original Date:		*9/10*
Revision Dates:		*9/14; 11/14*
Reviewed with no Changes Dates:		

附

录

MultiCare Health System Pharmacist Refill Authorization Flow Diagram

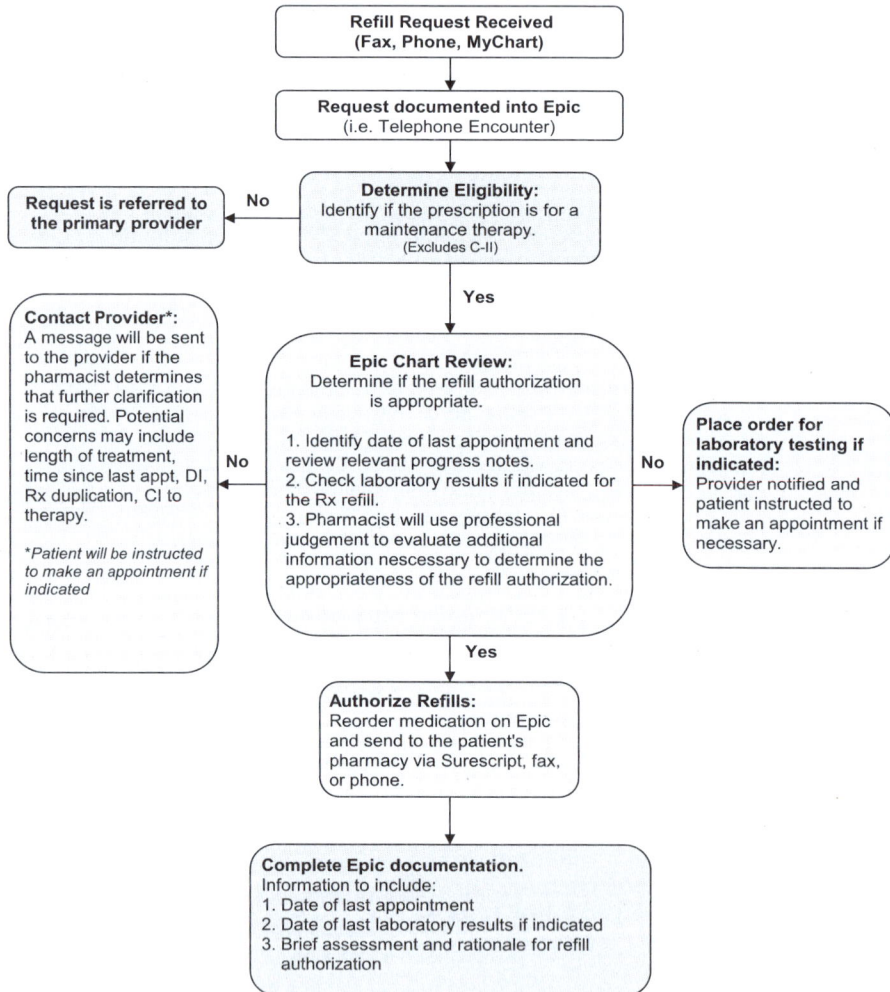

Refill Request Received
(Fax, Phone, MyChart)

Request documented into Epic
(i.e. Telephone Encounter)

Determine Eligibility:
Identify if the prescription is for a maintenance therapy.
(Excludes C-II)

No → **Request is referred to the primary provider**

Yes

Contact Provider*:
A message will be sent to the provider if the pharmacist determines that further clarification is required. Potential concerns may include length of treatment, time since last appt, DI, Rx duplication, CI to therapy.

*Patient will be instructed to make an appointment if indicated

No ←

Epic Chart Review:
Determine if the refill authorization is appropriate.

1. Identify date of last appointment and review relevant progress notes.
2. Check laboratory results if indicated for the Rx refill.
3. Pharmacist will use professional judgement to evaluate additional information nescessary to determine the appropriateness of the refill authorization.

No →

Place order for laboratory testing if indicated:
Provider notified and patient instructed to make an appointment if necessary.

Yes

Authorize Refills:
Reorder medication on Epic and send to the patient's pharmacy via Surescript, fax, or phone.

Complete Epic documentation.
Information to include:
1. Date of last appointment
2. Date of last laboratory results if indicated
3. Brief assessment and rationale for refill authorization

Based on Lexi-Comp and Micromedex

Medication Class or Indication	Laboratory Tests	Frequency	Additional Considerations
ACE inhibitor/ARB	BMP (K, Creatinine)[1-5]	1 year	Look for co-morbidities
Anticonvulsants	Drug Levels (i.e. Phenobarbital, phenytoin, Valproic Acid, divalproex, carbamazapine)[6-12]	1 year	
	CMP, CBC[6-12]	1 year	
Antipsychotics 2nd Generation	Hb A$_1$c, CMP fasting (glucose, lipids)[13]	At 12 weeks, then yearly	HEDIS focus on adherence
Bisphosphonates	Bone mineral density[14]	2 years	BMD for estrogens, calcitonin, denosumab, raloxifene, teriparatide and sex hormone combos if used for indication of osteoporosis
	CMP* (Serum calcium),	1 year	25(OH)D Levels when indicated. Check for duration – Bisphospanates should be stopped at 5 yrs.
Chronic Antibiotics	CMP, CBC[27]	1 year	
Depression Bupropion	CMP *(LFT's, Creatinine)[28]	Baseline then periodic monitoring	HEDIS focus on adherence
Diabetes Metformin, Thiazolidinediones (Pioglitazone)	Hb A$_1$c, CMP*(Fasting Blood Glucose, Creatinine)[15-17]	6 mo	If A1C<**7%** RFC fills 6 mo If A1C>**7%** RFC fills 3 mo- {simplified extraction of ADA guidelines}
	, Microalbumin (negative)	1 year	Evaluate GFR; Contact provider if sCr>1.5 for males or >1.4 for females
Digoxin	CMP* and magnesium (potassium, magnesium, calcium and creatinine) Drug Level, [18]	1 year	Closely monitor electrolytes in patients on diuretics and corticosteroids
Diuretics (all diuretics and antihypertensive combos)	BMP[4]	6 mo	
	BUN[4]	6 mo	
Hyperlipidemia	Fasting Lipid[19]		Lipid panel 4-12 weeks after statin initiation. Yearly lipid-provider to evaluate at time of annual physical

Medication Class or Indication	Laboratory Tests	Frequency	Additional Considerations
	LFT [19]	Baseline and if symptomatic myalgias CPK	Contact provider if ALT/AST >2x ULN
Thyroid Disorder	TSH[20]	1 year	Every 6-12 months (4-8 weeks after dosage adjustment)
Levothyroxine			
OCP	Younger than 21 yrs[21]	no PAP/ needs yearly appt.	
	21-65 years[21]	PAP Q 3yrs/ needs yearly appt.	If abnormal more frequent pap may be needed
Hormone Replacement Therapy (HRT)	> 65 years/or post hysterectomy[21]	no PAP/needs yearly appt.	
Lithium	Serum drug level BMP*(Creatinine Na+) TSH[22]	1 year	Renal function should be tested every 2–3 months during the first 6 months of treatment, and thyroid function should be evaluated once or twice during the first 6 months of lithium treatment
Iron/Folic acid	CBC/IRON[27]	1 year	
Gout	Uric acid, BUN, Creatinine, LFTs[23-24]	1 year	
Benign Prostate Hyperplasia	PSA[25]		Do not screen average-risk men under 54, those over age 70, or those with a life expectancy of less than 10-15 yrs
Testosterone	Testosterone level AM CBC, PSA[26]	1 year	PSA> 40yrs & baseline > 0.6ng/ml, at 3-6 mo. HCT 3-6 mo after initiation then yearly

*More cost effective for patient to get appropriate panel.

NHS
Warrington
Clinical Commissioning Group

Repeat Prescribing and Ordering Guidance

Version	1.0
Lead Author	Becky Birchall, CMCSU Medicines Management (MM) Team
Key Contributors	Pamela Soo, CWW Area Team Melanie Carrol, CPCW Local Pharmaceutical Committee Pauline Roberts, CMCSU MM Team (Care Home MM Lead) Joanne Goodwin, VR,E & S Cheshire CCG MM Team
Responsible Committee / Officers	Medicines Management Senior Team Cheshire and Merseyside Commissioning Support Unit
Issue Date	28/07/2014
Review Date	28/07/2016
Intended Audience	GP Practices, Community Pharmacies, Care Homes
Supporting organisations	Community Pharmacy Cheshire & Wirral (CPCW), Cheshire, Warrington & Wirral Local Pharmacy Network

Ratified By	Warrington Clinical Commissioning Group Primary Care Quality Committee
Date Ratified	28th May 2014

附

录

Repeat Prescribing and Ordering Guidance

This guidance provides good practice standards to facilitate GP practices, community pharmacies and care homes working in partnership to deliver safe and efficient management of repeat medication for patients

Repeat Prescribing and Ordering Guidance
Section Description
Forward
Glossary of terms
Introduction
Why Improve Current Systems?
Section 1 –Patients and Carers
Section 2 –GP practices
Section 3 –Pharmacy
Section 4 –Care Homes
Appendix 1
References
Consultation Group

Forward

I am pleased to be able to share this locally agreed and supported guidance document which we hope will help to provide assistance to all parties involved in the repeat ordering and dispensing of patient medication; care homes, practices and pharmacies.

This document will provide an understanding into the practical issues faced in the delivery of patient services from a number of perspectives within the overall processes required. Working together in in collaboration across all stakeholders to deliver the Medicines Optimisation agenda will be a key strategy for everyone involved in patient care. As such it is intended that this document will also act as a starting point in encouraging local discussions between practices, pharmacies and care homes, for the ultimate benefit of supporting the patient in managing their medicines.

Glenn Coleman, Head of Primary Care, Cheshire Warrington & Wirral Area Team

附录

Glossary of terms

The following terms are used in this document:

BNF	The British National Formulary is the key reference for prescribers, supplemented by local formulary recommendations
Care Quality Commission (CQC)	CQC is the regulator for all health and social care services in England.
Counterfoil	The right hand side of the prescription that should be used to re-order repeat medication at the appropriate time. These can also be called the 'repeat slip', 'ticklist' 'aside'.
Datix	Reporting system used in some areas for reporting of adverse events
Electronic Prescription Service (EPS)	Enables prescriptions to be generated, transmitted and received electronically
Medication	Indicates any medicines, dressings, appliances or equipment that can be prescribed on the NHS.
Medicine Managers/Medicines Co-ordinators	Member of the administration staff in a GP practice with responsibility for non- clinical medicine related issues.
National Patient Safety Agency (NPSA)	The National Patient Safety Agency was incorporated into the NHS Commissioning Board (NCB) from June 2012; the NCB intends to build on the expertise of the NPSA in learning from errors to improve patient safety.
Patient	Throughout this document, wherever 'patient' is noted, this refers to the patient or their authorised representative.
Repeat Prescribing	The traditional method of primary care prescribing. It involves prescribing regularly needed medicines to a patient that they have used before and can be renewed by the GP without the patient needing to be present. Standard practice allows patients to be able to collect their repeat prescriptions within 48-hours of taking their prescriptions to their GP.
Repeat Dispensing	Enables community pharmacists to dispense regular medicines to suitable patients, according to an agreed protocol, without the direct involvement of the GP surgery on each occasion a repeat is needed.

INTRODUCTION

- The aim of this guidance is to provide practices, pharmacies and care homes with a description of best practice and to highlight areas of risk. This document can be used in local discussions and development of protocols, in order to gain tighter control of repeat prescribing and ordering systems.

- Repeat prescribing enables patients to obtain further supplies of medicines without routinely seeing the prescriber, thereby reducing unnecessary consultations. It is an essential part of busy general practice, and accounts for about 60-75% of all prescriptions written by GPs, and 80% of their cost[1].

- The Kings Fund highlighted concerns in 2011, regarding inappropriate and unnecessary prescribing and the potential hazards for patients and wasted NHS resources. Their indicators for improving prescribing are set out in the executive summary of 'The Quality of GP Prescribing' www.thekingsfund.org.[2]

- Evidence shows a prescribing error rate of 7.5%, with 1 in 5 hospital admissions being medicines related, with two thirds of these being preventable.[3]

- The National Prescribing Centre commissioned a report summarising the evidence on medication errors in primary care and improvement strategies. *10 Top Tips for GPs- Strategies for Safer Prescribing*. NPC 2011[4]. This includes a table of 'Key points for safer repeat prescribing'.

- The Care Quality Commission (CQC) requires safe management of medicines (Outcome 9). Pharmacies are currently exempt from CQC registration, GP practices were registered from April 2013. A summary of the standards is available[5].

- This guidance is organised in three sections, from the perspectives of GP practices, pharmacies and care homes. Setting standards to improve repeat prescribing and ordering systems, and improving communication across these interfaces, will both improve patient care and maximise efficiencies.

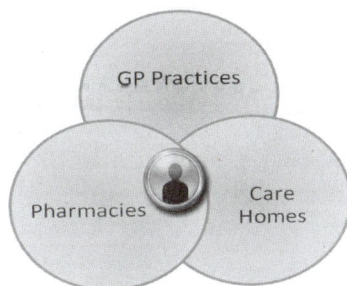

WHY IMPROVE CURRENT SYSTEMS?

✓ Clear and efficient systems enable GP practices, pharmacies and care homes to work together to improve patient care

✓ **Increased patient safety and high quality prescribing**

✓ Improved risk management to learn from near misses and avoid errors

✓ **Opportunities identified to improve patient/carer involvement and compliance with medication**

✓ Improved patient convenience and access to the medicines they need

✓ **Defined standards, roles and responsibilities for everyone involved, saving time by reducing queries**

✓ Appropriate use of skills for professionals and staff

✓ **GPs save time via efficient systems and develop their staff to identify and manage concerns early**

✓ Reduce wasted medication by controlling over-ordering and better use of NHS resources

✓ **Mitigate risks from prescription fraud**

✓ Compliance with standards, e.g., in contracts, from professional bodies and the Care Quality Commission

REPEAT PRESCRIBING GUIDANCE

Section 1

Patients and Carers

Benefits for Patients and Carers

Above all else an efficient and effective repeat prescribing and ordering process is of major importance to patients and carers. They want a convenient and accessible service that they have confidence in, and that protects them from harm.
A poorly designed system, or one that is not well managed, can cause frustration, waste precious time, as well as leading to an increase in the likelihood that mistakes can be made, thus putting patients' health at risk.

Benefits to patients and carers include[1]:

- Convenient and easy access to the medications they need.

- Clear understanding and appreciation of the process — knowing when and how to request the repeat, and knowing when, and from where, it can be collected. Reassurance that the system has a clear audit trail that can be tracked.

- Confidence that they are receiving the most appropriate medicines, tailored to their individual needs, provided through a system that conforms to good practice.

- Understanding of exactly how to take / administer medications as a result of receiving complete prescriptions with full instructions.

- An understanding of the importance and the process by which they have the opportunity to discuss their medication with a health care professional.

- Reduced potential for adverse incidents and adverse effects.

- Involvement in decisions about their health care, aiding self-management. This can improve concordance, resulting in improved outcomes of care, reduced hospital admissions, shorter hospital stays and fewer visits to the GP.

Patient/carer responsibilities

Patients and their carers are an important part of the repeat prescribing process and, within their level of competency, can take responsibility for:

- Making sure that they understand the repeat ordering system, and what help is available to enable them to obtain their medicines in a safe and timely way.

- Ensuring that they participate in medication reviews to discuss their medicines; including asking any questions that they have about how the repeat prescribing process works.

- Checking what is needed before placing an order for a repeat prescription, only ordering what will be needed before the next prescription is due, and then using it according the prescribers instructions.

- Placing the order for their repeat prescription using the most up to date counterfoil.

- Speaking to their doctor or pharmacist if any medicine is not suiting them, or they are not sure how and when to take the medicines.

- Checking that the medicines supplied are those that have been ordered, and that they are still needed, especially at times when things can change such as following a hospital admission.

- Letting their doctor and pharmacist know if they have a stock of medicines building up, and that they won't need to order for a while

- Planning ahead to allow sufficient time for the prescription to be checked, issued and dispensed, especially around holidays and Bank Holidays when there may be extra pressure on the system.

附

录

REPEAT PRESCRIBING GUIDANCE

Section 2

GP Practices

Index - Repeat Prescribing Guidance for GP Practices

附

录

4	**Re-authorising of repeats and medication reviews**
4.1	Clinical responsibility for re-authorisation
4.2	Medication review
5	**Collection and management of prescriptions**
5.1	Issue of prescriptions
5.2	Collection
5.3	Faxing prescriptions
5.4	Prescriptions to be posted
5.5	Uncollected/returned prescriptions
6	**Quality Assurance**
6.1	Repeat prescribing and ordering protocol
6.2	Improving the repeat prescribing and ordering system
6.3	Dealing with errors
6.4	Audit
6.5	Security of prescriptions
6.6	Contingency plan for hardware failure
7	**Repeat Dispensing**
8	**Electronic prescription Service (EPS)**

Standards for Repeat Prescribing and Ordering
GP Practices

These standards reflect best practice and will be aspirational in some cases.

Standard	Description
1	Only prescribers should authorise repeat status. If delegated to other members of staff this should be covered by a practice agreement and attached to the practice's Repeat Prescribing Policy.
2	All repeat items listed on the electronic medical records should be linked to an appropriate indication
3	Written criteria exist in the practice for drugs that are unsuitable to be issued on repeat prescription.
4	All drugs must have appropriate directions and be prescribed generically where appropriate.
5	Most repeat prescriptions should be written for 28 days' supply in line with best practice. Repeat medication for care homes must not exceed 28 days.
6	Drugs for each patient should be synchronised i.e. they should all last the same length of time.
7	Medication changes indicated on discharge and outpatient letters should only be entered onto the system by the prescriber.
8	The prescriber should update the patient's electronic medical records with an account of any consultations outside of the practice including details of handwritten prescriptions.
9	Repeat prescription requests are usually taken using the computer-generated counterfoil or via the web site. Telephone requests should not be accepted.
10	Only individual items that are ticked on the counterfoil should be issued. It must not be assumed patient needs all the items.
11	Each practice should have a system to inform patients how to order repeat prescriptions
12	There should be a practice protocol for dealing with controlled drug requests.

附

录

13	Practices should complete repeat prescription requests within 48 working hours.
14	Practices should have a clear protocol for processing repeat prescriptions and audit this annually.
15	Repeat prescriptions should be processed away from interruptions, by designated staff, who have received appropriate training.
16	Each practice should have a procedure in place so that the prescriber is informed when the medication review or monitoring requirements are overdue and no further repeats authorised.
17	Practices must have a procedure in place to ensure necessary monitoring has been done and assessed before a prescription is issued for high risk drugs.
18	All prescriptions that need re-authorising need to be passed to the prescriber. There should be a system in place to ensure this is done when the last available repeat is issued.
19	All people aged over 75 years should have medication reviews at least annually, and those taking four or more medicines should have reviews six-monthly, including an assessment of concordance.
20	A clear procedure should be in place to allow for the safe handing over of the correct prescription to the correct patient or representative and there should be a method of recording collection.

REPEAT PRESCRIBING IN GP PRACTICES

1. INITIATING REPEAT PRESCRIPTIONS

1.1 Authorisation of repeats

Repeat medications should only be set up once the patient is stable on a medication and efficacy and tolerability has been confirmed.

- Repeat dispensing should be considered.

- Only a prescriber can authorise repeat status. If setting up a repeat is delegated to other members of staff this should be covered by agreements specific to that practice and should be attached to the practice's Repeat Prescribing Policy e.g. in some practices the medicine managers/coordinators may add repeats after obtaining authorisation from a prescriber.

- All items should be linked to an appropriate indication. If a medication is used in an unlicensed manner, this should be fully documented in patient's notes and the patient informed that the medication is being used outside its license.

- Some medication is not suitable for repeat prescribing (see Appendix 1)

1.2 Recommended drug choices and generic prescribing

- In the majority of cases, prescribers should follow recommended drug choices agreed for the local health economy via local formularies and policies to improve prescribing quality and efficiency.

- If the drug dictionary allows, items prescribed should be written by generic name. Exceptions to this are:

  - Drugs specified in the BNF as unsuitable for generic prescribing, highlighted by clinical system or decision-support software. A list of medication to be considered for brand-name prescribing has been produced by UK Medicines Information[6].
  - Where a patient has proven documented intolerance to a generic form of a drug, the brand may be prescribed and should not be switched.
  - Where branded prescribing has been recommended locally to optimise cost savings.
  - Where there is a high risk of introducing dispensing errors by prescribing by the generic name, the prescriber may use their judgement and/or advice from the Medicines Management Team to prescribe by brand.

附

录

1.3 Number of days' supply

Most repeat prescriptions should be written for 28 days' supply because this repeat prescribing interval is recognised as being the best possible balance between patient convenience, good medical practice and minimal drug wastage. The number of units in total can be specified or the number of days' supply.

- GP practices that decide against adopting the default 28 day recommendation should still reduce intervals for individual patients where risks are apparent, or treatment is frequently changing and medicines waste is more likely. 56 day intervals may be more suitable for patients expressing a preference for convenience or financial considerations if they pay for prescriptions, however this should only be agreed when the risks of medication changing are low.

- Situations where intervals of **28 days or fewer** are more suitable:

  - Drugs liable to abuse
  - Situations where risks are perceived e.g., regarding storage in the home
  - Vulnerable patients prescribed complex regimens or with frequent hospital admissions and changeable therapy.
  - Terminally ill patients receiving palliative care support
  - Sip feeds
  - Dressings for short-term use or where likely to change
  - High cost medication
  - When necessary medication

- Situations where intervals of **more than 28 days** are suitable:
  - Oral contraceptives and HRT (supplied in 3 month packs)
  - Special packs
  - Where 28 days is not equivalent to the number of doses in a special pack i.e. a 200 doses inhaler as "1 OP" (original pack)

  These patients' other medication should be issued at more frequent intervals.

- Acute prescriptions should be used for the first prescription until treatment stabilised, particularly for drugs with a high incidence of adverse effects.

- On rare occasions, prescriptions for 7 days may be more suitable where risks are perceived or medication is frequently changing. Community pharmacies only require weekly prescriptions if the prescriber decides weekly dispensing is appropriate, and pharmacies must not issue more than one week at a time. Where the pharmacy is supplying medication in monitored dosage systems, 7 day prescriptions are not required unless the prescriber intends these to be dispensed and issued to the patient at 7 day intervals.

- The Misuse of Drugs Regulations 2006[7] makes a strong recommendation that 30 day intervals should be implemented for all schedule 2, 3 and 4 controlled drugs. A shorter interval may also be appropriate. This is one of the monitoring parameters for the Medicines Management Team and any concerns will be raised with practices.

- Repeat medication for care homes must not exceed 28 days

- A one-off synchronisation prescription is recommended where regular, stable items run out at varying times during the month. The time invested to synchronise medication will reduce wasted medication and staff time in dealing with the same patient several times a month.

1.4 Dosage instructions

- All new drugs added to the computer system must include clear dosage instructions. This includes liquid feeds, creams, dressings, nasal sprays, drops and all other external products. An absence of dosage instructions or "as directed" is not sufficient information for patients to use items appropriately and leads to problems for carers.

- Exceptions to specific directions may include gluten free foods, bath emollients, stoma and incontinence supplies and drugs requiring regular dose adjustments, particularly warfarin. For these the use of standard wording is advised.

1.5 The number of repeats to authorise

- The number of repeats authorised is a clinical decision and an important part of the repeat prescribing process. This should be low initially until the patient is stabilised, and compliance, monitoring requirements and chronic disease reviews should be taken into account.

- The number of days' supply should be set on the clinical system where possible, as this enables monitoring of early requests and over-use.

- Items not suitable for long-term use should only be authorised on repeat for short periods e.g. steroid creams. Procedures must be in place to ensure that excessive prescribing does not occur.

1.6 Authorising repeats for new patients

- There should be a system to ensure that information on previous medication is obtained before the first prescription is issued e.g., asking the patient for a current counterfoil from the previous GP, contacting the previous practice for clarification, inviting the patient for a consultation. It is often more appropriate to initially issue an acute script.

附

录

1.7 Medication initiated by hospitals and other agencies

- There should be a system for dealing with requests to start medication from other agencies e.g. hospital discharge notifications, outpatient appointments.

- All such notifications should be added by a prescriber who has access to the clinical record, before added to the system. Management systems should be in place to ensure these are dealt with efficiently and consistently and involve a prescriber. The prescriber should also ensure that any discontinued medication is removed from the screen and the reason documented in the patients notes. There is a significant risk of errors occurring if this guidance is not followed.

- Responsibility for prescribing in some cases should remain with secondary care. The RAG list defines Red and Amber drugs, where prescribing should remain with secondary care (Red) or responsibility should be shared (Amber).

- If prescribing is to remain with secondary care, details of these drugs should still be included on the practice system to enable prescriber awareness of any interactions with other drugs they may prescribe. The Medicines Management Team can advise on ways to do this.

- Patients should usually be discharged with at least 14 days' supply of medication/products in line with local agreements to allow for necessary information to be received and processed by the GP practice.

1.8 Consultations outside the practice and handwritten scripts

- The prescriber should update the patient's electronic medical records with an account of the home/care home visit in the same way as if the patient had been seen in a consultation at the practice. If available remote access should be used to ensure that the prescriber has full access to patient details and items can be added to the system.

- If a handwritten script is issued the medication should be added as an "acute" item and filed as a "hand written" prescription. Systems should be in place to ensure transfer to repeat if necessary. Any doses changed or medication discontinued should be added to the record.

1.9 Delegated authorisation

- Exceptions to prescriber authorisation must be by agreement with the practice and be supported by a written policy; this includes any policies written for the medicines managers/co-ordinators.

- With prior written agreement, Medicines Management pharmacists and pharmacy technicians may add new or discontinue medication; amend dosage instructions and quantities; re-authorise medication; and set review dates and monitoring requirements.

- Pharmacist or nurse supplementary prescribers may prescribe and authorise under an agreed clinical management plan.

- Non-medical independent prescribers may prescribe within their area of expertise and competence. Nurses with expertise in specialist areas who are prescribing for patients who have other chronic disease states outside of their expertise are not authorised to prescribe for those conditions. Contra-indications, disease and drug interactions of all the diseases and medications need to be considered before prescribing in the specialist area. Nurses should seek advice from the GP or pharmacist where they are unsure. Nurses must work within the boundaries of the Nursing Midwifery Council 'Standards for Medicines Management' 2008.

- To be able to prescribe in each practice all non-medical prescribers must be registered with the NHS Business Services Authority via a nominated person within the CCG. They must also deregister when they leave a practice.

2. ORDERING REPEAT PRESCRIPTIONS

2.1 Repeats ordered by the patient

- Patients should order medication using the counterfoil and individual items **MUST** be ticked. It must not be assumed that the patient needs all items. Where ordering is unclear, the patient must be contacted and the request remains unprocessed until this is clarified.

- When counterfoils are handed over in person and there is an opportunity to discuss what medicines are required, this should be utilised to reduce waste and identify any patient concerns.

- Where requests are not handed over in person these should be collected in a locked box in reception, sent by post, by fax or via the internet. Methods should be agreed by individual practices and included in their patient information. **Telephone requests should not be accepted.** The practice should ensure that any patient sensitive data is protected.

- Pharmacies may also act as a conduit for counterfoils completed by the patient but handed in by the pharmacy (refer to the Pharmacy section for recommended best practice). Pharmacies often offer longer opening hours that improve patient convenience for submitting counterfoils.

- Each practice should have a system to inform patients how to order repeat prescriptions. This is usually done by issuing a practice information leaflet and via their website. Further information reminders may be given by use of posters in the waiting room, electronic message boards and recorded messages on the answer machine/telephone. Arrangements should be made for patients with additional needs to be supported to understand and use the system.

- Although this should not be publicised surgeries should have a policy in place for dealing with urgent requests. If a patient consistently requests medication late, it should be brought to the Practice Manager's attention. The practice must not direct patients to the community pharmacy to obtain an emergency supply, as the pharmacist may legally refuse to supply.

2.2 Pharmacy involvement in repeat ordering and collection

- Where a patient is capable of ordering their own medication they should as a rule be encouraged to do so using the counterfoil. Pharmacy services can be particularly useful to improve access e.g. housebound patients.

- This guidance includes a definition of the types of ordering by community pharmacies, it is recommended GP practices and pharmacies describe systems in this way to avoid confusion:-

  — **Pharmacy accepting counterfoils** completed by patients

  — **Repeat ordering service**- where the pharmacy is involved in completing the counterfoil at the time the prescription needs to be ordered.

  — **Managed repeat ordering service**- where the patient completes their next order in advance via the pharmacy.

  — **Repeat collection service**- where the pharmacy submits the counterfoil and collects the prescription from the practice. This may or may not include delivery to the patient.

  — **Delivery services**

- GPs and practices may not direct patients to a particular pharmacy.

- Pharmacy requests should be made in line with the guidance included in the community pharmacy ordering section

- Practices should promote the need for pharmacy staff to stamp the counterfoil with pharmacy contact details, sign and date, when they have completed this on the patient's behalf, e.g., over the telephone. This is because pharmacy staff are responsible for checking whether each individual item is required.

- Counterfoils completed by the patient but dropped off by the pharmacy should be stamped if the pharmacy will be collecting, but not be signed/dated by pharmacy staff. Ideally they should be signed/dated by the patient. Alternatively another way of identifying these should be agreed between pharmacy and GP practice. The practice should ensure the pharmacy provides a list of the patients they collect for.

- It is best practice to obtain written permission from patients to allow a pharmacy to collect prescriptions on patients' behalf or manage their ordering. GP practices should keep records of prescriptions handed to third parties.

- In line with NPSA guidance, for medicines requiring closer monitoring, e.g., warfarin, methotrexate, lithium, ideally either a copy of the patient's record book or a copy of the latest results should be attached to the counterfoil.

- Pharmacies are guided to alert the practice to any feedback from the patient about discontinued items or items not regularly needed that remain on the counterfoil. Practices should operate a system to ensure this feedback is actioned, any compliance concerns addressed and the repeat medication list updated.

- **GP practices should become familiar with the section on pharmacy ordering guidance,** as further detail is included that underpins how these systems should operate to maximise safety and reduce wasted medication.

- There are examples of tightly managed pharmacy repeat ordering systems and they always result from a good relationship and ongoing communication between the pharmacy and the practice to ensure systems are mutually acceptable to both parties and the patients.

2.3 Third Party request

- For the purpose of this guidance a Third Party is defined as a supplier other than a pharmacy. This is often either a Dispensing Appliance Contractor (DAC) or Appliance Manufacturer or a manufacturer of supplementary feeds.

- The patient should order the items they require in the same way as medicines, but it is advisable to allow more than 48 hours as the prescription usually needs to be posted to the contractor.

- Prescriptions for appliances or enteral feeds should always be on a separate prescription.

- Retrospective prescriptions should not be issued routinely. Requests for new items from suppliers should be referred to the GP for a decision and confirmed by the specialist clinician involved in the patient's care.

附

录

2.4 Requests for controlled drugs

- There should be a practice protocol for dealing with controlled drug requests. Careful consideration should be given to deciding if the controlled drug should be available as a repeat.

- Prescribers can issue computer generated prescriptions for all controlled drugs. All details except the signature can be computer generated. Prescriptions for schedule 2, 3 and 4 controlled drugs are only valid for 28 days. Quantities should not exceed 30 days' supply and a shorter interval may be more appropriate.

2.5 Requests from nursing and residential homes

- Nursing and Residential Homes should request their medication on a monthly basis using the "Medication Administration Record" (MAR) sheet or counterfoil, by agreement between the GP practice, home and pharmacy.

- Medication should be ordered by the GP practice and not via the pharmacy.

- Twenty-eight days' supply ONLY should be given. Any requests for increased quantities should be referred to the prescriber.

- Items required that month should be clearly indicated, and only those should be processed. If over-ordering is suspected, the prescriber should be alerted.

- Any alterations to the MAR (for example new drugs, discontinued drugs, new doses) should be checked by the prescriber before changes are made to the patient's medication.

- Requests for dressings should be for current wound care that has been authorised by the prescriber and documented on the patient's records. These do not usually require repeat prescriptions. Practices should enforce arrangements so homes have to order dressings on the dedicated form, as this requires a reason for non-formulary choices and highlights this to the prescriber to check.

3.   GENERATING A REPEAT PRESCRIPTION

3.1 Period of notice

- Practices should complete repeat prescription requests within 48 working hours. In a normal week, a prescription ordered on a Friday will be ready on a Tuesday.

- Patients and community pharmacists should be informed of the notice needed when ordering prescriptions and when the prescription will be ready for collection. This can be via the practice information leaflet, information on the website or via a reminder notice close to the prescription request box.

3.2 Processing repeat requests

- All repeat prescriptions must be computer generated by designated staff, who have received training on the processes.

- Practices should have a clear protocol for processing repeat prescriptions and review this annually as minimum, to ensure there are no gaps between protocol and operating practice. The practice protocol should ensure that:

  - Repeat prescriptions are processed away from interruptions; no other duties should be performed whilst repeat prescriptions are processed.

  - The automatic prescription issue function must not be used. Where it is possible on the medical system this function should be disabled.

  - Request slips should be marked with the date processing started

  - The drug name, form, strength and dosage instructions should be checked, in order to highlight any discrepancies between the request and the repeat medication list to the prescriber.

  - Staff are clear about how to handle queries and documenting the query and outcome in the patient record, including requests for drugs not on repeat or re-issues from past drugs. There should be an audit trail of any communications regarding the request and therefore the clinical system functionallly should be utilised to do this electronically. The Medicines Management Team can provide advice specific to each clinical system.

  - Where the doctor wants to communicate a message to the patient this should be done electronically wherever possible and printed on the prescription. Separate notes may be used if attached firmly and a record made in the patient's clinical notes.

附

录

- When the medication review or monitoring requirements are overdue or there are no further repeats authorised, the prescriber should always be informed.

- Early or late requests may indicate over or under use of medication and this should be highlighted to the prescriber. Under use needs to be assessed with regard to risk of endangering the patient or others e.g., antipsychotics, asthma preventer inhalers. Over use is just as important clinically, e.g., for medication with addictive potential, or from a wasted medicines perspective. If early requests are processed, the reason should be documented in the notes.

- Items are discontinued that have not been ordered for over 12 months. Exceptions are medication required infrequently or seasonally, such as GTN spray, glucose oral gel, hayfever medication.

- There is a clear policy for dealing with private prescriptions to ensure these are not issued as an NHS item.

- There is a clear system for passing to the prescriber for signing. When the original prescriber is away there should be a system to identify who is responsible for signing and access to the clinical record is essential.

3.3 Requests for "High Risk" Drugs.

- "High risks drugs" include those that are toxic and require unusual dosing and those that require monitoring under a shared care agreement. Practices must have a procedure in place to ensure necessary monitoring has been done before a prescription is issued. Examples of high risk drugs are: Methotrexate, Warfarin, Lithium, DMARDs, insulin.

4. RE-AUTHORISATION OF REPEATS AND MEDICATION REVIEW

4.1 Clinical responsibility for re-authorisation

- Only the prescriber can re-authorise repeats. When a repeat is re-authorised it is the prescriber's responsibility to ensure ongoing need, repeat prescribing remains appropriate and necessary monitoring and medication review have been carried out. This is an essential part of the repeat prescribing system.

- All scripts that need re-authorising need to be passed to the prescriber. There should be a system in place to ensure this is done when the last available repeat is issued.

- Post-dating prescriptions is not recommended, as on some systems this will cancel reauthorisations.

- Re-authorisation is a good opportunity to align quantities so they all run out at the same time. This will avoid medicines waste and wasted staff time if multiple scripts are ordered each month for different items.

- Re-authorisation is a good opportunity to assess if the patient may benefit from repeat dispensing.

4.2 Medication review

- Patients with repeat medication should be regularly reviewed according to clinical need. The review date must be apparent on the counterfoil.

- Best practice supports that all people aged over 75 years should have reviews at least annually, and those taking four or more medicines should have reviews six-monthly, including an assessment of compliance.

- The medication review should be read coded and ensure that all medication is reviewed at the same time e.g. a practice nurse may have reviewed asthma therapy but no other drugs. A pharmacy medicines use review (MUR) is a useful concordance and compliance check involving the patient, however, this should not be read-coded as a medication review.

- The review should include:

  - the continued effectiveness and need for each drug
  - the appropriateness of the dose and presentation- e.g., if a dose has been titrated upwards it may be possible to give a higher strength preparation rather than two tablets.
  - the patient's understanding of the treatment
  - monitoring, tests, examinations and follow-up
  - a check for side-effects, drug interactions and contra-indications
  - discontinuing items not needed
  - appropriate frequency of requests
  - all prescriptions being for the same length of time
  - use of over-the-counter medications
  - consideration of whether repeat dispensing would be appropriate if medication is stable

附

录

5. COLLECTION AND MANAGEMENT OF PRESCRIPTIONS

5.1 Issue of prescriptions

- The issue of completed prescriptions to either the patient or the patient's representative can be by collection at reception, by post, via community pharmacist or via electronic transfer through the NHS spine.

5.2 Collection

- A clear timetable of when prescriptions will be ready for collection should be on display to the patients.

- A clear procedure should be in place to allow for the safe handing over of the correct prescription to the correct patient. Reception staff should check the identity and address of the patient collecting the prescription. If a patient's relative or friend can demonstrate proof they are collecting a prescription and the person is unknown to the reception staff, they should be required to sign for the prescription.

- Measures to determine the identity of a representative collecting a prescription are particularly important in the case of controlled drug prescriptions, and these must be signed for.

- Collection of prescriptions by children will be at the discretion of the Practice Manager or prescriber, and will need the permission of the parent or guardian or the person for whom the prescription is being collected.

- There should be a method of recording collection.

- There are a small number of patients who must collect their own prescriptions personally. These patients must have a screen message displayed on their computer record. This message should be clearly marked on the request form and transferred to the issued script. Staff should ensure that these prescriptions are given to no one other than the patient.

5.3 Faxing Prescriptions

- Prescriptions may be faxed to community pharmacies but ONLY in exceptional circumstances. A log should always be maintained of when and where the fax was sent and when the prescription was collected.

- Prescriptions faxed at the request of the prescriber must be given to the community pharmacy within a reasonable time. It is the responsibility of the GP practice to phone the pharmacy to let them know a prescription is being faxed.

- If a request for a prescription to be faxed is made by the community pharmacy it is their responsibility to collect the original prescription later.

5.4 Prescriptions to be posted

- The name and address of the patient should be checked against the addressed envelope in which it will be posted to ensure it is going to the correct person/ agency.

- Name, address and number of items on the prescription should be logged in the prescription log book, including the date of sending and the name of the person who prepared the post.

5.5 Uncollected/returned prescriptions

- Any prescriptions not collected after one month from date of issue must be reviewed by the prescriber. Where the issue is deleted from the computer, the prescription should be shredded and disposed of in the confidential waste, in the presence of a witness. A record should be made of the serial number within the practice records.

- If it was not possible to cancel the last issue, the serial numbers should be recorded on the patient records, and a comment to the effect that the prescription was not collected. Then the prescription should be shredded.

- Practices should have a procedure in place to deal with notifications from a community pharmacist that a prescription hasn't been collected.

6. QUALITY ASSURANCE

6.1 Repeat prescribing and ordering protocol

- Practices must have a clear, written protocol, describing the roles of each person involved in the production of prescriptions.

- This should be written by the practice and reviewed every two years.

- There should be a named person who is responsible for the policy and ensuring that all staff are adequately trained.

- All members of staff, including locum prescribers, need to be trained and fully aware of how the practice repeat prescribing system works, and are aware of their individual responsibilities.

- A system should be in place to ensure that all staff have read the procedure and it is included in the induction programme for new staff.

附

录

6.2 Improving the repeat prescribing and ordering system

- The Medicines Management Team are well placed to offer advice and spread best practice from other GP practices they work in, for example, how to maximise clinical system functionality or innovative improvement strategies.

6.3 Dealing with errors

- There should be a system in place to investigate and learn from any errors. The prescriber who signs the prescription takes ultimate responsibility for the prescribing of that medication and therefore needs assurance that the system is robust. Errors should be reported e.g. via the DATIX system. Errors should be discussed at practice meetings.

  In the event that unexpected or avoidable death or severe harm of one or more patient occurs, as a result of a prescribing error, this is classed as a serious incident. All serious incidents MUST be reported on the Strategic Executive Information System (StEIS) which the CCG can access and report on. All such incidents must be reported to the relevant CCG and an investigation conducted into the circumstances of the incident.

6.4 Audit

- The repeat prescribing system is required to be audited annually in order to ensure that patients and staff are kept safe by having systems to ensure that medicines are handled safely and securely.

- The practice manager will be responsible for ensuring the audit is carried out and learning and updates to the practice's protocol or additional training are followed through.

6.5 Security of Prescriptions

- All blank and completed prescriptions must be stored in a safe and secure manner. There are a wide range of aspects the practice must consider in line with national guidance and it is recommended that the practice have a Standard Operating Procedure (SOP) and all staff are trained.

- All staff must be aware of the process for dealing with missing/stolen prescriptions; this should also be detailed within the SOP.

- Risk assessment of prescription security should be carried out on a regular basis to ensure appropriate systems are in place.

6.6 Contingency plan for hardware failure

- The practice should have a contingency plan for power failure or system failure with degrees of time built in. They should ensure that prescriptions printed or handwritten are legible.

This process should include provision to record information on the clinical system once the problem is resolved.

7. REPEAT DISPENSING

- This offers an alternative way for patients with stable long-term conditions to access their medicines via the pharmacy without the need to contact the GP practice every time a new prescription is needed.

- Tightly managed repeat dispensing systems reduce GP and practice workload, improve services to patients, reduce medicines waste and enhance the role of community pharmacies.

- The patient is issued with a master copy of their authorised medication and up to a maximum of eleven copies allowing dispensing of medication at intervals without returning to the practice each time for a prescription.

- Repeat dispensing is not suitable for all patients. It is suited to patients with chronic conditions who are likely to remain stable on their medicines for the duration of the batch of repeat prescriptions. Patients prescribed significant numbers of items or who are likely to be hospitalised are less suited to inclusion in the repeat dispensing scheme.

- The prescriber must obtain the patients consent before commencing repeat dispensing.

- The practice must include repeat dispensing aspects in their practice's repeat prescribing and ordering protocol and staff training.

- Repeat dispensing prescriptions must be processed separately from standard repeat prescriptions.

- The receptionist must check that the master copy has been signed before handing it out.

- The patient's records must be clearly annotated to indicate repeat dispensing so that they are not issued as a standard repeat prescription as well.

- Schedule 2 and 3 Controlled Drugs cannot be prescribed via repeat dispensing. Repeat dispensing prescriptions for schedule 4 Controlled drugs can only be dispensed for the first time within 28 days of the appropriate date. After the first dispensing the repeats are legally valid within the normal periods of validity of the repeat prescription.

- At the point of dispensing each instalment, the pharmacist will be responsible for checking patient adherence and other clinical factors that are relevant to the appropriateness of the continued supply. Any issues of concern to the pharmacist will be reported to the practice[6].

8. ELECTRONIC PRESCRIPTION SERVICE (EPS)

- The Electronic Prescription Service (EPS) is currently being rolled out to practices. It is a service that allows GPs to generate and transmit electronic prescriptions using their computer system. The prescription can then be downloaded by a pharmacy that has also upgraded their computer system. This makes the prescribing and dispensing process more efficient and convenient for patients and staff.

- EPS will bring gains in both efficiency and safety for both patients and health professionals:
  - Improve patient safety by reducing the likelihood of dispensing errors due to unclear or illegible prescriptions.
  - Allow the instant cancellation of prescriptions thought no longer clinically appropriate.
  - Prevent the loss of prescription forms.
  - Reduce the number of fraudulent prescriptions.
  - Allows preparation of prescriptions in advance of collection, saving patient time at the dispensary, and making workflow and stock control easier for pharmacists to manage
  - Relieve patients of the need to collect prescriptions from the prescriber.
  - Eliminate the need for pharmacists to re-enter prescription information, thereby saving time and increasing dispensing accuracy.
  - For repeat dispensing, as the repeat dispensing regime is stored electronically this reduces the risk of a batch of prescriptions getting lost and improves accountability for prescriptions issued and dispensed. Pharmacies will no longer need to retain and store repeatable prescriptions and batch issues therefore decreasing workload and storage requirements.

- When electronic transfer of prescriptions is used it is important to remember that:

  - Prescriptions electronically sent to the NHS spine for access by the dispensing pharmacy, must be authorised by the prescriber and this is represented by the electronic signature

  - The signature must not be used by any other person than the authoriser.

  - The practice must have a robust protocol for electronic issue of prescriptions which meets clinical governance and risk management issues. This protocol must comply with the latest NHS IT standards.

Repeat Ordering Guidance

Section 3

Pharmacies

Index - Repeat Prescribing Guidance for Pharmacies

Section	Description
	Standards for Pharmacies
	Introduction
1	Patient communications
2	GP practice communications
3	Pharmacy processes
4	Pharmacy accepting counterfoils
5	Repeat ordering services
6	Managed repeat ordering service
7	Repeat Collection service
8	Delivery services
9	Electronic Prescription Service
10	Repeat dispensing

Standards for Repeat Prescribing and Ordering Pharmacies

All pharmacies should have Standard Operating Procedures (SOPs) that detail their repeat prescribing services; ideally the following recommendations should be covered by these SOPs.

These standards reflect best practice and will be aspirational in some cases:-

Standard	Description
1	The patient should initiate involvement in the services provided by the pharmacy.
2	An agreement should be signed by the patient; details of this agreement must be retained and also shared with the GP practice.
3	Patients should be asked and reminded wherever possible to inform pharmacy if any medicines are changed or stopped, for example after hospital admission.
4	Procedures should be in place so that messages from practices via counterfoils are passed on to patients as intended.
5	SOPs in the pharmacy should detail who can deal with verbal prescription requests and the training needed as these present additional risks.
6	All patients are asked on hand-out if they still require all the items they ordered, paying particular attention to PRN items.
7	Before a pharmacy offers services to their patients ideally they should agree the arrangements for the service they plan to offer with participating practices. This is particularly important in the case of repeat ordering and managed repeat ordering services.
8	For medicines requiring closer monitoring (e.g., warfarin, methotrexate, lithium etc.) the latest results and monitoring date must be available to the prescriber. Ideally a record of these should be attached.
9	Return any 'not dispensed' prescriptions to the practice with a brief explanation of reason.

10	Alert the practice if the patient provides feedback that they no longer require an item, this should be communicated back to the surgery for the attention of the prescriber.
11	Pharmacies should have an audit trail that identifies each request and supply of repeat prescriptions.
12	Any incidents, near misses or errors that occur as part of providing these services should be recorded and reported as per clinical governance requirements. The patient's GP practice should also be informed where appropriate.
13	Patients should be notified of when they should expect the prescription to be ready; timings should be in excess of the 2 working days the practice needs to generate the script.
14	When counterfoils are handed in that do not fully indicate what is required by the patient, suitably trained staff should clarify what items are to be ordered.
15	The counterfoil should be marked with the pharmacy stamp if they are to be collected by the pharmacy.
16	Medication ordered via a Repeat Ordering System should be requested from patients / carers no earlier than ten calendar days before medication is due to take account of the potential changes.
17	If patient request is via telephone the member of pharmacy staff who confirms which items are required with the patient should sign, date and add the pharmacy stamp on the counterfoil to indicate to the practice that they have provided this service.
18	Handwritten prescription requests are a particular risk and where unavoidable, must be accurate and legible.
19	A vital part of the Managed Repeat Ordering Service is that patients are asked at the point of hand-out whether all items are still needed including when prescriptions are delivered to patients.
20	When prescriptions are collected from the practice these should be checked against pharmacy records of items ordered. Any missing or excess items appearing on the prescription should be resolved with the practice.

REPEAT PRESCRIBING AND ORDERING GUIDANCE FOR PHARMACIES

INTRODUCTION

Pharmacies provide a range of services that offer benefits by increasing access for patients in need of support and also convenience regarding longer opening hours. These services offer an opportunity for pharmacies to manage the dispensing workload and therefore reduce risks, but they should only ever be initiated in the patient's best interest.

There are examples of tightly managed pharmacy repeat ordering systems and they always result from a good relationship and on-going communication between the pharmacy and the practice to ensure systems are mutually acceptable to both parties.

Community pharmacists can be involved in the repeat prescribing process in various ways. Confusion about level of involvement can lead to misconceptions. Therefore these services should be described in the following way to facilitate understanding and they should not be confused with repeat dispensing.

    i. **Pharmacy accepting counterfoils** completed by patients

    ii. **Repeat ordering service**- where the pharmacy is involved in completing the counterfoil at the time the prescription needs to be ordered.

    iii. **Managed repeat ordering service**- where the patient completes their next order in advance via the pharmacy.

    iv. **Repeat collection service**- where the pharmacy submits the counterfoil and collects the prescription from the practice. This may or may not include delivery to the patient.

    v. **Delivery services**

    vi. **Repeat dispensing**

1. PATIENT COMMUNICATIONS

- It should be the patient that initiates involvement in some or all of the services provided by the pharmacy. The agreement should be signed by the patient. Arrangements can be changed by the patient at any time. Agreement must be obtained from the patient before the pharmacy can take action on their behalf and details of this agreement must be retained.

- The patient/carer should be given information about their responsibilities. The risks from medication changing are a particular concern and therefore patients should be asked at the outset and reminded wherever possible to highlight if any medicines stopped or changed, for example after hospital admissions.

- Pharmacies will need to ascertain the identification of the person making the request and, if this is not the patient; that the person has authority to order on behalf of the patient. These aspects are particularly important for telephone communications.

- Where counterfoils are stored in the pharmacy due regard must be given to secure storage and patient confidentiality. Ensure the patient has an up to date copy of their counterfoil if they routinely leave these with the pharmacy. A photocopy should be provided if the patient does not already have a copy. Counterfoil information may well be needed by the patient for interaction with health professionals e.g. subsequent hospital admission, dental treatment etc. Counterfoils are also used by practices to pass on important messages e.g. reminders of tests required, booking flu injections etc. and these messages must be passed on by the pharmacy as intended.

- Verbal communications present additional risks that need to be managed e.g. where different strengths or forms of the same medication are on the counterfoil.

    i. The staff member should have access to the electronic Patient Medication Record or the counterfoil during these conversations.

    ii. A record of the conversation should be made e.g., who requested the order (patient / carers name), who from the pharmacy discussed the order with the patient/carer, the date and exact items ordered should be kept for internal audit purposes.

    iii. Phone calls should be taken in a manner with regard to patient confidentiality i.e., without the risk of patient details being overheard.

    iv. SOPs in the pharmacy should detail who can deal with verbal requests, the training needed etc. e.g., be able to show that there are enough staff suitably qualified and skilled, for the safe and effective provision of this service.

    v. Include in what situations telephone requests will be taken e.g., managed prescription service where there has been prior discussion with the patient.

- For MDS patients it would be recommended that medications not in blister packs (e.g., creams and inhalers) receive special attention with regard to suitability of reorder on each occasion to prevent stockpiling or waste

- Ensure that patients are asked on handout if they still require all the items they ordered and pay particular attention to PRN items.

2. GP PRACTICE COMMUNICATIONS

- Pharmacies are encouraged to use this as an opportunity to arrange a meeting to discuss processes with local GP practices and agree mutually beneficial systems that are safe, efficient, reduce waste and are flexible to patient choice. Ideally GP practices should participate in these meetings to ensure processes run efficiently and smoothly.

- Particularly in the case of repeat ordering and managed repeat ordering services, there should be co-operation with local prescribers. Before the pharmacy offers such services to their patients, they should agree the arrangements for the service they plan to offer with participating practices. GP practice guidance also encourages active communication of their views with pharmacies to avoid misunderstandings.

- For medicines requiring closer monitoring (e.g., warfarin, methotrexate, lithium etc.) the latest results and monitoring date must be available to the prescriber. Ideally a record of these should be attached.

- Any concerns over the patient's competency to reorder their medication should be discussed with the relevant GP and an appropriate strategy for reordering agreed in conjunction with the GP and the patient. This may be the case for patients with learning difficulties, dementia, confusion, as well as for patients whose medication is provided in Monitored Dosage System (MDS) or blister packs where they no longer know which medications are in their MDS packs. Details of such arrangements, the date the arrangement was agreed, details of the pharmacist and GP involved and appropriate review date should be recorded with the patient's agreement to these arrangements.

- Return any 'not dispensed' prescriptions to the practice with a brief statement (e.g. duplicate, not required by patient, discontinued medicines, not ordered by the patient etc.). This allows the practice records to be amended to reflect prescribed medicines that the patient did not receive.

- Alert the practice if the patient provides feedback when the medication is dispensed that they no longer require an item, this should be communicated back to the surgery for the attention of the prescriber such that any non-compliance concerns can be addressed, or repeat records updated. Any concerns regarding over or under ordering should be discussed with the

附
录

patient and if appropriate the GP. This could involve a Medicines Use Review if appropriate. Appropriate records of such interventions should be recorded and entered on the patient's PMR.

3. PHARMACY PROCESSES

- This guidance constitutes good practice and compromise to facilitate close working relationships with GP practices. GPhC Standards of Conduct, Ethics and Performance underpin a range of these aspects. Pharmacies must have standard operating procedures that detail these services. These must be in accordance with GPhC standards and it is strongly recommended they support the aims of this local guidance.

- Ensure that an audit trail exists to identify each request and supply. Record all interventions on the PMR, in order to be able to deal with any queries that may arise.

- Any incidents, near misses or errors that occur as part of providing these services should be recorded and reported as per clinical governance requirements. The patient's GP practice should also be informed where appropriate.

4. PHARMACY ACCEPTING COUNTERFOILS

- The pharmacy is effectively acting as a 'post-box' for counterfoils completed by patients. Many pharmacies have extended opening hours that may be more convenient to patients using this method. Patients return a few days later and their medication is dispensed ready for collection, or this may be delivered to the patient. Patients should be notified of when they should expect the prescription to be ready. Community pharmacists should not expect these prescriptions to be dealt with any differently by the surgery so timings should be in excess of the 2 working days the practice needs to generate the script.

- The pharmacy standard operating procedure should include the following points:

    i. If a counterfoil is handed into the pharmacy with no indication of what is required by the patient, suitably trained staff should speak to the patient to clarify what items are to be ordered. 'Blanket' ordering where the patient asks for 'them all' should be discouraged (especially for PRN medication) wherever the pharmacy is aware this is the case.

    ii. The counterfoil should be marked with the pharmacy stamp if prescriptions are to be collected by the pharmacy. Or an alternative system agreed with the practice to identify these from other requests awaiting collection by patients.

5. REPEAT ORDERING SERVICE

- Usually the patient provides consent to leave their counterfoil with the pharmacy until the next supply is due. The patient calls in, telephones or (in exceptional circumstances) the pharmacy telephones the patient to order their items a few days before their medication is required. This is different from the 'managed repeat ordering service', where orders are taken in advance, usually at the time the previous supply of medication is collected. The risks of medication changing between the repeat order and the prescription being generated are much lower.

- Where patients call in to the pharmacy they are asked to complete the counterfoil themselves. If a staff member completes the counterfoil within a telephone conversation the items required are recorded directly into the counterfoil. This system avoids the risk that patients use an out of date counterfoil to order their medicines.

- The pharmacy standard operating procedure should include the following points:

  i. Establish, at the time of each request, which items the patient or carer considers are required and ensure wherever possible that unnecessary requests are not made to exclude "blanket" ordering and possible waste or stockpiling. Special attention should be paid to medication which may not be required on a monthly basis e.g., PRN medication, inhalers, creams.

  ii. Orders for medication should be taken from patients / carers no earlier than ten calendar days before medication is due to take account of the potential for changes to regimes or patient status e.g., hospital admissions. Exceptional circumstances should be recorded and communicated to the GP practice. It is usually advantageous to agree the number of days in advance between the practice and pharmacy.

  iii. If the patient telephones the pharmacy, the member of pharmacy staff confirming which items are required with the patient should sign, date and add the pharmacy stamp on the counterfoil to indicate to the practice that they have provided this service. Any counterfoils received from pharmacies with no pharmacy staff details will indicate that the pharmacy has acted as conduit and has not participated in the actual ordering process for these patients.

iv. Ensure that requests are initiated by the patient/carer. A reminder system may be used but prescriptions may not be requested from a surgery before obtaining the patient's / carer's consent.

v. When prescriptions are collected from the practice these should be checked against pharmacy records of items ordered. Any missing or excess items appearing on the prescription should be resolved with the practice.

vi. There may be situations where the pharmacy does not have a counterfoil for the patient. This should not happen routinely and patients should be reminded of the importance of ordering via the counterfoil to reduce risks. In exceptional circumstances where this is unavoidable, the request must include the same level of information contained on the counterfoil. Medication must be ordered by the name it has been prescribed by and not by the brand that has been dispensed previously. Pharmacies should utilise their Patient Medication Record (PMR) to improve the accuracy of the order, although this may not be as up to date as GP records of recent changes. Caution is needed when using print outs from the PMR as medication is not listed in the same order as at the practice and may include one off or discontinued medication. Handwritten requests are a particular risk and where unavoidable, must be accurate and legible. Illegible handwriting and spelling mistakes reflect poorly on the pharmacy, this introduces risk for patients and will ultimately impact on the relationship with the GP practice.

vii. GP practices will have their own systems to manage the risk from patients occasionally needing to order without a completed counterfoil and therefore pharmacies are encouraged to discuss with their local GP practices to ensure these are aligned.

viii. When the patient requests medication that is not on repeat, it should be the patient that contacts the practice directly.

6. MANAGED REPEAT ORDERING SERVICE

- These managed repeat ordering systems are where orders are taken in advance, often at the time the previous supply medication is handed out. They represent the greatest area of concern for GP practices regarding risk management for medication changes and regarding the higher risk of wasted medication. **Pharmacies are urged to discuss with GP practices to agree a mutually acceptable way forward.**

- When patients collect their dispensed medicines, they are asked to mark the items required for the following month on their counterfoil. It is recommended that patients should sign the counterfoil. This differs from 'repeat ordering services' because the order is taken in advance and the risks of medication changing before the prescription is printed are higher.

- The following points should be considered for inclusion in the standard operating procedures:

    i. When patients sign-up to this service it must be emphasised that the patient is responsible for contacting the pharmacy if there are any changes to their medication mid-month or if they are admitted to hospital. Consider whether this is an appropriate system for patients that have frequent changes to their medication.

    ii. Establish, at the time of each request, which items the patient or carer considers are required and ensure against "blanket" ordering and potential for medicines waste or stockpiling. Special attention should be paid to medication which may not be required on a monthly basis e.g. PRN medication, inhalers, creams.

    iii. The patient is given a reminder card detailing when their medication will be ready for collection.

    iv. When prescriptions are collected from the practice these should be checked against pharmacy records of items ordered. Any missing or excess items appearing on the prescription should be resolved with the practice.

    v. A vital part of this service is that patients are asked at the point dispensed medicines are handed out whether all items are still needed. The SOP should detail how items returned to stock i.e., 'not dispensed items' should be managed and fed back to the practice. PSNC guidance states that scripts would be clearly annotated not dispensed and feedback should be provided to the GP practice for whole scripts and individual items.

    vi. A particular concern is patients on a managed repeat ordering system and also having medication delivered, because the interaction at the point medicines are handed out is via the delivery driver. Pharmacies should put systems in place to ensure this second check that all medication is needed at the point of dispensing is still carried out.

    vii. The longer the prescription duration the greater the concern regarding the potential for medicines waste and greater than 56 day quantities are inappropriate for the managed service.

    viii. Where these services are tightly managed in line with clear standard operating procedures, they do provide an opportunity for the

附

录

pharmacy to individually go through each item to ensure it is required, both at the ordering stage and when medicines are collected. This interaction may also generate discussion regarding the patient's concerns or questions and lead to overall improvement in the patient's knowledge and treatment.

7. REPEAT COLLECTION SERVICE

- Obtain and record the patient's consent to receive prescriptions during the Repeat Collection Service provision.

- Explain fully to the patient what the service involves including timescales to allow for collection / receipt of the prescription and dispensing of the medication.

- Counterfoils delivered to the practice from the pharmacy should show the pharmacy stamp as a guide to show practice staff that the pharmacy will be collecting the prescription.

  i. For patients who drop off counterfoils to the practice, the pharmacy should compile a list of patients they collect for that is taken to the practice when they collect prescriptions.

  ii. On receipt of prescriptions a check should be made that the pharmacy has authority to receive and dispense the prescriptions for each individual patient. Any prescriptions received for which this authority is not in place should be returned to the surgery or directed to the pharmacy authorised to receive it.

8. DELIVERY SERVICES

- Pharmacies should ensure that delivery drivers operate to same standard as medicines counter assistance in ensuring any concerns are fed back to the pharmacy and an audit trail ensures these are followed up.

- A particular concern is delivered items for patients on a managed repeat ordering service- pharmacies need to consider how the 2nd check happens, i.e., that all items are required. If the patient realises this after the delivery driver has left then the medication cannot be returned to stock which would avoid the prescribing cost.

9. ELECTRONIC PRESCRIPTION SERVICE (EPS)

- Electronic Prescription Service (EPS) is currently being rolled out to practices. It is a service that allows GPs to generate and transmit electronic prescriptions using their computer system. EPS enables prescriptions to be sent electronically from the GP to the pharmacy of the patient's choice. The prescription can then be downloaded by a pharmacy, this makes the prescribing and dispensing process more efficient and convenient for patients and staff.

NB The ordering of prescriptions would still be carried out in line with local agreements between GP surgeries, Pharmacies and Patients.

- EPS will bring gains in both efficiency and safety for both patients and health professionals:
    - Improve patient safety by reducing the likelihood of dispensing errors due to unclear or illegible prescriptions.
    - Allow the instant cancellation of prescriptions thought no longer clinically appropriate.
    - Prevent the loss of prescription forms reducing the risk of duplicate prescriptions being generated.
    - Reduce the number of fraudulent prescriptions.
    - Allows preparation of prescriptions in advance of collection, saving patient time at the dispensary, and making workflow and stock control easier for pharmacists to manage
    - Relieve patients of the need to collect prescriptions from the prescriber.
    - Eliminate the need for pharmacists to re-enter prescription information, thereby saving time and increasing dispensing accuracy.

- For repeat dispensing (batch prescribing) allows the prescriber to authorise a prescription with a specified number of issues and allows the pharmacist to prepare medicines for dispensing in advance of a patient visiting the pharmacy. As the repeat dispensing regime is stored electronically it makes repeat dispensing easier to use.
    - It reduces the risk of a batch of prescriptions getting lost
    - Any amendments can be made without the need for paper copies to be returned to the prescriber for reissuing.
    - Outstanding repeats can be cancelled to respond to changes in medicines, clinical condition or personal circumstances.
    - It improves accountability for prescriptions issued and dispensed with the pharmacist being responsible for checking patient adherence and other clinical factors that are relevant to the appropriateness of the continued supple.
    - The duration of the repeatable prescription can be aligned to a patient review, monitoring procedure or other clinical and administrative functions of the practice.
    - It reduces the workload issuing and re-authorising repeat prescriptions.

- When electronic transfer of prescriptions is used it is important to remember that:

- Prescriptions electronically sent to the NHS spine for access by the dispensing pharmacy, must be authorised by the prescriber and this is represented by the electronic signature

- The signature must not be used by any other person than the authoriser.

- The practice must have a robust protocol for electronic issue of prescriptions which meets clinical governance and risk management issues. This protocol must comply with the latest NHS IT standards.

10. REPEAT DISPENSING

- This offers an alternative way for patients with stable long-term conditions to access their medicines via the pharmacy without the need to contact the GP practice every time a new prescription is needed.

- The patient is issued with a master repeatable prescription of their authorised medication and up to a maximum of eleven identical copies allowing dispensing of medication at intervals without returning to the practice each time for a prescription.

- The master copy is the authority to supply the medicine and the pharmacy must safely and securely store a patient's master copy and, if requested by the patient, the related batch issues.

- At the point of dispensing each instalment, the pharmacist will be responsible for checking patient adherence and other clinical factors that are relevant to the appropriateness of the continued supply, for example, whether there are any problems the patient may be encountering with their medicines, whether the patient has recently been in hospital or had changes made to their medication regimen. Any issues of concern to the pharmacist will be reported to the practice.

- The outstanding repeats left on the prescription can be cancelled and the remaining batch issues destroyed or returned to the practice as and when required, to respond to changes in medicines, clinical condition or patient circumstances.

- When GP practices implement release 2 of the electronic prescription service (EPS), an electronic version of the repeat dispensing model will be available to GPs.[8]

Repeat Prescribing Guidance

Section 4

Care Homes

This section of the policy gives guidance to care homes on ordering repeat medication. Community pharmacies and GP surgeries will have policies for handling the repeat prescriptions and care home policies must be written in conjunction with the community pharmacy and the GP surgeries. Good communication between GP, Pharmacist and Home is essential.

附

录

Index- Repeat Prescribing Guidance for Care Homes

Section	Description
	Standards
	Legal issues and national guidelines
	Guidance
1.	Self-administration of medication
2.	Relationship with GPs and community pharmacies
3.	Administration systems
4.	Training and education
5.	Patients with swallowing difficulties
6.	Ordering repeat prescriptions
7.	Exceptions for 28 days' supply
8.	Checking existing stock
9.	Prescriptions
10.	Delivery and checking medications
11.	Recording systems

Standards for Repeat Prescribing and Ordering
Care Homes

These standards reflect best practice and will be aspirational in some cases:-

Standard	Description
1	For the efficient ordering and supply of medication ideally a care home should deal with one pharmacy.
2	A suitably trained member of staff in a care home should be responsible for all aspects of the repeat ordering process.
3	If possible the home should identify a named person in the pharmacy and surgery they can deal with, with regards to any queries.
4	Medication administered in an unlicensed manner e.g., crushed must be authorised by the prescriber and detailed on the MAR chart.
5	The prescription ordering system should highlight any changes made to the medication in the last month to the pharmacy.
6	Creams, ointments and oral liquids must be marked with the date of opening and can usually be used up to 6 months once opened unless otherwise stated on the label/information sheet.
7	Prescriber should be consulted about reducing quantities of creams, ointments and liquids that last for more than 3 months after opening.
8	Unused PRN medication that is in date should be carried over for the next month rather than being removed to reduce waste.
9	Dosage instructions for 'when required' medication should include an indication for use, dose, frequency and if appropriate, a maximum daily dose. Any medicines received with instructions such as 'as directed' or 'when required' should be referred back to the pharmacist for clarification.
10	The care home should ensure that the pharmacy is made aware of any medication that has been discontinued and any discrepancies on the MAR/counterfoil.
11	Medicines should be ordered on a 28 day cycle

附

录

12	The care home should allow adequate time to for the surgery and pharmacy to process prescriptions and supply medicines. A minimum of two weeks is recommended.
13	The pharmacy cannot organise ordering of medication on behalf of the home.
14	Records of the medication requested should be kept by the home.
15	New medication needed part way through a 28 day cycle should be requested in a quantity that will ensure that this medication will then fit in with future 28 days cycles of prescribing and be recorded on a MAR chart.
16	It is good practice for care home staff to keep written records of all queries so there is a clear audit trail.
17	Care staff must not transfer medication to other containers; this is called secondary dispensing and is illegal.
18	If medication that hasn't been ordered for 6 months or more the GP should be notified to see if this item can be discontinued
19	A trained member of staff should check the prescriptions received from practice for each resident against MAR chart and list of requested medicine, before sending it to the pharmacy. They will check they have all medication ordered, any anomalies and for any items which are not required, these should be clearly marked 'not required'.
20	The community pharmacy should deliver all medications and MAR charts for the next 28 day cycle at least two days before the start of the cycle.
21	Trained care home staff need to check the medicines against their records of what they ordered, identify any problems and discuss any discrepancies with the pharmacist/GP surgery as appropriate.
22	The home should have product information leaflets available for all medications received. If missing follow up with pharmacy.
23	The MAR chart is a legal document and should be kept by the home for a period of at least 3 years from the last date of entry.

Management of medicines in care homes is identified as a regulated activity in The Health and Social Care act 2008 (regulated activities) regulations 2010[9]. Regulation 13 states:

"The registered person must protect service users against the risks associated with the unsafe use and management of medicines, by means of the making of appropriate arrangements for the obtaining, recording, handling, using, safe keeping, dispensing, safe administration and disposal of medicines used for the purposes of the regulated activity."

The act also states that the Care Quality Commission is the responsible regulatory body. The care qualities document "Guidance about compliance; essential standard of quality and safety"[5] gives guidance to care homes on how to comply with this act. Outcome 9 applies to management of medicines.

Outcome 9b states that the home should have:

"Systems in place to ensure they comply with the requirements of the Medicines Act 1968 and the Misuse of Drugs Act 1971, and their associated regulations, the Safer Management of Controlled Drugs Regulations 2006, relevant health technical memoranda and professional guidance from the Royal Pharmaceutical Society of Great Britain and other relevant professional bodies and agencies."

Therefore any guidelines for care homes must be mindful of these constraints and we advise that not only care home staff but community pharmacists and any GP practice staff who deal with care homes have a basic knowledge of the guidelines from the Royal Pharmaceutical Society. Pharmaceutical Society guidance on pharmaceutical services to social care settings[10] and 'The Handling of Medicines in Social Care' is available on its website[11].

Guidance

1. SELF ADMINISTRATION OF MEDICATION

Residents in care homes should be actively encouraged to self-administer their own medicines, where possible. In some situations this means they will be responsible for obtaining their own medication. In the majority of situations the care home will order supplies. The following policy applies to residents where the home has taken over responsibility for ordering medication for the resident.

2. RELATIONSHIPS WITH GPs AND COMMUNITY PHARMACIES

The emphasis in the CQC (Care Quality Commission) standards is to ensure person centred care and that the resident is consulted on all aspects of care and their views are taken into account when decisions about their treatment are made. These views have to be taken into account with all aspects of the medication cycle.

Care homes often have a number of different GP practices to deal with e.g., a 40 bed home may deal with 10-12 GP practices. In this situation the resident will decide which GP practice to register with (if the GP is in agreement). In some areas Clinical Commissioning Groups have developed locally enhanced services for care homes. In this situation one GP surgery will take over the care for the entire home and most residents will be registered with that practice. Residents still have the right to be registered with another surgery if they wish.

For the efficient ordering and supply of medication it is recognised that a care home should deal with one pharmacy.

Therefore care home staff may deal with a number of GP practices but routinely only with one community pharmacist. Wherever possible the same community pharmacy should be used for both acute and repeat scripts.

It would be good practice for any GP who has a financial interest in the care home where they also prescribe for residents; or for any community pharmacist who has a financial interest in a care home where they supply medicines for residents, to declare that interest through the normal route, it is also good practice to inform the Medicines Management Team.

3. ADMINISTRATION SYSTEMS

The system of administration used in most homes is a monitored dosage system (MDS). There are a number of different MDSs in use, Nomad (which is a 7 day system in a plastic tray) and the Venalink and Manrex systems which are often referred to as blister packs. They are perceived by some care homes as a 'safer' means of medicines administration than traditional containers. However in practice all homes have to also administer from bottles and cartons, as liquid medication, and some solid dose medications are not suitable for a blister pack.

> The CQC Inspection **does not require** that medicines for Care Homes are dispensed in a monitored dosage system.

The use and funding of MDS in care homes is an arrangement between the care home and the pharmacy. When this decision is made both parties should consider the following points:

- There is no legal requirement to use MDS.
- Only certain medication can be put in an MDS so some medication will still need to be dispensed in other containers.
- Homes will need to have procedures in place to deal with changes in dose, because the use of MDS can lead to delays in doses being changed and extra waste. In certain situations e.g., end of life medication MDS may not be appropriate.
- Only regular medication should be dispensed in a MDS. As required medication should be dispensed separately to give flexibility of dosing and reduce waste.
- If a MDS is used the person administering the medication is still responsible for ensuring that the right medication is given to the right patient and that they are aware of side effects, special dosing requirements such as before food etc.
- Patient information leaflets should be available.

Community pharmacists should comply with professional guidance on MDS.

4. TRAINING AND EDUCATION

For the repeat ordering system to run smoothly it is essential for staff to be trained and competent in all aspects of the process. A suitably trained member of staff in a care home should be responsible for all aspects of the repeat ordering process. This should be a nurse (in a nursing home) or a senior carer (in a residential home).

The manager should keep a list of suitably trained staff and ensure that training is up to date. It helps with the smooth running of the process for the pharmacy and surgery to have a named person within the home they can contact with queries relating to prescriptions. However the manager should ensure that there is adequate cover for holidays etc. and that the system isn't reliant on one member of staff. If possible the home should identify a named person in the pharmacy and surgery they can deal with, with regards to any queries etc.

5. PATIENTS WITH SWALLOWING DIFFICULTIES

If a patient is unable to take their medication in the prescribed form the prescriber should be notified, so that a medication review can be carried out. This may involve simplifying the regime, prescribing an alternative medication or prescribing an alternative preparation. Although it is good practice to only used medication that is licensed it is sometimes necessary to use it in an unlicensed way (e.g., crush, open capsule) or on the rare occasion prescribe an unlicensed product (special). Some medication cannot be crushed etc. The community pharmacist or medicine management team will be able to offer advice on whether medication can be crushed or dissolved in water but it is the prescriber that must authorise this.

> **Medication may need to be crushed or dissolved in water before administration, if the patient is unable to swallow tablets/capsules and there is no licensed liquid preparation available. This can only be done if authorised by the prescriber. If a medication is to be given in this way the MAR chart should be annotated appropriately.**

6. ORDERING REPEAT PRESCRIPTIONS

Community pharmacies and care homes need to develop a robust system for ordering medication to ensure the following points are taken into account:

- Checks are made to highlight any changes made to the residents' medication in the previous month.
- Creams, ointments and oral liquids can usually be used up to 6 months once opened unless otherwise stated on the label/information sheet.
- They should be marked with the date of opening. If the product is lasting more than 3 months consult with the prescriber about reducing quantity.

> **When necessary (PRN) medication, creams and ointments etc. should be retained and used for the next month if still in date. There is no need to discard as this is a waste.**

- Any instructions which state "when required" should be clarified with the GP surgery. The instructions for when required must include an indication for use, dose, frequency and if appropriate a maximum daily dose. The use of 'as directed' should be avoided.

- The home and GP surgery should agree whether the counterfoil should be used or whether the carbon medication request form which is part of the MAR chart may be used. Whichever system is used the home should ensure that the community pharmacy is aware of any discontinued medication and that the GP is aware of any discrepancies between the MAR and the counterfoil.

> **If discontinued medication has been left on repeat notify the surgery that this medication has been discontinued so it can be taken off repeat.**

- Medicines should be ordered on a 28 day cycle (see exceptions below).

- Allow adequate time for the surgery and pharmacy to process prescriptions and supply medicines, a minimum of two weeks is usually needed.
- **The pharmacy cannot organise ordering of medication on behalf of the home as this is unethical and carries a higher risk of error because the pharmacy may not be aware of changes that have occurred during a previous month.**
- Records of the medication requested should be kept by the home.
- New medication needed part way through a 28 day cycle should be requested in a quantity that will ensure that this medication will then fit in with future 28 days cycles of prescribing.

> **It is good practice for care home staff to keep written records of all queries e.g., telephone conversations and action taken in the course of managing medication for care home residents. There should be a clear audit trail.**

7. EXCEPTIONS TO 28 DAY'S SUPPLY

Supply of medication in care homes should be for 28 days, however some exceptions apply:

- If an item is started mid-cycle it is good practice for a prescriber to issue a prescription for amount needed until the start of the next cycle, to avoid waste.
- Patients who require palliative care or who are terminally ill, often have frequent changes of medicines, especially those to relieve pain and nausea. During this phase of a patient's care, the home should arrange with the GP and community pharmacist that medicines are prescribed in 7 day amounts (taking into account supply over a weekend) and dispensed by the community pharmacy in bottles or cartons to allow for greater flexibility when frequent changes are made.
- At other times the home may request unusual quantities of medication to cover residents going on holiday etc. The home should try to make such requests to the surgery in writing with an explanation for such a request. If a resident regularly goes out for a day the home should discuss the options with the prescriber. It may be possible to change the timing of medication or to issue a separate prescription.

> **Care staff must not transfer medication to other containers; this is called secondary dispensing and is illegal.**

8. CHECKING EXISTING STOCKS

- Before starting the ordering process it is important to establish the quantity of medication left from the previous cycle.

> **If you don't need it, don't order it.**

附

录

- Particular attention must be made to quantities of dressings, topical products (creams, ointments, and scalp applications bath/shower products), stoma and continence products. If available use dressings order form. As some PRN medication can be kept for several months, care should be taken with storage especially with items like dressings that may be supplied individually.

> **Creams, ointments and oral liquids must be marked with the date of opening and can usually be used up to 6 months once opened unless otherwise stated on the label/information sheet.**

- Checks should be made to see if when required medication is needed. If this hasn't been ordered for 6 months or more the GP should be notified to see if this item can be discontinued.

> **Always inform the GP if a resident is regularly refusing medication**

- Any recent deliveries should be taken into account when ordering medication.

9. PRESCRIPTIONS

- All drugs issued on a prescription must include clear dosage instructions. This includes liquid feeds, creams, dressings, nasal sprays, drops and all other external products. "As directed" is not sufficient information for patients to use items appropriately and leads to problems for carers.
- Once issued the prescription should be sent to the care home. A trained member of staff should check the prescription for each resident against MAR chart and list of requested medicine, before sending it to the pharmacy. They should have a process in place to ensure they have a prescription for all the items they ordered.
- Any anomalies or omissions should be rectified with the surgery at this stage.
- Systems should be in place to ensure that any changes to medication made in the previous month are highlighted to the community pharmacist.
- Any items which have been printed on the prescription which are not in fact required should be clearly marked 'NOT REQUIRED'. The home should then send all the prescriptions to the community pharmacy for dispensing.
- The GP must also be notified of any items not required so they can amend their systems accordingly. If a prescribed item has previously been discontinued this should be highlighted to the GP so it can be removed from the repeat screen to save confusion in the future.

> **Time spent sorting out discrepancies at this stage will enable the repeat process to run smoothly and save time in the future**

- All prescriptions should be issued for the quantity required for 28 days. Issuing of larger quantities can cause practical and safety issues for care homes. Contact the GP surgery and ask them to reduce quantities on repeat if necessary.

10. DELIVERY AND CHECKING MEDICACTION

- The community pharmacy should deliver all medications and MAR charts for the next 28 day cycle at least two days before the start of the cycle.
- Trained care home staff need to check the medicines against their records of what they ordered, identify any problems and discuss any discrepancies with the pharmacist/GP surgery as appropriate.
- This includes checking the amount received the accuracy of the labels and the accuracy of the information recorded on the MAR charts. Any medicines received with instructions such as 'as directed' or 'when required' should be referred back to the pharmacist for clarification.
- The home should have written information available for all medications received. Check all new medications to ensure product information leaflets are available. If not follow up with the pharmacist.

> **It is good practice for care home staff to keep written records of all queries e.g., telephone conversations and action taken in the course of managing medication for care home residents. There should be a clear audit trail.**

11. RECORDING SYSTEMS

The community pharmacist will usually supply printed Medicine Administration Record (MAR) charts as part of the service to the home. This is an additional service not remunerated by the NHS. Production of an accurate up to date chart is only possible if there is adequate communication between the prescriber, care home and pharmacist.

> **It is essential to inform the pharmacist of any medication that is discontinued so it can be deleted from the MAR.**

Community pharmacists who provide MAR charts should comply with the practice guidance for 'Provision of printed medicine administration record charts (MAR) by community pharmacists for use in health and social care settings.' from the RPharmS[12]

The MAR chart is a legal document. The Care Quality Commission document, "Guidance About Compliance: essential standards of quality and safety" states that people should be confident that records are kept for a period of at least 3 years from the last date of entry.

If a new medication is prescribed part way through the cycle the community pharmacist should provide a new MAR chart. However, if this is not possible, it may be necessary for care staff to hand write the new medication on the MAR chart. They should have a supply of blank MAR charts from the community pharmacist for those occasions when there is not sufficient room on the chart of an existing resident, or to hand write medication for a new resident.

Any additions/ amendments to the MAR chart should be signed, dated and the reason for the change clearly stated. It is good practice for the member of staff who adds information to the MAR chart to sign and date it and for a second member of staff to check, countersign and date it too. It is also be good practice to attach a photocopy of the original prescription to the MAR chart, to evidence the details of the hand written record.

There should be a clear audit trail for any changes made to a MAR sheet, it is a legal document.

APPENDIX 1

EXAMPLES OF ITEMS NOT SUITABLE AS REPEAT MEDICATION

Drug group	Specific drugs or groups of drugs
Antibacterials / antifungals	Oral antibiotics / antifungals Topical antibiotics / antifungals
Corticosteroids	Oral corticosteroids Very potent topical steroids
Drugs subject to misuse	Hypnotics and anxiolytics Controlled drugs Cyclizine pseudoephedrine
Drugs limited to one treatment course	Varenicline
Weight Loss treatment	Orlistat

This list is not exhaustive – please consult the prescribing formulary or the BNF for advice about specific drugs / preparations.

附录 4　Cumbria Repeat Prescribing a Practice Guide（第三章附件 2）

NHS
Cumbria
Clinical Commissioning Group

Repeat prescribing
A practice guide

January 2014

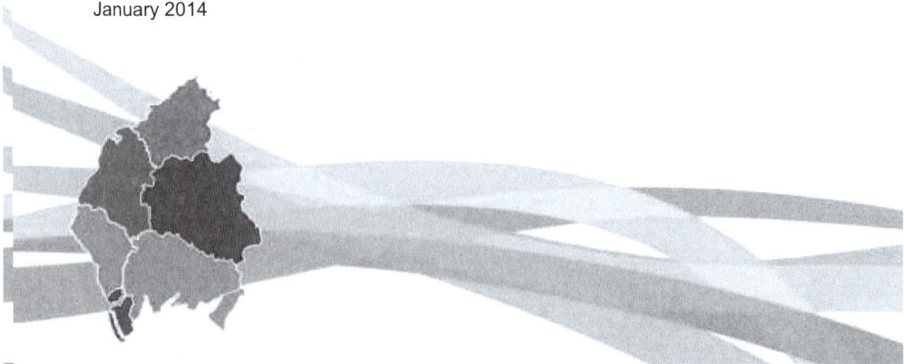

Repeat Prescribing Systems

Introduction

Repeat prescribing plays a significant part in the supply of medicines to patients in primary care. Two-thirds of prescriptions generated in primary care are for patients who have requested a repeat supply of medicines they take regularly; this represents some 80% of medicines costs. It is estimated that 2.4 million prescriptions are issued each day in England, meaning that approximately 1.92 million prescriptions are issued each day for repeat items[1]. It is therefore important to general practice staff and patients that an efficient and effective repeat prescribing system is in place.

A poorly designed system, or one that is not well managed, can cause frustration to patients, practice staff and other health care professionals. It can waste precious time, as well as leading to an increase in the likelihood that mistakes could be made, thus putting patients' health at risk.

The new General Medical Service (nGMS) Contract recognises the need for an effective and efficient repeat prescribing system by the inclusion of several quality indicators relating to medicines management[2]. Benefits of a well-managed system include:

- Improved quality of prescribing
- Improved patient convenience and access to the medicines they need
- Improved patient safety
- Better and more appropriate use of relevant professional and practice staff skills and time
- Decreased GP and practice workload
- Optimal efficiency in the processes involved
- Increased patient / carer involvement and responsibility
- Better use of NHS resources

To reduce unnecessary burdens on general practice, it is important for repeat prescribing systems to adapt and evolve to meet the demands of a changing demography and developments in the NHS. In addition, the impact of supplementary and independent prescribing, the implementation of new IT systems and extended opportunities for community pharmacies need to be considered.

What is a repeat prescribing system?

Repeat prescribing is a partnership between patient and prescriber that allows the prescriber to authorise a prescription so it can be repeatedly issued at agreed intervals without the need for a GP consultation at each prescription request
An essential component of this process is that the authorising prescriber ensures that arrangements are in place for any necessary monitoring of usage and effects, and for the regular assessment of the continuing need for the repeat prescription — which should be considered within the context of the clinical review of the patient.

附

录

The figure below shows a simplified diagram of what this system might look like.

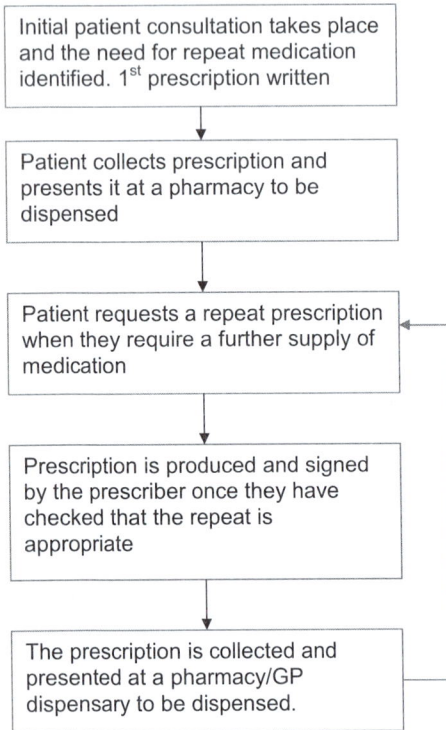

Figure 1 — A simplified repeat prescribing system

The way in which a request for a repeat prescription is made can vary, and may include electronic ordering, using the right hand side of the prescription itself, or making a telephone or written request or via Electronic Prescription Service (EPS).

There are also different ways in which the prescription can be collected from the surgery, ranging from the patient collecting it directly to it being sent electronically to a community pharmacy. In fact, repeat prescribing systems can vary considerably from practice to practice and, whilst there are good practice examples and ideas for improvement to systems, it is important to adapt each change to a practice's local situation and check that it will work first.

Benefits to patients and carers of a well run system

- Convenient and easy access to the medications they need
- Clear understanding and appreciation of the process — knowing when and how to

request the repeat, and knowing when, and from where, it can be collected
- Confidence that they are receiving the most appropriate medicines, tailored to their individual needs, provided through a system that conforms to good practice
- Understanding of exactly how to take / administer medications as a result of receiving complete prescriptions with full instructions
- An understanding of the importance and the process by which they have the opportunity to discuss their medication with a health care professional
- Reduced potential for adverse incidents and adverse effects
- Involvement in decisions about their health care, aiding self-management. This can improve concordance, resulting in improved outcomes of care, reduced hospital admissions, shorter hospital stays and fewer visits to the GP.

Benefits to practices of a well run system

- Earlier recognition of problems, reducing the risk of patient harm and for potential complaints and litigation. Demonstrating that there is a properly organised system for issuing and monitoring repeat prescriptions may help to defend the prescriber from criticism, or worse, if there is an adverse event
- More manageable workload resulting from improved efficiency across all systems
- Fewer queries to practice staff, reduced 'traffic' at the reception counter and enhanced reputation of the practice
- Appropriate and efficient use of professional and practice staff time and skills
- Greater understanding of the process by everyone involved, including roles responsibilities and timelines
- Improved professional and staff morale through knowledge of a job well done
- Achievement of quality goals in the nGMS Contract, maximising practice income
- Improved co-operation and working relationships with other health care professionals, such as non-medical prescribers, nurses and community pharmacists
- Easier implementation of new initiatives that will further reduce work burden and improve quality of care, e.g. Electronic Transfer of Prescription, repeat dispensing.

Benefits to the NHS of a well run system

- Assurance that medicines are used in a safe, effective and appropriate manner
- Efficient use, with reduced waste, of resources available to the NHS
- Appropriate use of individuals' particular skills and knowledge, and a broadening of responsibilities
- Reduced potential for 'near misses' and adverse incidents. Facilitated shared learning across the NHS to help prevent them occurring again

Making improvements

Repeat prescribing is a complex system involving many people and processes, and accuracy is essential. There are many opportunities for things to go wrong or for potential
'near misses'. The entire system needs to be reviewed regularly with input from those integral to the process, to help practices assure the quality of their service, and minimise the risks of inefficient and unsafe systems. Regular audits, as part of clinical governance activities, can help.

When making improvements to a repeat prescribing system we need to balance speed with safety. Whilst recognising and maintaining this balance, however, more efficient systems may be achievable.

Mapping the system

Reviewing and redesigning the repeat prescribing process is about providing a better service for patients. Practices may find process mapping a useful exercise to identify exactly how their own repeat prescribing system works, and any areas of inefficiency or weakness. There will be many common elements, but all systems will have local variables included.

Process mapping the repeat prescribing system is an excellent way of identifying potential problems or bottle-necks and allows a review of those parts of the system that have been identified.

Mapping out a system is not a difficult task, but it does need some protected time and the involvement of the entire team including users and carers, and others outside the practice environment, e.g. community pharmacists.

When making any changes to a system it is important to be clear about what you want to achieve and to think about how you will recognise an improvement.

There are many successful initiatives that we already know about that have led to significant improvements in medicines management within Repeat Prescribing Systems. Here are some examples:

- Some practices have developed web based systems for the ordering of repeat prescriptions. These reduced GP practice workload and increased patient choice. Patients no longer had to fit ordering their repeat medication around when it was convenient for the practice.

- One PCT made it possible for selected patients to order their repeat prescriptions using a text message service. This service proved very popular with patients who had certain disabilities such as poor hearing.

- Synchronising a patient's repeat prescriptions can save time for both the practice and patient as well as potentially helping to reduce waste. Several sites from the NPC medicines management programmes have looked at different ways of increasing the number of synchronised prescriptions and more information is available on the website.

- To make better use of GP time and to improve patient satisfaction some practices had a dedicated member of staff for the repeat prescribing system.

- Introduction of EPS 2 has   reduced the workload generated by patients requesting and   collecting individual prescriptions and the ability to make wider use of the repeat dispensing service.

- Reduction in workload by the ability to review electronic prescriptions on screen, and either sign electronic prescriptions individually or select multiple electronic prescriptions to sign. Making the prescribing process more efficient.

- Ability to cancel electronic prescriptions at any point up until they are dispensed and to record the reason they were cancelled.

- Where currently a GP practice, operates a prescription collection service, staff will no longer need to sort (or post) prescriptions saving both time and resource.

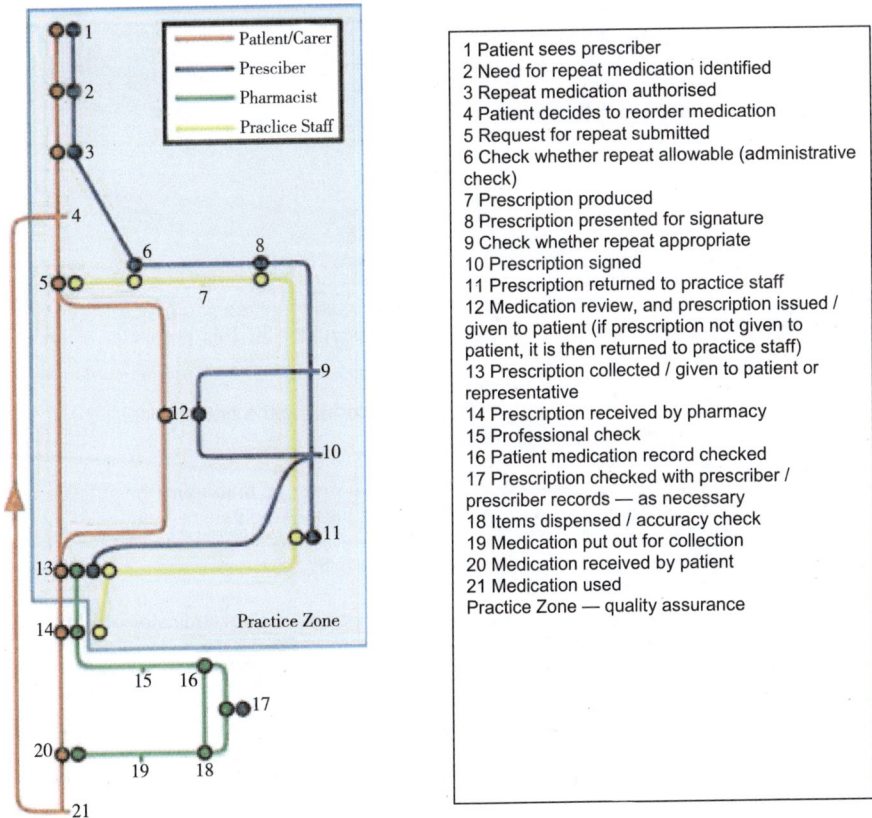

Legend:
- Patient/Carer
- Presciber
- Pharmacist
- Praclice Staff

1 Patient sees prescriber
2 Need for repeat medication identified
3 Repeat medication authorised
4 Patient decides to reorder medication
5 Request for repeat submitted
6 Check whether repeat allowable (administrative check)
7 Prescription produced
8 Prescription presented for signature
9 Check whether repeat appropriate
10 Prescription signed
11 Prescription returned to practice staff
12 Medication review, and prescription issued / given to patient (if prescription not given to patient, it is then returned to practice staff)
13 Prescription collected / given to patient or representative
14 Prescription received by pharmacy
15 Professional check
16 Patient medication record checked
17 Prescription checked with prescriber / prescriber records — as necessary
18 Items dispensed / accuracy check
19 Medication put out for collection
20 Medication received by patient
21 Medication used
Practice Zone — quality assurance

Figure 2 A map of the main elements of the repeat prescribing process

To aid understanding of the repeat prescribing process, and what needs to be done to improve the quality of its management, it can be divided it into nine key areas for consideration.

> Authorising repeat prescriptions
> Requesting repeat prescriptions
> Should we generate the prescription?
> Prescription production and signing
> Medication review
> Patient gets the prescription
> The community pharmacist's role
> Using the medication
> Quality assurance of the process

However, Zermansky[3] offered a model of repeat prescribing that many practices have used when developing practice policies. A brief description of this model is given below.

1. **Production**: involves receiving requests and producing the prescription. Usually delegated to a practice receptionist.

2. **Management control**: generally an area of the practice manager's or practice medicines manager's responsibility, comprising four elements:

   I. Authorisation check
   II. Compliance check
   III. Review date — ensuring that every patient has a clear indicator of when therapy should be reviewed
   IV. Flagging — ensuring that each patient due for review is brought to the prescriber's attention.

3. **Clinical control**: this is the doctor, or other qualified prescriber's responsibility, and involves two tasks:

   I. Authorisation — the decision that a repeat prescription is appropriate, the prescriber being satisfied that the drug is effective, well tolerated and still needed
   II. Periodic review — a review of the patient and the medication to ensure that treatment is still effective, appropriate and well tolerated. The prescriber makes an informed decision as to whether to continue, change or stop medication.

Further information on developing and improving repeat prescribing systems can be obtained from the National Prescribing Centre legacy website. The NPC is now part of

NICE but maintain their library of previous resources on the legacy website.
http://www.npc.nhs.uk/repeat_medication/repeat_prescribing/index.php

Characteristics of a model repeat prescribing system – checklist

- It is clearly defined by written policies and procedures that are regularly reviewed to take into account changes in prescribing arrangements (e.g. supplementary prescribing, repeat dispensing arrangements) and practice developments.
- It is overseen and managed by an appropriately trained individual, with deputy and cover arrangements
- All members of staff, including locum prescribers, are trained and fully aware of how the practice repeat prescribing system works, and are aware of their individual responsibilities
- It maintains comprehensive, up-to-date and accurate repeat prescribing information for each patient
- It keeps all information secure and confidential, and all staff are regularly trained in the use of any computerised system
- Computerised systems are kept secure using confidential individual passwords for all users, in line with the security policy of the practice including Caldicott Policies, other requirements of the Data Protection Act and the Freedom of Information Act. Regular backups of the repeat prescribing information are made
- Information on screens is not visible to unauthorised personnel, patients or representatives, unless specifically designed for that purpose, e.g. Clinical Knowledge Summaries 'shared' screens
- It only allows addition of medications to a repeat prescription when the medication has been shown to be beneficial for the patient, and then only by a qualified prescriber
- It only allows the issue of medications that have been appropriately authorised by a qualified prescriber
- All prescriptions are reviewed and signed by an appropriately qualified prescriber who knows the patient or at least has direct access to the patient's medical records
- It explicitly states which medications are not considered suitable for routine repeat prescribing, e.g. controlled drugs, hypnotics, bearing in mind the needs of particular groups of patients such as the terminally ill
- A clear audit trail exists for the inclusion / removal of all medications to the patient'srepeat prescribing list
- There is an agreed process for reviewing all changes in medication following hospital inpatient or outpatient attendance, etc., before making changes to the repeat prescription
- It clearly defines an appropriate interval of reauthorisation for repeats, with a proper system to call patients for review. Regular clinical and medication reviews take place, including an assessment of concordance
- Prescriptions are produced accurately, providing full administration instructions, also maximising the synchronicity of items and avoiding therapeutic duplication
- The frequency of medication supply is kept within auditable limits so that any abuse of the system can be quickly identified, investigated and eliminated where appropriate

附

录

- Quantities prescribed take into account what each patient needs, the nature and stability of their clinical condition, patient safety and convenience, avoidance of waste, likely complications of treatment and any necessary monitoring
- Regular assessment of the patient's condition(s) is made; the continuing need for the medication being prescribed; continued benefit from treatment being derived; adverse drug reactions and drug interactions are picked up; and all necessary monitoring is being carried out
- Partnership with the patient is utilised to ensure maximum concordance and satisfaction with the treatment option, and early feedback of any potential problems
- Information is readily available to help patients and carers understand the system (ordering, collecting prescriptions, how to request help, reviews, etc.), and considers the needs and convenience of carers, including those looking after more than one patient. Comments received are carefully considered and, where appropriate, acted on
- Quality is regularly assessed. Learning from adverse incidents, including complaints and 'near-misses' are used to improve and evolve the system.
- Adverse incidents involving black triangle drugs are reported via the 'Yellow Card Scheme'.

The Repeat Risk Assessment (Appendix 1) provides an easy method of identifying areas of your repeat prescribing system which could be reviewed and change implemented to improve the system.

Appendix 1

Repeat Risk Assessment Tool

Question	Score	
Is there a written protocol?	Yes = 0 No = 1	
PRODUCTION		
1. Request		
How is the request taken?	Telephone = 2 Telephone for housebound = 0 Written/ e-mail / post / fax = 0	
If the request is hand-written is it presented on:	Backslip = 0 Other = 1	
If the request is taken verbally does the same person generate the script?	Yes = 0 No = 1	
Are the required items marked?	Yes = 0 No = 1	
Are the items requested on repeat?	Yes = 0 No = 1	
2. Production		
Is the member of staff doing the repeats designated and trained?	Yes = 0 No = 1	
Are the scripts computer generated?	Yes = 0 No = 2	
What is the turnaround time?	< 48 hours = 0 ≥ 48 hours = 1	
Is there designated time set aside for doing the repeats?	Yes = 0 No = 1	
3. Signing		
Is there a set time for signing?	Yes = 0 No = 1	
Are the appropriate resources available (e g computer) when signing?	Yes = 0 No = 1	
Does the doctor perform a check before signing?	Yes = 0 No = 1	
4. Miscellaneous		

附

录

What happens when a prescription is lost?	Reprint = 0 Re-issue = 1	
What happens when prescriptions are not collected?	Recorded = 0 Not recorded = 1	
If a prescription is reprinted, is this documented?	Yes = 0 No =1	
	Production total	
MANAGEMENT		
1. Authorisation		
Who authorises the repeats?	Receptionist = 2 Nurse = 0 Doctor = 0 Nurse Specialist = 0	
What is the process for reauthorisation?	GP notified = 0 GP not notified = 2	
How many issues are made?	0-6 = 0 6-12 (for stable patients) = 0 6-12 (for unstable patients) = 1 > 12 = 2	
2. Compliance		
Is compliance checked before prescription issued?	Yes = 0 No =1	
Is there a standard written procedure for over / under compliance?	Yes = 0 No =1	
3. Housekeeping (Use a sample of 20 patients)		
Out of the sample were there any branded items that should be generic?	Yes = 1 No =0	
Out of the sample were there any items that required dose optimisation?	Yes = 1 No =0	
Out of the sample were there any duplicated items?	Yes =2 No =0	
Out of the sample were there any items that had not been collected for 6 months or more?	Yes = 1 No =0	
Out of the sample were there any dosage instructions missing?	Yes = 1 No =0	
Are the drug monitoring tests up to date?	Yes = 0 No =1	
Are all quantities equivalent?	Yes = 0 No = 1	
	Management total	

CLINICAL		
1. Acute requests		
Who issues acute requests?	Receptionist = 2 Receptionist from agreed protocol = 0 Doctor = 0	
Can previously authorised acutes be issued by receptionists?	Yes = 2 No=0 Yes from agreed protocol = 0	
2. Discharges		
Who makes the decision to add / delete medication from the repeat?	Doctor = 0 Other =2	
Who updates the repeat screen?	Doctor = 0 Receptionists not checked by doctor after update = 2 Receptionist but doctor checks after update = 0	
3. Medication review		
Who carries out medication reviews?	Doctor = 0 Pharmacist = 0 Nurse = 0 Not been reviewed at appropriate intervals = 2	
Is there a procedure for highlighting when medication review is due?	Yes = 0 No =1	
	Maximum Risk Score = 46	

NHS
Cumbria
Clinical Commissioning Group

Contact Details:
Name: Sally Styles
Medicine Optimisation Pharmacist for NHS Cumbria CCG
North of England Commissioning Support (NECS)
Tel: 07799478747
E-mail: Sally.Styles@cumbria.NECSU.nhs.uk

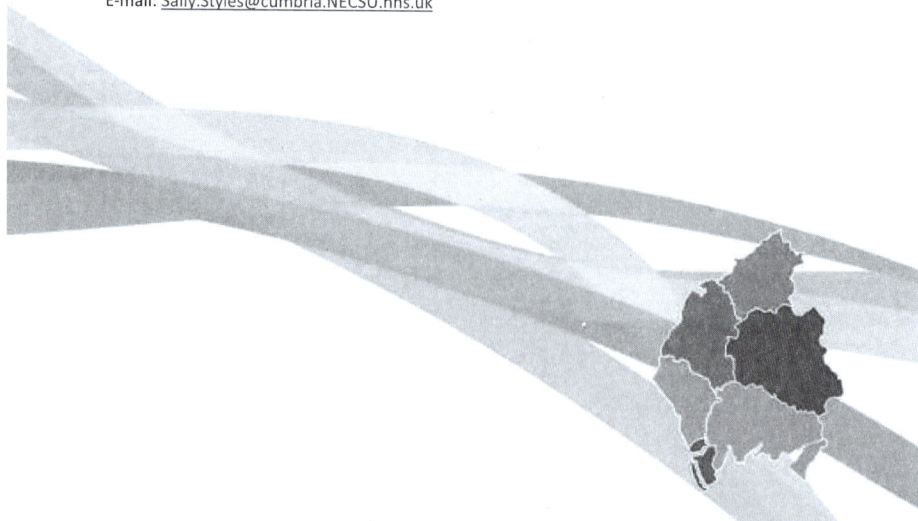

附录 5　Canada Health Professions Act – BYLAWS SCHEDULE F（第四章附件 2）

Health Professions Act – **BYLAWS**

SCHEDULE F

PART 1 - Community Pharmacy Standards of Practice

Table of Contents

附

录

Application

1.   This Part applies to all registrants providing pharmacy services in a community pharmacy.

Definitions

2.   In this Part:

        "community pharmacy" has the same meaning as in section 1 of the bylaws of the college under the *Pharmacy Operations and Drug Scheduling Act*;

        "drug therapy problem" means a potential or actual adverse consequence of drug therapy that interferes with achieving the goals of the drug therapy;

        "**incentive**" means money, gifts, discounts, rebates, refunds, customer loyalty schemes, coupons, goods or rewards;

        "patient's representative" means a person who is authorized to act on a patient's behalf;

        "personal health number" means a unique numerical lifetime identifier used in the specific identification of an individual patient who has any interaction with the BC health system;

        "prescription copy" means a copy of a prescription given to a patient by a registrant for information purposes only;

        "prescription transfer" means the transfer via direct communication from a registrant to another registrant of all remaining refill authorizations for a particular prescription to a requesting community pharmacy;

        "refill" means verbal or written approval from a practitioner authorizing a registrant to dispense additional quantities of drug(s) pursuant to a prescription;

        "renewal" means authorization by a full pharmacist to dispense additional quantities of drug(s) pursuant to a previously dispensed prescription, in accordance with section 25.92 of the *Act*;

        "*Residential Care Facilities and Homes Standards of Practice*" means the standards, limits and conditions for practice established in Part 3 of this Schedule.

Patient Choice

3.   Registrants, owners and directors must not enter into agreements with patients, patient's representatives, practitioners, corporations, partnerships, or any other person or entity, that limit a patient's choice of pharmacy, except as required or permitted under the bylaws.

Community Pharmacy Technicians

4.   (1)   Pharmacy technicians in a community pharmacy may prepare, process and compound prescriptions, including

(a) receiving and transcribing verbal prescriptions from practitioners,

(b) ensuring that a prescription is complete and authentic,

(c) transferring prescriptions to and receiving prescriptions from other pharmacies,

(d) ensuring the accuracy of a prepared prescription,

(e) performing the final check of a prepared prescription, and

(f) ensuring the accuracy of drug and personal health information in the PharmaNet patient record.

(2) Despite subsection (1), a pharmacy technician in a community pharmacy may dispense a drug but must not

(a) perform the task of ensuring the pharmaceutical and therapeutic suitability of a drug for its intended use, or

(b) do anything described in

(i) sections 6(5), 6(10), 10(2), 11(3), 11(4), 12, 13(2), 13(3) or 13(4) of this Part, or

(ii) Part 4 of this Schedule

(c) dispense a drug pursuant to HPA Bylaws Schedule F, Part 5

(3) A pharmacy technician must identify his or her registrant class in any interaction with a patient or a practitioner.

Pharmacy Assistants

5. A registrant may delegate technical functions relating to the operation of the community pharmacy to a pharmacy assistant if the registrant directly supervises the pharmacy assistant and implements procedures, checks and controls to ensure the accurate and safe delivery of community pharmacy services.

Prescription

6. (1) A registrant must ensure that a prescription is authentic.

(2) Upon receipt from the practitioner, a prescription must include the following information:

(a) the date the prescription was written;

(b) the name of the patient;

(c) the name of the drug or ingredients and strength if applicable;

(d) the quantity of the drug;

(e) the dosage instructions including the frequency, interval or maximum daily dose;

(f) refill authorization if applicable, including number of refills and interval between refills;

(g) the name and signature of the practitioner for written prescriptions;

(3) For the purpose of subsection (4), "prescription" includes a new prescription, a refill, a renewal or a balance owing.

(4) At the time of dispensing, a prescription must include the following additional information:

(a) the address of the patient;

(b) the identification number from the practitioner's regulatory college;

(c) the prescription number;

(d) the date on which the prescription was dispensed;

(e) the manufacturer's drug identification number or the brand name of the product dispensed;

(f) the quantity dispensed;

(g) written confirmation of the registrant who

(i) verified the patient identification,

(ii) verified the patient allergy information,

(iii) reviewed the personal health information stored in the PharmaNet database in accordance with section 11(4),

(iv) performed the consultation,

(v) performed the final check including when dispensing a balance owing, and

(vi) identified and addressed a drug therapy problem, if any.

(5) A full pharmacist must

(a) review prescriptions for completeness and appropriateness with respect to the drug, dosage, route and frequency of administration,

(b) review patient personal health information for drug therapy problems, therapeutic duplications and any other potential problems,

(c) consult with patients concerning the patient's drug history and other personal health information,

(d) consult with practitioners with respect to a patient's drug therapy unless s.25.92(2) of the *Act* applies, and

(e)   take appropriate action respecting a drug therapy problem.

(6)   A registrant may receive verbal prescription authorizations directly from a practitioner or from a practitioner's recorded voice message.

(7)   A registrant must make a written record of a verbal authorization, and include his or her signature or initial.

(8)   A registrant must not dispense a prescription issued for more than one patient.

(9)   For refill authorizations, a registrant

(a)   may

(i)   accept a refill authorization for Schedule I drugs from a practitioner's agent if confident the agent consulted the practitioner and accurately conveyed the practitioner's direction,

(ii)   retain the current prescription number for a quantity change if the software system is capable of retaining a record of the quantity dispensed on each previous occasion, and

(iii)   document the refill authorization on the original prescription if

(A)   a computerized transaction log is maintained, or

(B)   a new prescription number is assigned, and

(b)   must

(i)   cancel any unused refill authorizations remaining on any previous prescription if a patient presents a new prescription for a previously dispensed drug,

(ii)   advise the other pharmacy of the new prescription if unused refills are at another pharmacy, and

(iii)   create a new prescription number if a renewal authorization involves a different drug identification number, practitioner or directions for use.

(10)   If a full pharmacist authorizes a prescription renewal, he or she must

(a)   create a written record,

(b)   assign a new prescription number, and

(c)   use his or her college identification number in the practitioner field on PharmaNet.

Transmission by Facsimile

7.   (1)   Prescription authorizations may be received by facsimile from a practitioner to a pharmacy, if

附

录

(a) the prescription is sent only to a pharmacy of the patient's choice,

(b) the facsimile equipment is located within a secure area to protect the confidentiality of the prescription information, and

(c) in addition to the requirements of section 6(2), the prescription includes

    (i) the practitioner's telephone number, facsimile number and unique identifier if applicable,

    (ii) the time and date of transmission, and

    (iii) the name and fax number of the pharmacy intended to receive the transmission.

(2) Prescription refill authorization requests may be transmitted by facsimile from a pharmacy to a practitioner, if the pharmacy submits refill requests on a form that includes space for

(a) the information set out in section 6(2),

(b) the name, address and 10 digit telephone number of the pharmacy, and

(c) the practitioner's name, date and time of transmission from the practitioner to the pharmacy.

(3) A registrant must not dispense a prescription authorization received by facsimile transmission for a drug referred to on the Controlled Prescription Drug List.

(4) Prescription transfers may be completed by facsimile transmission if

(a) the transferring registrant includes his or her name and the address of the pharmacy with the information required in section 8(4), and

(b) the name of the registrant receiving the transfer is known and recorded on the document to be faxed.

Prescription Copy and Transfer

8. (1) If requested to do so, a registrant must provide a copy of the prescription to the patient or the patient's representative, or to another registrant.

(2) A prescription copy must contain

(a) the name and address of the patient,

(b) the name of the practitioner,

(c) the name, strength, quantity and directions for use of the drug,

(d) the dates of the first and last dispensing of the prescription,

(e) the name and address of the community pharmacy,

(f) the number of authorized refills remaining,

(g) the signature of the registrant supplying it, and

(h) an indication that it is a copy.

(3) Upon request, a registrant must transfer to a pharmacy licenced in Canada a prescription for a drug if

(a) the drug does not contain a controlled drug substance, and

(b) the transfer occurs between a registrant and another registrant or an equivalent of a registrant in another Canadian jurisdiction.

(4) A registrant who transfers a prescription to another registrant under subsection (3) must

(a) enter on the patient record

(i) the date of the transfer,

(ii) the registrant's identification,

(iii) identification of the community pharmacy to which the prescription was transferred, and

(iv) identification of the person to whom the prescription was transferred, and

(b) transfer all prescription information listed in subsection (2) (a) to (f).

(5) A registrant must make prescriptions available for review and copying by authorized inspectors of Health Canada.

Prescription Label

9. (1) All drugs dispensed pursuant to a prescription or a full pharmacist-initiated adaptation must be labeled.

(2) The label for all prescription drugs must include

(a) the name, address and telephone number of the pharmacy,

(b) the prescription number and dispensing date,

(c) the full name of the patient,

(d) the name of the practitioner,

(e) the quantity and strength of the drug,

(f) the practitioner's directions for use, and

(g) any other information required by good pharmacy practice.

(3) For a single-entity product, the label must include

附

录

      (a)   the generic name, and

      (b)   at least one of

            (i)   the brand name,

            (ii)   the manufacturer's name, or

            (iii)   the drug identification number.

(4)   For a multiple-entity product, the label must include

      (a)   the brand name, or

      (b)   all active ingredients, and at least one of

            (i)   the manufacturer's name, or

            (ii)   the drug identification number.

(5)   For a compounded preparation, the label must include all active ingredients.

(6)   If a drug container is too small to accommodate a full label in accordance with subsection (2),

      (a)   a trimmed prescription label must be attached to the small container,

      (b)   the label must include

            (i)   the prescription number,

            (ii)   the dispensing date,

            (iii)   the full name of the patient, and

            (iv)   the name of the drug, and

      (c)   the complete prescription label must be attached to a larger container and the patient must be advised to keep the small container inside the large container.

(7)   All required label information must be in English, but may contain directions for use in the patient's language following the English directions.

Dispensing

10.   (1)   A registrant may adjust the quantity of drug to be dispensed if

      (a)   a patient requests a smaller amount,

      (b)   a manufacturer's unit-of-use standard of package size does not match the prescribed quantity,

      (c)   the quantity prescribed exceeds the amount covered by the patient's drug plan, or

(d)   a trial prescription quantity is authorized by the patient.

(2)   A full pharmacist may adjust the quantity of drug to be dispensed, if

    (a)   he or she consults with a practitioner and documents the result of the consultation, and

    (b)   if

        (i)   a poor compliance history is evident on the patient record,

        (ii)   drug misuse is suspected, or

        (iii)   the safety of the patient is in question due to the potential for overdose.

(3)   If a registrant doubts the authenticity of a prescription, the registrant may refuse to dispense the drug.

(4)   All drugs must be dispensed in a container that is certified as child-resistant unless

    (a)   the practitioner, the patient or the patient's representative directs otherwise,

    (b)   in the registrant's judgment, it is not advisable to use a child-resistant container,

    (c)   a child-resistant package is not suitable because of the physical form of the drug or the manufacturer's packaging is designed to improve patient compliance, or

    (d)   child-resistant packaging is unavailable, or

    (e)   the drugs are prescribed for medical assistance in dying.

(5)   A registrant must not dispense a prescription more than one year from the prescribing date, except for oral contraceptives which may be dispensed for up to two years.

Patient Record

11.   (1)   A patient record must be established and maintained for each patient for whom a Schedule I drug is dispensed.

    (2)   The patient record must include

        (a)   the patient's full name,

        (b)   the patient's personal health number,

        (c)   the patient's address,

        (d)   the patient's telephone number if available,

(e)　　the patient's date of birth,

(f)　　the patient's gender,

(g)　　the patient's clinical condition, allergies, adverse drug reactions and intolerances if available including the source and date the information was collected,

(h)　　the date the drug is dispensed,

(i)　　the prescription number,

(j)　　the generic name, strength and dosage form of the drug,

(k)　　the drug identification number,

(l)　　the quantity of drug dispensed,

(m)　　the intended duration of therapy, specified in days,

(n)　　the date and reason for discontinuation of therapy,

(o)　　the directions to the patient,

(p)　　the identification of the prescribing practitioner,

(q)　　special instructions from the practitioner to the registrant, if appropriate,

(r)　　past and present prescribed drug therapy including the drug name, strength, dosage, frequency, duration and effectiveness of therapy,

(s)　　the identification of any drug therapy problem and the description of any action taken,

(t)　　the description of compliance with the prescribed drug regimen, and

(u)　　Schedule II and III drug use if appropriate.

(3)　　If a full pharmacist obtains a drug history from a patient, he or she must request and if appropriate record the following information on the patient record:

(a)　　medical conditions and physical limitations,

(b)　　past and current prescribed drug therapy including the drug name, strength, dosage, frequency, duration and effectiveness of therapy,

(c)　　compliance with the prescribed drug regimen,

(d)　　Schedule II and III drug use.

(4)　　A full pharmacist must review the patient's personal health information stored on the PharmaNet database before dispensing a drug and take appropriate action if necessary with respect to any concern regarding the appropriateness of the drug or any drug therapy problem.

Pharmacist/Patient Consultation

12.   (1)   Subject to subsection (2), a full pharmacist must consult with the patient or patient's representative at the time of dispensing a new or refill prescription in person or, where not practical to do so, by telephone.

      (2)   Where a patient declines the consultation, the full pharmacist must document that the consultation was offered and declined.

      (3)   The full pharmacist must conduct the consultation in a manner that respects the patient's right to privacy.

      (4)   The pharmacist/patient consultation for a new prescription must include:

          (a)   confirmation of the identity of the patient,

          (b)   name and strength of drug,

          (c)   purpose of the drug,

          (d)   directions for use of the drug including the frequency, duration and route of therapy,

          (e)   potential drug therapy problems, including any avoidance measures, and action recommended if they occur,

          (f)   storage requirements,

          (g)   prescription refill information,

          (h)   information regarding

              (i)   how to monitor the response to therapy,

              (ii) expected therapeutic outcomes,

              (iii) action to be taken in the event of a missed dose, and

              (iv) when to seek medical attention.

          (i)   issues the pharmacist considers relevant to the specific drug or patient.

      (5)   The pharmacist/patient consultation for a refill prescription must include:

          (a)   confirmation of the identity of the patient,

          (b)   name and strength of drug,

          (c)   purpose of the drug,

          (d)   directions for use of the drug including frequency and duration,

          (e)   whether the patient has experienced a drug therapy problem.

      (6)   If a drug therapy problem is identified during patient consultation for a new or refill prescription, the full pharmacist must take appropriate action to resolve the

附

录

problem.

(7) If an adverse drug reaction as defined by Health Canada is identified, the full pharmacist must notify the patient's practitioner, make an appropriate entry on the PharmaNet record and report the reaction to the appropriate department of Health Canada.

Schedule II and III Drugs

13. (1) A registrant must not attribute a new prescription or refill for a Schedule II or Schedule III drug to a practitioner without the authorization of the practitioner.

(2) A pharmacist must offer to consult with the patient or the patient's representative regarding the selection and use of a Schedule II drug at the time of purchase.

(3) The pharmacist/patient consultation for a Schedule II drug must include potential drug therapy problems, including any avoidance measures, and action recommended if they occur.

(4) A pharmacist must be available for consultation with a patient or patient's representative respecting the selection and use of a Schedule III drug.

Sole Pharmacy Services Provider

14 The manager of a pharmacy may enter into an agreement with another person to be the sole provider of pharmacy services in a premise or part of a premise, if

(a) pharmacy services are provided in a manner that is consistent with the *Residential Care Facilities and Homes Standards of Practice,*

(b) patient therapeutic outcomes are monitored to enhance patient safety, and

(c) appropriate provision has been made for safe and effective distribution, administration and control of drugs.

Prohibition on the Provision of Incentives

15 (1) A registrant must not provide or distribute, or be a party to the provision or distribution of, an incentive to a patient or patient's representative for the purpose of inducing the patient or patient's representative to

(a) deliver a prescription to a particular registrant or pharmacy for dispensing of a drug or device specified in the prescription, or

(b) obtain any other pharmacy service from a particular registrant or pharmacy.

(2) Subsection (1) does not prevent a registrant from

(a) providing free or discounted parking to patients or patient's representatives,

(b) providing free or discounted delivery services to patients or patient's representatives, or

(c) accepting payment for a drug or device by a credit or debit card that is linked to an incentive.

(3)   Subsection (1) does not apply in respect of a Schedule III drug or an unscheduled drug, unless the drug has been prescribed by a practitioner.

附录6　Australia National Health (Continued Dispensing) Determination 2012（第七章附件2）

National Health（Continued Dispensing）Determination 2012

Dated 29 June 2012

Part 1　Purpose

This determination specifies the pharmaceutical benefits that may be supplied, and the conditions that must be satisfied when those pharmaceutical benefits are supplied, by an approved pharmacist without a current prescription, but on the basis of a previous prescription from a PBS prescriber.

Part 2　Conditions

2.01　General

（1）For paragraph 89A（3）（b）of the Act, this Part sets out the conditions that must be satisfied when making a supply（the requested supply）of a pharmaceutical benefit to a person under subsection 89A（1）of the Act.

（2）An approved pharmacist must consider the PSA Guidelines when:

（a）satisfying the conditions set out in this Part; or

（b）deciding whether those conditions are satisfied.

（3）In this Part:

（b）a reference to the PBS prescriber is a reference to the PBS prescriber who most recently prescribed the supply of the pharmaceutical benefit to the person.

2.02　Not practicable to obtain prescription

A condition is that the approved pharmacist is satisfied that it is not practicable for the person to obtain a prescription for the pharmaceutical benefit from a PBS prescriber before the person needs the supply of the pharmaceutical benefit.

2.03　Previous supply of pharmaceutical benefit

A condition is that the approved pharmacist is satisfied that:

（a）the person has previously been supplied the pharmaceutical benefit on the basis of a prescription from a PBS prescriber; and

（b）the PBS prescriber prescribed the supply of the pharmaceutical benefit for the person in at least one of the circumstances determined for that pharmaceutical benefit under paragraph 85（7）（b）of the Act.

2.04　Stability of therapy

A condition is that the approved pharmacist is satisfied that the person's therapy is stable.

2.05　Prior clinical review by PBS prescriber

A condition is that the approved pharmacist is satisfied that:

（a）the person has been taking the pharmaceutical benefit regularly for an uninterrupted period; and

（b）since the start of that period, the PBS prescriber has assessed the person's condition and decided that there is a need for ongoing treatment with the pharmaceutical benefit.

2.06　Prescription for last supply of pharmaceutical benefit

A condition is that the approved pharmacist is satisfied that the person had a valid prescription under Part Ⅶ of the Act for the last supply of the pharmaceutical benefit to the person before the requested supply.

2.07　No continued dispensing in previous 12 months

A condition is that the approved pharmacist is satisfied that the person was not supplied with the pharmaceutical benefit under subsection 89A（1）of the Act in the 12 months before the requested supply.

2.08　Declaration by person supplied with pharmaceutical benefit

A condition is that the person, or an agent of the person（other than the approved pharmacist）, signs a declaration acknowledging that the person is being supplied with the pharmaceutical benefit without the presentation of a valid prescription under Part Ⅶ of the Act.

2.09　Maximum quantity of supply

A condition is that the approved pharmacist supplies a maximum quantity or number of units of the pharmaceutical item in the pharmaceutical benefit determined under paragraph 85A（2）（a）of the Act.

2.10　Preparing and recording information

（1）A condition is that, when the pharmaceutical benefit is supplied, the approved pharmacist:

（a）records the information that the pharmacist used to support his or her decision to supply the pharmaceutical benefit; and

（b）prepares information about the supply that the pharmacist will send to the PBS prescriber.

（2）The information that must be recorded and prepared includes the following:

（a）a statement that the pharmaceutical benefit supplied is a pharmaceutical benefit determined under paragraph 89A（3）（a）of the Act;

（b）a statement that the conditions mentioned in sections 2.02 to 2.05 are satisfied;

（c）a statement that the approved pharmacist is satisfied that the pharmaceutical benefit needs to be supplied to the person to facilitate continuity of treatment.

MOH CLINICAL PRACTICE GUIDELINES　2/2008
Prescribing of Benzodiazepines

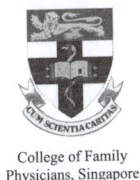

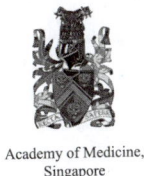

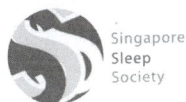

College of Family
Physicians, Singapore

Academy of Medicine,
Singapore

Singapore
Sleep
Society

MINISTRY OF HEALTH
SINGAPORE

Executive summary of recommendations

Details of recommendations can be found in the main text at the pages indicated.

Pharmacological considerations

Appropriate facilities, equipment and drugs (including flumazenil) for respiratory or cardiovascular assistance should be readily available whenever benzodiazepines are administered intravenously. Close observation is required until the patient recovers fully from sedation.

Grade D, Level 4

Neither benzodiazepines nor zolpidem/zopiclone should be used in acute narrow angle glaucoma, acute pulmonary insufficiency, respiratory depression, sleep apnoea syndrome or marked neuromuscular respiratory weakness including unstable myasthenia gravis and in the presence of known hypersensitivity (to the drug or any excipients) .

Grade D, Level 4

Patients should be routinely warned that hypnotics/anxiolytics cause drowsiness and may impair ability to perform hazardous activities that require mental alertness or physical coordination (e.g. operating machinery or driving a motor vehicle). As such, the concomitant use of alcoholic drinks should also be avoided .

Grade B, Level 2++

Patients should be warned about possible effects on memory (e.g. amnesia) and report to their doctor any behavioural or mental changes (e.g. depression) that develop during treatment with benzodiazepines or zopiclone/zolpidem

Grade B, Level 1+

附

录

Psychiatric uses - insomnia, schizophrenia, depression and anxiety

Prescription of zolpidem and zopiclone should be treated with the same cautions as benzodiazepines.

Grade A, Level 1+

Judicious use of hypnotic medications (e.g. benzodiazepines) may be indicated for short-term (up to 2-4 weeks) relief of insomnia symptoms after considering non-pharmacological treatments. Instructions are necessary concerning side effects (including tolerance and dependence), follow-up for efficacy and discontinuation.

Grade A, Level 1+

If treatment does not work with a shorter-acting benzodiazepine, zolpidem or zopiclone, the doctor should not prescribe one of another shorter-acting benzodiazepine, zolpidem or zopiclone.

Grade A, Level 1+

Patients with insomnia should be referred to an appropriate specialist if physical, psychological or benzodiazepine/substance abuse/dependence problems are suspected.

Grade D, Level 4

If acute insomnia (of less than 4 weeks) is severe, distressing and disabling, and is expected to resolve quickly, a short course of a benzodiazepine or a similar hypnotic drug (up to 2-4 weeks) may be considered.

Grade A, Level 1+

When a benzodiazepine is indicated as a hypnotic, the minimum effective dose should be used for the shortest duration so as to minimize side effects and risks of dependence.

Grade D, Level 4

For chronic insomnia (longer than 4 weeks), non-pharmacological therapies are the mainstay of management.

Grade A, Level 1+

Hypnotic drug use in patients with chronic insomnia (longer than 4 weeks) should be avoided as far as possible because efficacy is not clearly established.

Grade A, Level 1+

Benzodiazepines should not be used as monotherapy in the treatment of schizophrenia, schizophrenia-like psychoses and acute psychotic behaviour.

Grade A, Level 1+

A short-term trial of adjunctive benzodiazepines may be considered only in psychotic patients with persistent and clinically significant symptoms of anxiety, dangerous or assaultive behaviour.

Grade A, Level 1+

Benzodiazepines may be added (for less than 4 weeks) to an antidepressant in a depressed patient with anxiety and/or insomnia in the initial phase of treatment.

Grade A, Level 1+

Benzodiazepines should not be used as monotherapy for depression

Grade A, Level 1+

Benzodiazepines are indicated for the short-term relief (2-4 weeks only) of anxiety that is severe, disabling or subjecting the individual to unacceptable distress, occurring alone or in association with insomnia or short-term psychosomatic, organic, or psychotic illness.

Grade D, Level 4

As an adjunct to antidepressant treatment in anxiety disorders, the use of benzodiazepines should be limited to 2-4 weeks in the lowest effective dose. The dose should be gradually tapered off. Benzodiazepine use should be closely monitored for adverse effects, abuse, tolerance, dependence and withdrawal symptoms.

Grade D, Level 4

Benzodiazepines prescribed for anxiety may be abused by some patients with co-morbid alcohol/substance abuse or dependence and are best avoided where possible in such patients.

Grade D, Level 4

附

录

Patients with panic disorder and co-morbid depression should not be treated with benzodiazepine monotherapy.

Grade A, Level 1+

Medical uses

Benzodiazepines such as clonazepam and clobazam may be used as add-on therapy in refractory focal and generalized epilepsy.

Grade D, Level 3

Intravenous lorazepam and diazepam are effective first-line treatments for prolonged seizures in adults.

Grade A, Level 1+

For treatment of prolonged seizures in adults, an initial dose of 5-10 mg diazepam is given either intravenously or rectally. If there is no response, the same dose can be repeated after 10 minutes. Respiratory or circulatory effects should be monitored for and usually occur with doses greater than 20 mg .

Grade D, Level 4

Benzodiazepines (e.g. chlordiazepoxide, diazepam, lorazepam) are the drugs of choice for treatment of acute alcohol withdrawal (including alcohol withdrawal delirium) (pg 23). (Refer to Annex A. Table A1 for suggested dosage ranges)

Grade A, Level 1+

Patients with complicated alcohol withdrawal should be referred to general hospitals.

GPP

Benzodiazepine abuse and dependence

Long-term chronic use of benzodiazepines (e.g. for the treatment of insomnia or anxiety symptoms) is not recommended because efficacy is not clearly established. In view of this, for any continued or repeat benzodiazepine prescription, there must be appropriate clinical review, clear indications and adequate documentation.

Grade A, Level 1+

Benzodiazepine use should be limited to short-term relief (between 2-4 weeks), at the lowest dose and be taken intermittently (e.g. 1 night in 2 or 3 nights).

Grade D, Level 4

Extended use of benzodiazepines (especially those with short half-lives) beyond 2-4 weeks is not recommended, even when prescribed at the therapeutic dosages.

Grade A, Level 1+

All patients receiving benzodiazepines should be routinely advised about the risk of developing dependence.

Grade A, Level 1+

Patients receiving prescription for benzodiazepines should be advised to obtain all such prescriptions from the same doctor wherever possible, so that risk of abuse and dependence may be monitored.

Grade D, Level 4

Avoid prescribing benzodiazepines to known polydrug users.[48] In view of this, medical practitioners should examine for any signs of intravenous drug use before considering prescribing benzodiazepines.

Grade D, Level 4

Oral midazolam (e.g. Dormicum®) and nimetazepam (e.g. Erimin®) are not recommended for routine outpatient prescription as they are highly addictive and commonly abused by drug addicts in Singapore.

Grade D, Level 3

Benzodiazepines should be gradually tapered, monitored and titrated to minimize withdrawal symptoms.

Grade A, Level 1+

Propanolol, dothiepin, buspirone or progesterone should not be used in the primary management of benzodiazepine withdrawal.

Grade A, Level 1+

Patients may be switched to a long half-life benzodiazepine (e.g. diazepam), then taper gradually to facilitate smoother withdrawal.

Grade A, Level 1+

附

录

Supervised gradual discontinuation of benzodiazepines with brief intervention strategies may be used. It has been shown to be more effective than discontinuation alone.

Grade A, Level 1+

For patients on less than 4 weeks of benzodiazepine therapy, the dose can be discontinued or reduced over 1-2 weeks.

GPP

Patients who have been on high dose for over 4 weeks or on regular doses for longer than 12 weeks may be switched from a short acting to a long-acting benzodiazepine (e.g. diazepam). The slower elimination of diazepam creates a smoother taper in blood level. (See Table A3 in Annex A for approximate diazepam equivalent dose)

Grade C, Level 2++

A suggested withdrawal protocol for patients with more than 4 weeks of benzodiazepine therapy is as follows:
1. Calculate the approximate equivalent oral daily dose of diazepam.
    (a) For those whose daily dose exceeds 30 mg/day, start reduction from half of this amount or 30 mg/day, whichever is lower.
    (b) For those on 30 mg/day or less, reduce from this dose.
2. Reduce oral diazepam dose every 1-2 weeks in steps of 2-5 mg.
3. If withdrawal symptoms are severe, reduce dose in smaller steps.
    If patients are unable to stop completely by 4-8 weeks, or if complications arise, consider referral to the appropriate specialist or general hospital.

GPP

Patients who are undergoing benzodiazepine discontinuation, especially those with concurrent medical or psychiatric conditions, should be closely monitored. Patients who develop complicated withdrawal symptoms (e.g. seizures, delirium) or serious psychiatric complications (e.g. psychotic symptoms, suicidal tendency) during benzodiazepine discontinuation should be referred to the specialist or general hospital.

GPP

Special populations: elderly, child and adolescent, pregnancy and breast-feeding

Non-pharmacological interventions, which have been shown to be effective for management of insomnia in older adults, should be initiated first before prescribing a benzodiazepine. (See Annex B, Tables B1-3)

Grade A, Level 1++

Benzodiazepines may be used with caution on a short-term basis in the elderly to improve sleep although the magnitude of improvement is modest compared to the risk of adverse events.

Grade A, Level 1++

Long-term use of benzodiazepines should be avoided in the elderly in view of the increased risk of cognitive impairment and fractures.

Grade C, Level 2+

The dose of benzodiazepines in the elderly should generally be only one-quarter to half of the normal adult dose.

Grade D, Level 4

Benzodiazepines with long half-lives (such as diazepam, flurazepam, clorazepate, chlordiazepoxide) should be avoided in the elderly.

Grade D, Level 4

Benzodiazepines should be gradually withdrawn in the elderly as this may produce improvement in cognitive functions.

Grade B, Level 1+

Children and adolescents are at increased risk of disinhibition with benzodiazepines; first-line treatment with benzodiazepines should be avoided

Grade D, Level 3

Benzodiazepines should be avoided during pregnancy and breast-feeding

Grade C, Level 2+

附

录

Appendix 2 ADMINISTRATIVE GUIDELINES ON THE PRESCRIBING OF BENZODIAZEPINES AND OTHER HYPNOTICS

All registered medical practioners:

1. There is a need for every medical practitioner to ensure that benzodiazepines are used appropriately. These drugs are sometimes inappropriately prescribed to treat insomnia, anxiety and other psychiatric and medical conditions. Tolerance and drug dependence can be the undesired result.

2. To assist medical practitioners in prescribing the benzodiazepines appropriately, the 'Guidelines for Prescribing Benzodiazepines' which were developed in 2002 to guide doctors on the proper prescribing of benzodiazepines have been updated and revised by the Ministry of Health, which had worked in conjunction with relevant experts and professional organisations.

3. All medical practitioners are advised to familiarise themselves with the 2008 revised guidelines on the prescribing of benzodiazepines and other hypnotics and to comply with the guidelines.

4. In addition, all medical practitioners are requested to comply with the administrative guidelines (enclosed as Annex A) with immediate effect for the purpose of assisting the Ministry of Health in monitoring the appropriate use and documentation of all benzodiazepines prescribed to each patient. Your strict cooperation is appreciated.

5. All medical practitioners are reminded that under Regulation 19 of the Misuse of Drugs Regulations, a medical practitioner who attends to a person whom he considers, or has reasonable grounds to suspect, is a drug addict shall, within 7 days of the attendance, furnish to both the Director of Medical Services and the Director of the Central Narcotics Bureau the following particulars of that person:

(a) Name;

(b) Identity Card number;

(c) Sex;

(d) Age;

(e) Address; and

(f) The drug to which the person is believed to be addicted.

A sample of the notification form is attached as Annex B.

PROF K SATKU

DIRECTOR OF MEDICAL SERVICES

ANNex A ADMINISTRATIVE GUIDELINES ON THE PRESCRIBING OF BENZODIAZEPINES AND OTHER HYPNOTICS

Documentation and maintenance of patient medical records

(a) All information relating to a particular patient must be consolidated as one medical record relating only to that patient. Such information must be legibly documented.

(b) Each patient's medical record must be entirely reproducible upon request by the Ministry of Health or Singapore Medical Council.

(c) The following information must be documented in the medical record of every patient who is prescribed with benzodiazepines/ other hypnotics:

(i) Comprehensive history, including psychosocial history and previous use of benzodiazepines or other hypnotics;

(ii) Comprehensive physical examination findings, including evidence of misuse of benzodiazepines or other drugs; and

(iii) Withdrawal symptoms to benzodiazepines/ other hypnotics previously experienced by the patient, if any.

(d) The following information must be documented in the medical records of every patient each time he/she is prescribed benzodiazepines / other hypnotics either

附

录

initially or as repeat prescriptions:

（ⅰ）The prescribed type/name of benzodiazepine/hypnotic，its dosage and duration of use;

（ⅱ）Indication（s）and/or justification（s）for prescribing benzodiazepines/ other hypnotics; and

（ⅲ）Physical signs or evidence of tolerance，physical/psychological dependence or any illicit use or misuse of benzodiazepines or other drugs（eg. needle tracks on skin，inappropriate lethargy）.

Use of benzodiazepines

（e）Medical practitioners are strongly discouraged from prescribing highly addictive benzodiazepines such as midazolam and nimetazepam（except for midazolam use in surgical procedures）.

（f）Benzodiazepines / other hypnotics，when used for treating insomnia，should be prescribed for intermittent use（eg. 1 night in 2 or 3 nights）and only when necessary.

（g）Medical practitioners should routinely warn patients about rebound insomnia with the use of benzodiazepines and document such warning accordingly.

（h）The dosage of benzodiazepine / other hypnotic used should be the lowest effective dose necessary to achieve symptomatic relief.

（ⅰ）The concurrent prescribing of two or more benzodiazepines should be avoided.

（j）Repeat prescriptions for benzodiazepines / other hypnotics should not be provided without a clinical review.

（k）Where there are doubts about dosage prescription or tapering of benzodiazepines/ other hypnotics，a psychiatrist or other specialists should be consulted.

（l）Care should be taken when prescribing benzodiazepines / other hypnotics to avoid excessive sedation（which may pose a risk to the patient who drives，operates heavy machinery, etc).

(m) Caution should be exercised when prescribing benzodiazepines for patients with a history or evidence of alchohol or other substance abuse.

Specialist referrals

(n) The following categories of patients should not be further prescribed with benzodiazepines / other hypnotics and must be referred to the appropriate specialist for further management[a]

(i) Patients who require or have been prescribed benzodiazepines / other hypnotics beyond a cumulative period of 8 weeks;

(ii) Patients who are already on high-dose and/or long-term benzodiazepines from their specialists or general hospitals; where possible, these patients should be referred back to their respective specialists for further management until they are weaned off benzodiazepines / other hypnotics; and

(iii) Patients who are non-compliant with professional advice or warning to reduce intake of benzodiazepines/ other hypnotics.

(o) Patients who refuse to be referred to a specialist should be counselled appropriately. Such refusal should be documented in the patients' medical records. Patients who refuse referrals and turn aggressive should be reported to the police.

Annex B

Notification to MOH and CNB   * fields are mandatory

1.   I, Dr _____, MCR number _____ of

_____ (clinic name) hereby certify that I am treating the

following patient for the following:

* **Drug to which
the person is
believed to be
addicted**   _____

2.   The particulars of the patient is given as follows:

* **Name**   _____

* **IC Number**   _____

* **Age**   _____

* **Sex**   ☐ Male ☐ Female

* **Address**

_____

_____

Postal Code: _____

Please complete the form and fax one copy to MOH at fax number 6325 1744, and one copy to CNB at fax number 6227 3978.

Incomplete form will not be entertained.

Appendix 3 Good Pharmacy Practice Guide（Excerpts）

（F）DISPENSED MEDICINES

Pharmacists should always undertake or directly supervise all dispensing activities including the selection and compounding of medicines as well as counselling.

1）Receipt of Drug Order or Prescription

A pharmacist should review and interpret every drug order or prescription and resolve any problems or ambiguities before it is processed. The pharmacist must ensure that:

i) The prescription or medication order is not forged or tampered with. For forged or tampered prescriptions, the pharmacist should gather enough information and inform the police as well as the Compliance Branch of the Health Science Authority immediately.

ii) All legal requirements have been complied with.

iii) The medication is indicated for the condition being treated.

iv) The drug regimens (dosage, duration and frequency) are appropriate.

v) There is no therapeutic duplication in the patient's drug regimen.

vi) There are no contraindications e.g. allergies.

For any drug order or prescription that is not clear or the pharmacist believes is unacceptable (e.g. very high dose or being used beyond the labelled indications), appropriate interventions with the doctor to be done and documented before processing.

2) Interventions

Any form of intervention should be documented on the drug order or prescription. Details of the recording should include the following:

i) The name of the doctor involved or clinic assistant if the doctor is unavailable

ii) The reason (s) for clarification

iii) The outcome

iv) The time and date of the intervention

v) The name of the pharmacist who did the intervention and signed by him or her

3) Packaging and Labelling

i) Information on Labels

For all dispensed medicines, the label must contain the following information:

a) The generic or proprietary name, form, strength, and quality of the medicine

b) The dosing instructions

c) The name of the patient, or in the case of an animal, the name of the owner of that animal

d) The date of dispensing

e) The prescription number or any identification number

f) The name, address and telephone number of the pharmacy where the medicine is dispensed

g) The directions for the correct storage (where appropriate) and expiry date (where applicable) of the medicine

h) The relevant cautionary instructions (e.g. as listed in the British National Formulary) and any other special precautions.

ii) Legibility of Labels

All labels should be printed using computer or typewriter to produce a neat, even, legible print. In the event of a typing error, a new label should be prepared.

iii) Language and Expression

a) Care should be taken to ensure that the wording used is not ambiguous or confusing.

E.g. Separate dose from frequency–

"Take **ONE** tablet **THREE** times a day"

Avoid using decimals–

"Take $1\frac{1}{2}$ml" rather than "Take 1.5ml"

b)Use layman terms whenever possible, e.g. "ear" rather than "otic" or "aural", "eye" rather than "ophthalmic".

c) Use appropriate language, e.g. "each night" is not necessarily the same as "at night"; "when needed" is not necessarily the same as "if necessary".

d) Use descriptive language when appropriate, e.g. "rub in" liniments, "dab on" lotions, "sip" linctuses.

iv) Dosing Instructions for Pharmacy Only Medicines

The labels for counter–prescribed medicines must bear the indications for use and dosages for all age groups.

v) Dispensing Containers

a) The manufacturer's original container should be used as far as possible.

b) When repackaging medicines, dispensing containers used should comply with the manufacturer's specifications or official monographs.

vi) Placement of Labels on Containers

a) All labels should be firmly attached to the primary container of the medicine with the exception of metered aerosols where the labels may be attached to the outer containers or boxes.

b) Care should be taken to ensure that labels when placed on containers are not wrinkled or crooked.

The following information should be made visible:

· The manufacturer's name

· The instructions on usage, storage and indications for use

· Generic and proprietary names

· Expiry date (unless inappropriate e.g. reconstituted antibiotic mixtures and eye drops)

· Batch number

4) Counselling

It is considered professional and an essential pharmacy practice for pharmacists to impart sufficient information to patients about their medicines to ensure that the medicines are used safely, correctly and effectively.

To perform this task effectively, both oral and written means must be employed in all cases since the use of written means without oral explanation may lead to miscommunication and confusion. Oral counselling without written information can be easily forgotten.

The following points must be emphasised to the patients during counselling:

ⅰ）Drug name and its indication

ⅱ）Drug regimen（dosage，frequency and duration）

ⅲ）Special directions for preparation（e.g. freshly boiled and cooled water for reconstitution of antibiotic suspensions）

ⅳ）Special directions for administration （e.g. correct use of inhalers and transdermal patches）

ⅴ）Potential drug–drug or drug–food interactions and other contraindications

ⅵ）Common side effects that may be encountered，including their avoidance and the action required if they occur

ⅶ）Adverse drug reactions

ⅷ）Action to be taken in the event of a missed dose

ⅸ）Proper storage

ⅹ）Any other information that is peculiar to the specific patient or drug

Patient information leaflets of the various medicines and manufacturer's patient instruction leaflets should also be routinely used. The product insert（s）for professionals should preferably be removed when dispensing to patients.

◇ 后 记

随着我国工业化、城镇化、人口老龄化进程不断加快，以及疾病谱变化、生态环境和生活方式变化，慢性病已成为严重威胁我国居民健康的一类疾病，成为影响国家经济社会发展的重大公共卫生问题。《中共中央 国务院关于深化医药卫生体制改革的意见》《"健康中国2030"规划纲要》《"十三五"深化医药卫生体制改革规划》对慢性病防治工作给予高度关注。但是慢性病影响因素的综合性、复杂性决定了防治任务是长期而艰巨的。如何更好地为慢性病患者服务、方便其治疗、提高患者生活质量是一项亟待研究攻克的重要课题。

本书比较系统地整理了国际慢性病长期用药处方项目。通过对比研究与总结借鉴，编写专家都感觉到慢性病长期用药处方项目能在平衡药品可获得性和用药安全性以及加强医药合作等方面取得很好的社会效果。我们建议在深化医药卫生体制改革工作中，在国际借鉴的基础上，能将慢性病长期用药处方项目尽快纳入慢性病综合防控工作机制；在提供全人群生命全周期的慢性病防治管理服务的国家慢性病综合防治工作中，能进一步发挥医院药房和社会药房在慢性病防控网络中的重要社会功能，进一步发挥药师在加强药品质量管理、提供合理用药指导等方面的作用；在医药卫生相关政策中，应尽快落实药师权利和责任，支持药师开展更多处方相关服务、临床用药指导、规范用药等工作。

当然，我们也意识到，推行慢性病长期用药处方项目是一个非常复杂的过程，不少问题需要进一步研究解决。我们开展相关制度研究并出版本书的主要目的也是为了抛砖引玉，希望引起更多的部门重视，并有更多的志同道合的专业人士参与问题的解决和方案的建设工作。

　　本书编写组是一支特别优秀的精英团队，在北京协和医院药剂科副主任朱珠教授、和睦家医疗总药剂师 Helen Zhang 教授两位主编的带领下，有多位国内国际优秀的中青年药师参与，以严谨的学术态度和负责精神，高标准、高效率地共同完成了项目研究和编写工作，国内复旦大学药学院叶桦教授、西安交通大学医学院方宇教授、国家食品药品监督管理总局执业药师中心陈皎副主任、加拿大的罗红教授、McMaster 大学谢锋教授等不少专家学者，为项目研究提供了重要研究材料和指导意见；此项目研究中，我们还引用了很多国内外专家学者的理论、研究成果和学术观点。中国医药科技出版社为本书的设计、编辑、出版倾注了大量精力，在此一并表示诚挚谢意！

　　本项目研究工作，还得到优时比中国的资助和支持，在此郑重表示感谢！

　　最后，需要特别说明的是，由于时间和研究对象专业性等问题，书中疏漏和错误之处，请读者多多批评指正。

中国药师协会

2017 年 5 月